The Holistic Handbook
of Sauna Therapy

The Holistic Handbook of Sauna Therapy

Nenah Sylver, PhD

The Center for Frequency
PO Box 952
Stone Ridge, New York 12484-0952

845-687-0963

www.NenahSylver.com

The Center for Frequency
PO Box 952
Stone Ridge, New York 12484-0952
845-687-0963
www.NenahSylver.com

Library of Congress Catalogue Number: 2003104169
ISBN: 0-9672491-7-1

Cover and book design by Craig R. Smith / www.smithcraft.org

Photo and illustration credits:

Sweaty skin, cover, courtesy of Don Dement
Diagram of cross-section of skin on page 29 by Craig Smith
Diagrams of the electromagnetic spectrum on pages 94 and 95 by Craig Smith
Electric light bath on page 136 courtesy of Bernarr Schaeffer, U.S. Health Equipment Co., Inc.
Sauna cabinets on page 137 courtesy of John Doty, Battle Creek Equipment
Saunex sauna cabinets on page 138 courtesy of Bernarr Schaeffer, U.S. Health Equipment Co., Inc.
AromaSpa, Infra-Therapist, Finn Haven, and HealthMate saunas on pages 139–141 courtesy of BNH Corporation
White poplar sauna cabinet on page 140 courtesy of Bob Morgan, Heavenly Heat Sauna
Sauna cabins, heaters, and sauna bathers on pages 142–145 courtesy of Stephen Johnson, Northernlight Sauna
Photo of Nenah Sylver on page 333 by Paul Silverfox

Dedicated to

Bernarr Schaeffer

resourceful inventor
ethical human being
and dear friend

Contents

I came to know Dr. Nenah Sylver through a physician friend of mine who is a sauna expert. The minute Dr. Sylver and I started talking about sauna therapy, I could tell that she is well-versed in the subject. Later, when I had the privilege of previewing *The Holistic Handbook of Sauna Therapy*, I was delighted to discover the thorough research and fact-collecting she has accomplished to produce this authoritative work. Dr. Sylver's description of how the body perspires, various types of saunas, indications and contra-indications of sauna therapy, and how to take a sauna, are exhaustive and complete. The facts she presents are not hearsay statements, but are based on scientific documentation.

Using the sauna to raise body temperature provides numerous health benefits; the list is endless. Regular sauna, along with good exercise and wholesome food, is one of the primary components of maintaining good health and preventing disease. In fact, sauna therapy is one of the most important prophylactic measures one can take to stop acute and chronic conditions before they start—including heart diseases and cancers. In the early stages before both cancer and heart disease take root, sauna therapy can actually repair the damages done to the body.

Sauna therapy is also the most efficient way to eliminate toxins and metals from the body. Pesticides, petroleum-based and organic chemicals, drugs, toxins of all kinds are eliminated through sweat produced in the sauna. Dr. Sylver cites research showing that 15 minutes of sauna, through sweat, eliminates the same amount of heavy metal that would take the kidneys 24 hours to excrete. Mercury loss by sweating may be even more substantial. It is my opinion that most of today's practicing physicians have become pill pushers of pharmaceutical products that are toxic to the body. They have forgotten that an ounce of prevention is worth more than a pound of cure.

It was therefore a joy to read Dr. Sylver's book, which is filled with step-by-step guidelines on how to use this extraordinary natural healing method. It is written in simple language and will be appreciated by medical professionals, paramedical personnel, and the general public. Every health care provider, health club, bath house, sauna club, exercise and physical fitness center, weight watching group, medical school, and public library should carry this book. The preservation of health is our duty. Using sauna in a daily routine should be an integral part of your program, whether you are a healer, a health promoter, or an individual who desires to preserve your own health.

Sauna is an island of hope in a sea of hopeless health habits. As the saying goes, "If money is lost, you can make more. If character is lost, you can build it back. But if health is lost, everything is lost."

The information you are about to read is a refreshing eye opener for those who have forgotten the natural ways of healing. This book is a must for everyone who wants to maintain good health!

Dr. T. R. Shantha, MD, PhD, FACA
Medical director, Integrated Medical Specialists of Atlanta
Visiting professor, JJM Medical College, Davanagere, India

Acknowledgments

This book would not have been possible without the input and support of many people. First and foremost, I extend my loving gratitude to Bernarr Schaeffer, whose inventions and ideas have been the inspiration for this project. Bernie's enthusiasm, encouragement, and support never wavered. He also generously supplied a large quantity of out-of-print publications.

Early in the project, William A. MacKay, PhD, Associate Professor in the Department of Physiology at the University of Toronto, graciously offered to become my "sweat mentor." I deeply appreciate the many hours he patiently devoted to answering my endless questions, as well as to reviewing numerous portions of the manuscript.

For their critiques of the manuscript, thanks go to Oscar Abraham Jaeger, JD, Lorene Schaeffer, and Nicholas Vittum. Lawrence Wilson, MD, deserves special mention for reviewing a very early draft of the manuscript and suggesting organizational changes, and for contributing research materials. Others who commented on the manuscript, either portions or its entirety, are David Carpenter, MD, Professor of Environmental Health and Toxicology at SUNY at Albany; Roger Chown; Huy Hoang, MD; Joan Neilsen, MD, PhD, of Health Care for the 21st Century; Saul Pressman, DCh; and Abbas Qutab, MD, of Élan Vitál Medical Centers and Spas (who also provided research materials). It is not possible to name all of the sauna enthusiasts who gave me input on the manuscript; I hope they know they are appreciated.

I also want to acknowledge the following health care professionals who consented to be interviewed about their detoxification programs: Walter Crinnion, ND, of SpiritMed in Seattle, Washington and Tempe, Arizona; Jeff Gates, MD, and Bruce Hyde, MD, of the Battle Creek Lifestyle Health Center in Battle Creek, Michigan; William Rea, MD, of the Environmental Health Center in Dallas, Texas; David Root, MD, of HealthMed in Sacramento, California and New York City, New York; and T. R. Shantha, MD, PhD, FACA, of Integrated Medical Specialists in Stockbridge, Georgia (who also sent research materials and kindly commented on the manuscript).

For providing additional information, thanks go to Mary Bukhari; Marie Cecchini, MS; Pat Gurnick; Tom Harrelson; John Hood; John Oster; Stephen Johnson; Marian Porter, ND; John Shultz; and Dick Wullaert, PhD, John W. Doty, and LNF Books deserve special mention for supplying out-of-print books by John Harvey Kellogg. And a big round of applause goes to Robin Walsh, head librarian at Ulster County Community College, who on several occasions used her amazing sleuthing skills to unearth and acquire some hard-to-find journal articles for me.

I feel blessed for having the considerate help of Carol Nichols and Craig Smith, who helped the book reach its final stage of production. With great dedication, Carol edited a final version of the manuscript and labored many long hours to help me create a beautiful, functional index. Craig was immensely helpful with the index preparation as well. He also worked with me closely and respectfully to create the brilliant diagrams, artistic photo layout, readable format, and lovely cover, all of which transformed the manuscript into a real book.

As always, my dear companion Paul Silverfox was gracious and generous with his loving support on so many levels, enabling me to write undisturbed. Paul was always willing to listen to my ideas and offer common-sense advice on matters large and small. True friendship is priceless. Its special place in one's heart cannot always easily be expressed in words.

The word "research" conjures an image of someone sitting for long hours, reading and taking notes. All this was done, true—but during the last two years of manuscript preparation, I also had the opportunity to enjoy sauna bathing right in my own home. I extend my deepest thanks to Bernarr Schaeffer, Jim Schaeffer, BSME, and Wayne Schaeffer of U.S. Health Equipment Co., Inc., who created the superb far infrared sauna cabinet that I used almost daily, for periods ranging from twenty minutes to two hours. No amount of reading could ever take the place of real life sweating—"hands-on," practical experience that transformed this book from an intellectual study into a rewarding healing program. I cannot emphasize enough the value of empirical evidence.

Last but not least, I sincerely thank you, the reader, for your interest in healing and holistic living. In healing ourselves, we more effectively help and enrich others.

Introduction

It is more elegant to pontificate than it is to sweat.

HAROLD EVANS, BRITISH JOURNALIST AND PUBLISHER,
AT A MEMORIAL SERVICE FOR JOURNALIST DAVID BLUNDY, JANUARY 24, 1990.

In the year 2000, archaeologists from Boston University trekking through the lowlands of Central America came upon an unusual structure. In an ancient, simple Mayan village of thatched roofs, where natives had grown corn and manioc and hunted deer and wild pig, someone had taken the trouble to construct a partially closed building with a domed roof and a fire pit.

What could it be? the excavation team wondered. This building was in the center of the village, occupying a position of obvious importance. But it was only eight feet wide—surely not large enough for a meeting place, nor comfortable enough for a home of even just one occupant. In one corner of the hut the walls were red and gray, obviously burned by a very hot fire of long duration. For what purpose would such a fire be needed? Then the team saw another puzzling sight: near the ash deposits of the fire pit, low benches of stone had been erected. Obviously, whoever had built this structure had wanted to make sure that the furniture inside would not burn up. But why would someone want to sit so close to a roaring fire—in tropical heat of 90°Fahrenheit (32.2°Celsius), or higher?

Perplexed, the archaeologists tossed ideas back and forth one day as they erected a tarp over part of the excavation site to protect themselves from the fierce sun. Suddenly, "a chance remark suggested the answer." As one of the researchers wrote later, "It was hot and humid—like a sauna, someone said—and we suddenly realized what we had was a *pib na*, or sweat house." This was a historic find, the remains of "the earliest known Maya sweat house, a place for therapy and ritual"[1]— built 3,000 years ago.

Throughout history, people all over the world have gone out of their way to build heating chambers of various sizes so they could go inside and sweat. The temperatures used for these rooms range between 175°F and 205°F (79.4°C and 96.1°C), although sometimes the temperature climbed even higher. Today, we call this practice of therapeutic body heating, as well as the space in which the heat bath is located, sauna.

Why would anyone enter a cubicle, sometimes the size of a small closet, to deliberately perspire? In some cultures in this modern age, people in so-called polite society have an aversion to sweating, and will do anything to hide it. Yet body heating is enjoying a tremendous renaissance now, and the reason is simple: people want to experience the tremendous relaxation and health benefits that it provides.

Although sauna bathing is one of the oldest therapeutic modalities in human history, our forebears did not always understand exactly how or why it works. Now, with modern scientific methods available, we are privileged to know in detail what our ancestors sensed intuitively: that when used properly, heat—a major life-giving force of nature—will heal.

"The History of Saunas," the theme of Chapter 1, introduces sauna bathing as both a cultural and medical phenomenon. When I began my research, I had no idea that body heating had so many forms, or so many rituals connected to it. You may be as surprised as I was, at how various cultures have used the sauna, and under what circumstances—and how the practice was eventually adopted as a medical procedure by some sophisticated physicians. "How and Why We Sweat," the topic of Chapter 2, describes in detail how and why the body produces sweat, and explores why deliberate sweating can induce such powerful and positive results. Chapter 3, "What We Sweat, and Why We Need to Get Rid Of It," discusses toxins—which take the form of biological wastes, heavy metals, and organic chemicals—and why it's a matter of life or death to pay attention to them.

Chapter 4, "The Three Types of Heat," addresses the mechanics of heat transfer and how these principles apply to traditional and modern sauna methods. Both dry and moist heat are explored. Chapter 5, "Construction of the Sauna," focuses on the materials used for the heat source and for the sauna chamber itself. Taken together, Chapters 4 and 5 will help you to decide which method of body heating is best for you, and to select the appropriate sauna building materials and heating system that will deliver the desired results.

Chapter 6 provides valuable information on "Who May Use the Sauna and Who Should Not." Whether you are being treated by a physician for chronic or acute illness, have general wellness issues, or simply want to use the sauna to relax, you need to understand how heat affects the ways in which your body functions. There are actually very few conditions that contraindicate the use of a sauna. However, since this therapy might not be suitable for everyone all the time, it is important to know when not to heat the body.

Chapter 7 provides step-by-step instructions on "How to Take a Sauna." Knowing how to use the sauna can make the difference between having a pleasurable and healing experience or possibly hurting yourself. This chapter is packed with practical advice gleaned from data collected over many years by doctors, clinics, spas, and sauna manufacturers. Our "how-to" focus continues in Chapter 8 with "Detoxification Programs for Getting Well and Staying Well." You will learn what to expect when the sauna therapy starts to work, and get an overview about some successful detoxification programs used by respected doctors, some of them experts in the environmental medicine field.

A number of health care professionals as well as laypeople feel that a sauna session is incomplete without the addition of ozone. If you are curious about ozone and its benefits, or how to use it in conjunction with sauna therapy, read Appendix A, "A Brief Summary of Ozone."

If you want to know where to find a doctor, clinic, or spa that features some form of body heating as part of an overall treatment regimen or general wellness program, see Appendix B, "Resources." Appendix B also contains a listing of sauna manufacturers, spa and service organizations, and products related to sauna therapy. (The entries were carefully culled from many sources. If you are a manufacturer, doctor, or other service provider and feel that you should be included in the next edition of this book, please contact me.)

Finally, the Bibliography provides an extensive list of books, journal and magazine articles, and a few websites devoted to the science of body heating. Although some of these primary sources date back to the 1800s, the scientific methodology and degree of accuracy they display is impressive; these materials have as much relevance today as they did one hundred years ago.

This book covers all aspects of sauna *therapy*—as well as advice on how to choose a sauna suited to your needs, based on the materials of which it is constructed, and how those materials influence the quality of the sweat. But *instructions* on how to *build* your own sauna are not included. If you are handy with tools or need to make your own unit due to financial considerations, instructions for the design and construction of saunas can be found in Marilyn McVicker's *Sauna Detoxification Therapy: A Guide for the Chemically Sensitive*, in Bert Olavi Jalasjaa's *Art of Sauna Building*, and in Mikkel Aaland's *Sweat* (whose chapter "Build Your Own Sauna or Sweatlodge" is reproduced on Aaland's website and sold as a separate booklet). In addition, Dr. Lawrence Wilson offers plans for an inexpensive infrared light bulb heating unit and sells a kit of hard-to-find parts. See Appendix B for detailed contact information on all of these do-it-yourself ventures.

This book is devoted primarily to the obviously physical aspects of wellness. However, since my background is also in psychology, I want to comment here on the difference in attitudes toward body functions that often exist between Americans and people in other countries. These differences were hard to miss as I immersed myself in the multicultural aspects of body heating. Quite a few other cultures are much more comfortable with sweating and nudity than are Americans. The reasons for our cultural aversion to natural bodily processes and odors are many—some understandable, others not—but we as a culture pay a steep price for indulging in this body hatred, for by denying ourselves the right to sweat, we keep ourselves ill.

The aversion to sweating is often related to a negative attitude toward nakedness, and the repression of sexuality in general. I was surprised and a bit saddened to discover how many people do not use a sauna because it would involve getting undressed in front of strangers (unless one can afford to purchase a sauna to use in the privacy of one's own home). Sauna bathing, even if done in a mixed gender group, should never be confused with flirting, foreplay, an orgy, or some other sexual behavior. A sauna chamber is sacrosanct to people who use it. In fact, combining sex with sauna bathing is considered an insult to—and distortion of—the entire sauna culture. Not surprisingly, people raised to incorporate sauna therapy into their daily lives have a much more relaxed and natural relationship with their bodies than those who do not. (There are studies that show this, but it should be self-evident from simple observation.) Americans would benefit greatly—and would certainly enjoy their sauna experience more—by adopting the more relaxed attitude of our European friends about group nudity.

A few editorial comments: first, out of respect for both American readers and those across the oceans, temperature readings are given in both Fahrenheit and Celsius. Second, in the text that I write I keep spelling, numerical notation, and capitalization consistent, according to modern rules of grammar and punctuation. However, when quoting other authors, I leave their passages alone and do not make corrections for consistency; so the quoted remarks do not always correspond to the style of my own text. Third, when referring to people suffering from various health problems, I use terms like "people with cancer" or "people with multiple sclerosis" as opposed to "cancer patients" or "multiple sclerosis patients." Although this can be a bit cumbersome, I avoid the word "patient" because all too often it reflects and reinforces a hierarchical medical model that relegates the seeker of health services to a role that is subordinate to the doctor. Since one theme of this book is self-empowerment, I want the words I use to reflect this.

The ancient and respected tradition of sauna bathing has survived because *it works*. In the United States, the Food and Drug Administration approves saunas as therapeutic devices, and some insurance companies even reimburse claimants for the cost of sauna therapy or the saunas themselves. But as with any modality that promises relief from what ails you, it is wise to use some common sense by learning what sauna therapy actually can and cannot do, instead of blindly believing any affirmative claim made by a sauna manufacturer—or any negative comment made by a detractor.

The Holistic Handbook of Sauna Therapy is designed to help people who are considering sauna therapy, but first want to educate themselves about why it is effective, and how it may be used safely. It has been written for both the health care professional and the layperson—so that anyone can, with a little effort, improve their health and the health of those they care about. This book is also directed to those who already use saunas, and want to enrich their experience with practical suggestions on how to make the most of what they are already doing. It serves as a brief introduction to holistic health as well, so that even if you don't have access to a sauna, you can still learn what detoxification really means, and why it's important. And, it is hoped, that based on what you learn, you'll be tempted to try a sauna at least once.

The ancient Greek physician Hippocrates is thought to have declared, "Give me a chance to create fever and I will cure any disease." An exaggeration? Maybe not. This statement is closer to the truth than one might think—especially today, with high levels of pollution contributing to problems far more complex than anyone might have imagined two millennia ago. In the following pages, I will show you how sweating can make a huge difference in the way you feel—whether you are sick or well.

Nenah Sylver, PhD
Stone Ridge, New York
February 2004

Notes

1. Wilford, John Noble, "Before Rome's Baths, There Was the Maya Sweat House," *The New York Times*, March 20, 2001, -F5.

CHAPTER I

The History of Saunas

The sauna is Finland's medication…
and a poor [person's] apothecary.
(Finnish Proverb)

JOHN O. VIRTANEN,
THE FINNISH SAUNA: PEACE OF MIND, BODY AND SOUL, 1998

All over the world, whenever people hear the word "sauna" they think of the Finns. "Sauna" means "bathhouse" in Finnish. Pronounced "sow'-na" (or sometimes "saw'-na" in English), it is the only Finnish word used by English-speaking countries. "Sauna" has been borrowed by many other languages as well. This is appropriate, because the Finns seem to have been the most influential of anyone in spreading the 2000-year-old tradition of sauna bathing across the globe. Some researchers believe that the sauna was invented during the Byzantine or Scythian empires, carried by the Slavs when they migrated to the lands of the ancestral Finns, and then brought by the Finns when they relocated to the rest of Scandinavia and to Russia, Germany, Australia, Canada and the United States. Whether or not the Finns actually invented the sauna, they are rightly credited with being the worldwide connoisseurs of body heating.

Although people associate the sauna with Finland, sometimes they are not always clear about what comprises a sauna. In *The Finnish Sauna: Peace of Mind, Body and Soul,* John O. Virtanen, who was born in a sauna in his native Finland, writes that it is a "common mistake" to equate the Finnish sauna with a Turkish or Russian steam bath. "In an authentic Finnish sauna, the heat emanating from the special stones feels velvety soft to the skin, and it is more penetrating than the heat in a cloud of steam. The difference is so important that sometimes a person must experience more than one sauna to fully appreciate the distinction between genuine and imitation saunas."[1] Nevertheless, since many people do associate the two—or alternate between both when they visit spas or receive medical treatments—throughout this book I will be discussing the wetter modalities along with pure saunas.

In all of history, in virtually every culture in the world, the wealthy did not consider their houses complete unless they were equipped with a body heating facility. Following is a brief overview.

Popularity in Early Cultures

Finland

According to some estimates, the Finns have been using saunas for 2000 years. "The very oldest saunas," the website of the Finnish Sauna Society reads, "were probably only pits dug in a slope in the ground and primarily used as dwellings in winter….Buildings used as both a sauna and a home were still found in Finland as late as in the 19th century. These were exceptions, though…[due to] either poverty or temporary use of the building. Other than the very earliest times, saunas have always been separate from homes."[2]

These early structures in the earth were lined with either stone, wood, or both. An article called "Traditional Use of the Sauna for Hygiene and Health in Finland" explains how these sauna pits were used.

> [An Arab traveler] visited the Mordvians [sic], a tribe related to
> the Finns. [The traveler] Ibn Dasta wrote that "this tribe lives
> during the winter time in dwellings dug in the earth. And into
> these cellars moved whole families; they take some wood and
> stones with them and heat the stones in the fire to the point
> that stones get red. Then they pour water on them which makes
> the water turn to vapour, which warms up the room to such an
> extent that people take their clothes off."[3]

Water, when poured onto hot rocks, creates a sudden burst of vapor called a *löyly* (pronounced low-lū; the "low" rhymes with "cow")—which in Finnish means "spirit of life," as Mikkel Aaland writes in his book *Sweat*.[4] This process moistens the air by as much as 40%—not enough to see vapor, but enough to prevent dry hot air, which can irritate the lungs.

Often, in between sweat cycles, Finnish sauna bathers completely immerse themselves in water (usually cold, but occasionally hot). They are known for taking freezing cold showers or rolling in the snow; but any cold tub, cool sponge bath or rubdown with ice will do. Ancient peoples intuited what modern science has recently learned: that there are many therapeutic benefits of alternating heat with cold. I will discuss this later in various parts of this book.

The Finns developed the practice of slapping the skin with a *vihta* (or *vasta*)—a whisk of twigs and leaves usually made from birch but sometimes other woods—to stimulate the circulation in the capillaries and tone the skin. Often the *vihta* was dipped into a bucket of warm water before being applied to the skin. Today, people use a washcloth, scrub brush, or brush the skin with a loofah "sponge"—the rough, fibrous sponge-like inner portion of the loofah gourd.

The sauna was utilized in many ways by the versatile Finns. It was an ideal smokehouse. The frequent heating and sterile coat of soot (charcoal) on the walls rendered it more hygienic than other parts of the home, which made it ideal for simple medical procedures such as wound cleansing. The sauna was also a popular place to give birth, as the warmth was welcomed and needed by both mother and newborn.

Before Finland became a sovereign nation, it was controlled by France and then Russia—which, in the 1800s, heavily censored or outright banned political discussion and printed material. Under those circumstances, the sauna had yet another use, that of a political meeting place.

Egypt

There is a very old Egyptian document, dated at about the 17th century BC and called the Edwin Smith Papyrus, which scholars have reason to believe was copied from yet another, much older manuscript from about the 30th century BC. The Egyptian Orthopedic Association's website describes the painstaking medical chronicling contained in the papyrus:

> There are 48 cases in all, starting with injuries of the head, then those of the face, temporal region, mandible and chin, cervical vertebrae, clavicle, humerus [sic] and sternum. In every group of cases such as the eight cases of the head he [the author] starts with the simpler, more superficial and less dangerous cases, going on to describe lesions which are deeper, more complicated and more dangerous. The writer was undoubtedly endowed with a rare talent for classification.[5]

Another remarkable aspect of the Papyrus is its recommendation of the use of heat for tumors:

> If thou examinest a man having tumours with prominent head in his breast, (and) thou findest that the swellings have spread with pus over his breast, (and) have produced redness, while it is very hot therein, when thy hand touches him…Thou shouldst burn for him over his breast (and) over those tumors which are on his breast.[6]

India

An Aryuvedic medicine document from India, dated at 568 BC, is slightly reminiscent of its ancient Egyptian predecessor. As described by Virtanen:

> Generally, it was considered important to perspire before bathing….The Indians classified thirteen methods of inducing perspiration. Among them, for example, was covering a sore with hot cow manure, sand, or some similar substance in order to raise the temperature of the affected portion of the body. The use of steam was also commonplace. In one form, heated pieces

of iron or hot rocks were dropped into a pan of water placed beneath the sickbed.[7]

In India today, and at some spas and clinics in many parts of the world, a favorite way of heating the body is massage with smooth hot stones covered in warm oil. Besides the benefit of heat from the stones, oil conditions the skin and massage helps relax the body.

Ancient Greece and Rome

For many of the world's peoples, dry saunas and the therapeutic benefits of bathing in wet pools coexisted under one roof, or side by side as complementary therapies. (See the section in this chapter on "Hydrotherapy in Austria" on page 11.) The warm Mediterranean climate spawned the famous baths of ancient Greece and Rome—architectural masterpieces carved from magnificent marble whose adjoining pillared rooms featured steam chambers, hot baths, and cold pools. We know about body heating in ancient Greece thanks in part to Herodotus, who was among the first to chronicle their use of therapeutic steam. "The steam baths," Virtanen describes,

> were usually heated by open fireplaces made of charcoal pans filled with hot rocks over which water was poured to make steam. This sort of bathing was common among athletes. Rather sophisticated gymnasiums had special areas for cold baths, warm baths, massage and dressing. Those buildings were usually round and built so that the roof narrowed toward the highest point leaving a bronze plate that could be opened and closed for ventilation.[8]

The Greeks also used steam therapy for mourners at funerals. Bathhouses were created from three tall sticks in the ground, meeting at the center like a teepee, around which a woolen blanket was wrapped. "The bather then entered and threw hemp seeds on the hot rocks, creating steam," writes Virtanen. "The bather howled with fear, or was it joy?"[9]

Roman baths, writes medical doctor Sidney Licht in *Therapeutic Heat and Cold*, had many "special rooms, with water or air baths at different temperatures, and these were used in varying patterns of increasing and decreasing exposures to heat and cold." People too weak for a full, heated bath were given a "partial" one. "Although the baths were used largely for cleansing and pleasure, physicians did prescribe the various forms of available heat for hygiene and in illness."[10] The very wealthy were given baths of heated milk or oil, while the poor people had to be content with plain water. So much water was used—for fountains as well as the bathhouses—that the aqueducts bringing it to Rome were spacious enough to accommodate a man on horseback.

As might be expected, body heating and bathing were commonly used by the ill, frail, and post-childbirth women for therapy, cleansing and rejuvenation. But the communal bathhouse was often a social center as well—indeed, the *only* social center—of the village or town. Early Roman bathhouses, impressive in their own right (they were large enough to contain 35 dwellings), evolved into a giant sculptured complex with shops, a library, gymnasium, theaters for poetry readings and music, and even a restaurant and sleeping quarters for overnight guests. In short, the baths gave birth to a community where every social and recreational need was met. Interestingly, prostitution and various other forms of sexual behavior were allowed in various Mediterranean bathhouses as long as nobody complained, and depending on whether someone permissive was in political power at the time. This is an unusual exception that contrasts with the strict separation between sex and sauna bathing that has existed—and continues to exist—in most cultures.

In ancient Greece and Rome, as with many other cultures, a ritual was made of massages and oil rubs after the sauna.

Turkey

The Islamic *hamman* in Turkey was a faithful, though smaller, model of a Roman bathhouse, built from marble and bricks and containing lavish water fountains. First intended as a place of hygiene, the *hamman* became a meeting place as well after Muhammad himself told his followers that the heat would enhance fertility. As in Greece and Rome, massage and shaving were administered by attendants. Aaland writes that the benefits of the *hammam* were so valued, and it was recognized as such an important part of Moslem women's lives—especially since they "had virtually no other opportunity to socialize with anyone outside the home"—that the men begrudgingly allowed them their visits "after an illness or after they had given birth." Before long, the women's "privilege" became a "right." "If a husband were to deny his wife her visits to the *hammam*, she had grounds for divorce."[11] (The political and social climate in the Middle East is of course different today than when Aaland wrote *Sweat* in 1978; but even if this partial softening of attitude no longer exists, it is still a good illustration of people's regard for the bath.)

Central America

Some researchers believe that the sauna migrated up through Mayan culture along the entire western coast of Central America into North America. In the Guatemalan city of Piedras Negras alone, archaeologists found several ruined buildings that they recognized as saunas. One excavation site yielded the remnants of a sauna that was 1200 years old.

Mexico

Native Mexicans made their *temescal* from wood and perhaps mortar, with thatch for the roofs. A man named Fray Diego de Duran, author of a 1567 book called *New Spanish Indian History*, is quoted by both Aaland and Virtanen. Virtanen writes:

> The *temescalli*, a low building into which at most ten people will fit, is heated with a fire. One cannot sit and can hardly stand, and the door is very low so that only one person may pass at a time [Aaland adds, "creeping on all fours"]. In the rear is a stove which is so hot that it is difficult to bear. These are called dry baths. The bathers sweat only from heat and not from the effect of any medication. Indians, sick or well, bathe there regularly. To the outsider this looks horrible, for after they have sweated for a time they emerge from the sauna nude, wash, and then pour ten to twelve buckets of water over themselves without any fear of chilling or sickness. If a Spaniard tried this method of bathing, he would surely faint and be paralyzed.[12]

Aaland, who apparently used a different translation of Duran's words, adds: "Although this [procedure] seems terribly brutal, it is my opinion this is not so. When the body becomes used to this, it becomes quite natural."[13] Whichever translation is correct, it is clear that the Mexicans relished their saunas.

North American Native Cultures

Among the many other cultures that have also enjoyed body heating are the North American Eskimos and Native Americans—mostly from the central plains, southwest and eastern wooded areas—who built sweat lodges. Their portable lodges generally consisted of curved branches in a dome or igloo shape covered with animal skins. Other lodges were stationary, built with logs, bark, and sod cement. For all sweat lodge ceremonies, carefully selected large stones were heated in a fire outside the lodge; and after the rocks became intensely hot, they were carefully placed into a hollow in the dirt floor in the middle of the lodge. For those following native traditions, the sweat lodge was a place of purification, not only of the physical body, but of the spiritual and emotional bodies as well. Outer cleanliness represented inner peace and mastery of one's emotional and mental energies, and vice-versa.

Early Colonial America

The earliest non-native saunas in America were built before 1638 by Finnish and Swedish immigrants in the Delaware River Valley. In Alaska, which was widely colonized by Russians and Finns, saunas were built in the 1830s, either (it is speculated) by a wealthy Russian who had lived near the Finnish border, or a Finnish sea captain. The Alaskan Indians reported using Finnish saunas before 1867. "The last known sauna in Sitka, located at the foot of Castle Hill," writes Virtanen, "was a modern type of Finnish sauna, rather than the more primitive smoke sauna; it included two rooms, the outer of which served as a dressing room."[14]

In the 1880s and 90s, saunas were built in Michigan, Minnesota, Ohio, Wisconsin and Massachusetts, among other states. "Americans who chanced to see the sauna in use were puzzled," Aaland relates.

> [The Americans were asking,] "What is this strange nocturnal
> rite?" Farmers in Minnesota, neighbors to Finns, [were]

complaining to authorities that Finns were worshipping pagan gods in strange log temples—seen from time to time cavorting naked in the moonlight in what seemed to be ritualistic dances. A sauna went on trial in Wright County, Minnesota in 1880. An American homesteader…went to court in an attempt to rid the countryside of "that pagan temple."…But it was proved to the judge's satisfaction that the Finns were law abiding, American citizens of a staid Lutheran caliber when it was explained the sauna was a place for cleaning and not for worshipping pagan gods. The judge ordered the plaintiff to pay the defendant thirty dollars for damages to his reputation plus forty dollars to have the sauna moved to a more isolated location.[15]

According to Aaland, some historians believe that Sauna was the first name of the city that became Philadelphia. Whether or not this is true, in the Philadelphia Navy Yard there is a plaque marking the site of the first sauna.

Canada

"Canadian use of the Finnish sauna dates principally back to the time of the logging camps in the rugged Canadian forests, although some kind of sweat baths existed in early times," Virtanen states.

> The story of the Canadian loggers defrosting themselves in their sauna parallels the story of the early use of the sauna in Finland. There, too, natural circumstances forced people to do exceptionally heavy physical work for their living. The physical stress and the cold environment created a need for the sauna, and the available timber supplied both the sauna buildings materials and the fuel.[16]

Japan

The Japanese have their own traditional hot room called a *mushi-buro*. Assembled from wood or clay, it is sometimes so small that one must crawl into it. A 19th century Japanese poet praises the benefits of *mushi-buro*: "The power of this kiln bath equals hundreds of medicines."[17] To the Japanese, relaxation has been an important part of being healthy, the physically therapeutic effects of their heating chamber intertwined with emotional and spiritual aspects.

Africa

Saunas also have an honored heritage in Africa, where today, many of the original customs still survive. In Eastern Africa, Aaland reports,

> a tribal doctor will instruct his assistants to dig a hole, about the size of a grave. A fire is built in the hole and, after it has almost burned down, is smothered with large green leaves. The patient is then laid on poles over the hole until he is thoroughly smoked. Another Ugandan method is to shut the patient in a hut with a large fire until those outside decide to let him out.[18]

Russia

In some parts of the world, variations of dry body heating and bathing in pools of water evolved into steam baths. In Russia it was called the *bania* (or *banya*), a room of steam that was more humid than even the Turkish vapor bath. (In Moscow today, there are more than 50 *banias* that are so large, they can accommodate 70 people at a time.) The rooms were not as luxurious as their marble predecessors, but people wrote enthusiastically of the virtues of body heating. Like the Finns, the Russians used various sticks and branches to slap the body and bring circulation to the surface of the skin. Meanwhile, the Turkish bath was exported to America, Germany, Australia, and the British Isles.

England

In 1679, as chronicled by Virtanen, a stylish Turkish bathhouse was opened in London. The building had a domed roof embedded with round glass balls that allowed light to enter, marble on the walls, ten compartments containing benches, and pools of hot and cold running water. By the mid 1800s, there were several Turkish baths. Although some people insisted that the therapeutic baths were worthless, this may have been due to prudery rather than legitimate medical objections. There were plenty of supporters, Aaland writes:

Medical journals were full of glowing accounts for…the Turkish baths. Pamphlets were published, lectures held, and discussion groups assembled. General Sir George Whitlock said, "I was confined to my bed as a result of a kidney and liver infection, but after the third bath, I could ride my horse home at 3:00 in the morning all by myself." Some doctors claimed the Turkish bath was a good treatment for mental illnesses. And Dr. Robertson from Essex said the bath was good for "constipation, bronchitis, asthma, fever, cholera, diabetes, edema, syphillus [sic], baldness, alcoholism, and not to mention the fact that the health of the average bather was improved."[19]

Hydrotherapy in Austria

Hydrotherapy is used in conjunction with hot air heating so often, and is such a valued therapeutic modality in its own right, that it deserves a brief mention. Hydrotherapy treatments consist of baths, showers, moving or bubbling water in tubs, and compresses to promote healing and prevent disease. The water can be hot, warm, cool or cold, and different temperatures of water can be used in succession for different effects.

Water therapy has been used to lower fevers (one can be given a cold sponge bath on rubber sheets); relieve soreness, spasms and inflammation from muscles and joints (underwater exercise is used by physical therapists for people suffering from paralysis and muscle and joint problems); treat burns and frostbite (the person is immersed in water for long periods); ease labor pains (note the current interest in underwater births); and of course, help induce relaxation and eliminate stress. "The temperature of water used affects the therapeutic properties of the treatment," according to the *Gale Encyclopedia of Alternative Medicine.*

> Hot water is chosen for its relaxing properties. It is also thought to stimulate the immune system. Tepid water can also be used for stress reduction, and may be particularly relaxing in hot weather. Cold water is selected to reduce inflammation. Alternating hot and cold water can stimulate the circulatory system and improve the immune system….Adding herbs and essential oils to water can enhance its therapeutic value. Steam is frequently used as a carrier for essential oils that are inhaled to treat respiratory problems.[20]

In *The Columbia Encyclopedia*, a passage on hydrotherapy states that skin temperature water—approximately 93°F or 33.9°C—"prevents [the] loss of body heat."[21]

The Roman physicians Galen and Celsus are reported to have used hydrotherapy in the first century AD for a variety of maladies, including joint pain, hysteria, convulsions, and kidney disease. However, the medical art of hydrotherapy as we know it today originated with Vincent Priessnitz, who was born in Austria in 1799. Priessnitz, according to the *Columbia Encyclopedia*, "is credited with a number of inventions still in use, including the sponge bath, the douche, and the wet sheet pack, and he is acknowledged as an important contributor to the rise of the health spa movement in Europe."[22]

In Gräfenberg, Priessnitz built a large stone house to treat people with cold spring water in the form of baths, packs, and showers. By the end of 1839, the spa's first year in operation, Priessnitz had seen more than 1500 guests. Of this number, 120 were European doctors who had come to study his therapeutic methods so that they could establish hydrotherapy centers in their own countries.

In 20 years, the Gräfenberg spa enjoyed such an extraordinary reputation, reports Priessnitz historian Dr. Miloš Kočka, that "the Emperor's commission from Vienna declared Priessnitz's hydrotherapy a 'new remarkable discovery in the area of medicine.'" Hydrotherapy facilities were started at the Universities in Vienna and Munich by doctors Wilhelm Winternitz and Ed Schnitzlein. "The Prussian King enacted regulations regarding the approval for the establishment and managing of hydrotherapeutic institutes by doctors as well as by laymen under the supervision of doctors." Moreover, Priessnitz "was so famous he received a letter from South America with an address of only: 'Vinzenz Priessnitz—Europe.'"[23] Monuments were built in many countries to honor this innovative healer, and by 1905, more than four hundred books had been published about Priessnitz and his hydrotherapy.

A number of people, including the British physician Sir John Floyer, are credited with helping to publicize the benefits of water treatments. However, the hydrotherapy movement was given an even more dramatic boost when Bavarian priest Sebastian Kneipp (born in 1821) was cured of tuberculosis through cold water applications based on Priessnitz's methods. Kneipp wrote abundantly on the subject and opened a series of hydrotherapy centers known as the Kneipp clinics, which are still in operation today. The Spa that Priessnitz founded in Gräfenberg is still operating as well. Today, thousands of spas all over the world provide hydrotherapy as well as sauna bathing.

WORLDWIDE POPULARITY IN RECENT TIMES

Sauna Treatments in Early Medical Science

By the 1800s, when the formalized medical profession gained a strong foothold across the globe, some early published reports of the benefits of hot air therapy became rather technical and scholarly in nature as opposed to anecdotal. According to Sidney Licht,

> The first scientific clinical study in thermotherapy occurred in France before 1840....Jules Guyot, a young Parisian surgeon, began in 1833 to meditate on the value of heat in wound healing. He selected some rabbits and dogs and went to his house in the country, where he set up an animal hospital and for three months devoted himself to experiments and observations on therapeutic heat. He constructed a hot air cabinet, very similar to one that Bier devised about a half-century later, heated with alcohol lamps in such a manner that he could maintain, at will, an environmental temperature anywhere between 30 and 70 degrees Celsius [86° and 158°Fahrenheit]. He found that when the temperature was maintained at about 30 degrees [86°F], the healing of wounds was more rapid. When Magendie saw the results, he insisted that the method be tried on his patients at the Hôtel Dieu. Guyot began with the treatment of ulcers, white tumor (tuberculosis) and sciatica. "Each new trial confirmed my belief that heat incubation was a powerful therapeutic agent...." Eventually he was allowed to work on the kind of wound he felt could be helped most—the fresh wound following amputation.[24]

"As might have been expected," Licht notes, "the new treatment with heated air was used by many in different countries with glowing reports."

> Hollaender found currents of hot air under pressure of value
> in lupus (1897); Cabitto found the warm air bath effective in
> relieving attacks of epilepsy (1897); and Schmeltz used thermal
> insufflations of the vagina in pelvic inflammations (1899). The
> most glowing reports were on joint disease. Sarjeant, using a
> temperature of 240°F [115.6°C] for 40 minutes, wrote of eight
> cases of arthritis and sprain in which the "pain is generally not
> only relieved but entirely removed."[25]

Of historical interest is an article called "On Hydrophobia and Its 'Treatment': Especially by the Hot-air Bath, Commonly Termed the Bouisson Remedy," which appeared in the June 9, 1888 edition of the *British Medical Journal.* "Hydrophobia" literally means "fear of water," one of the symptoms of rabies and an early name for that disease. The article refers to the hot air sauna promoted by Etienne Frederic Bouisson (who was also known, in the 1850s, for conclusively identifying cancer of the mouth with pipe smoking, based on a statement made by a John Hill in 1761 that certain cancers were caused by smoking). It should be noted that the "hydrophobia" author categorically denounced the hot-air bath, writing that "All those patients who have been reported by respectable practitioners to have been suffering from genuine hydrophobia have died in spite of the Bouisson treatment." Rabies is deadly; anyone suffering from the disease should *not* self-treat but see a doctor immediately. Nevertheless, the author's objectivity is called into question when one also reads, "As might be supposed, its [the hot-air bath's] adoption is principally urged by those who are, for obvious reasons, opposed to the progress of medical science, the paid anti-vivisectionist agitators."[26] It is clear that the medical community was very aware of the widespread use of saunas, even if there appeared to be political reasons for not condoning their use.

Dr. John Harvey Kellogg's Heat Therapy

All early saunas and baths were made from natural materials such as wood, stone, clay, skins, and cloth. The heat source of these saunas was fire, rocks that had been placed in the fire, and/or water that was heated by fire. With the advent of modern technology, saunas were heated by gas-burning stoves, and later electric light bulbs and electric heaters. Although modern saunas deviate from centuries of tradition, they have produced consistent health benefits.

Perhaps the most radical changes in sauna construction, the greatest number of changes, and the most profound healing as a result of those improvements, were launched by John Harvey Kellogg in Battle Creek, Michigan in the late 1880s. Dr. Kellogg, a renowned and highly successful surgeon whose neat stitches became his trademark, performed over 22,000 operations in his lifetime until the age of 88. Most people today associate Kellogg solely with the name of the company that manufactures "empty calorie" junk food cereals, not realizing that the breakfast food Kellogg did in fact design was whole grain and sugarless, intended for sick people who needed a high-energy, nourishing morning meal. (What eventually became Kellogg's corn flakes was soaked grain accidentally left in the oven over-night and flattened to a crisp. The public liked it so much that a multi-million dollar, multi-company breakfast cereal industry was consequently born in Battle Creek.) But Kellogg was essentially a holistic doctor. Realizing the importance of diet, exercise, fresh air and pure water in the prevention of disease, he established a serious healing center in the late 1800s called the Battle Creek Sanitarium, which people from all over the world visited to receive hydrotherapy and other holistic treatments.

Dr. Kellogg was a prolific scientist and inventor, always searching for ways to improve people's health. Although he was already getting excellent results with hot and cold water baths and the steam cabinets he had built for the sanitarium guests, he wanted an even more efficient modality. So he began administering ozone in his steam cabinets. He was the first American to therapeutically utilize ozone in medical treatments, as reported in his book *Diphtheria: Its Nature, Causes, Prevention, and Treatment.* (A discussion of ozone combined with sauna therapy can be found in Appendix A.) Then in 1891, Kellogg started constructing horizontal cabinets large enough to hold the entire body.

The design of Kellogg's upright cabinets was not totally original—such structures had already been produced and sold for some 30 years—but at least Kellogg's saunas were not the renovated caulked barrels heated with small wood fires or hot bricks that others were using. They were far more sophisticated than the method offered in the *Encyclopedia Britannica* of that era: "heat a brick in the oven and place it in a metal basin; then pour water over it to produce steam. The bather, wrapped in a towel, should sit on a chair above the brick." Kellogg's cabinets were also far less cumbersome than the "elaborate steam bath, patented in 1814" that "included an impressive boiler to feed steam under a bed cover, and a four-posted canopy with curtains to form a roomy steam tent." And Dr. Kellogg's saunas were more advanced than the five-dollar mail-order so-called Quaker model, "a fabric cylinder enclosing a chair and spirit lamp. The bather sat for 15 minutes or so, sweating in the hot, dry air."[27]

Instead, Kellogg's cabinets were sturdy, roomy, and quite attractive. (A photo of one of his original saunas is on page 136.) However, as Kellogg himself emphasized, it was not the cabinet that did the work, it was what they contained: Thomas Edison's new electric light bulbs. The story of how Kellogg came to invent his electric light bath is not well known. As chronicled in *Physical Therapy in Nursing Care,*

> It was left to a nurse, who later was graduated as a physician from the University of Michigan in 1875, Dr. Kate Lindsay, to recognize the value of radiant heat. Doctor Lindsay suffered much from asthma, and in one of these attacks she improvised a means by which she could use an electric-light bulb in such a way that she might benefit from the heat which it gave off. She received such benefit from this simple experiment that the attending physician, Dr. J. H. Kellogg, at once conceived the idea of developing apparatus so that this form of heat could be applied with more effectiveness than by the improvised measure used by Doctor Lindsay. The present radiant-heat apparatus is the outgrowth of this observation of the benefit of heat radiated from an electric-light bulb.[28]

Once Kellogg was able to observe this simple but elegant cure, it was a natural next step to invent the electric light bath, which, writes Licht, "represented an effective substitute for sunlight."

> He began to work with the electric light because he believed that, since sunlight was so important to life and nutrition in plants and animals, it might be beneficial in certain illnesses. In 1891 he built a rectangular cabinet with 40 lamps of 20-candle power, and interior reflectors....He used it on many patients in the Battle Creek Sanatorium [sic]...He had his patients sit

in the cabinet completely nude, with the head outside as in the vapor baths or sweat cabinets...[29]

Kellogg's new sauna was unique in its effects as well as the materials of which it was constructed. Although the body perspired profusely within a matter of a few minutes, the temperature of the air in the cabinet was not much higher than the temperature of the body itself. This was because many of the heat emissions from the light bulbs were in the far infrared radiation range. Far Infrared radiation (FIR), which is emitted by the sun, is the range of wavelengths in the electromagnetic spectrum that warms solid bodies without significantly heating the air, and has distinct biological effects on living organisms. I will discuss the three ways in which heat is transmitted, as well as infrared and far infrared radiation, in Chapter 4.

Dr. Kellogg's new invention was introduced at the 1893 Chicago World's Fair. However, writes Kellogg biographer Richard Schwartz, the electric light bath "aroused little interest there. Even though the Battle Creek Sanitarium installed a number of them and patients used them regularly, little widespread public demand developed for the cabinet baths in the United States." Fortunately, Dr. Wilhelm Winternitz—who was one of Dr. Kellogg's teachers and had already established a hydrotherapy clinic in Europe—visited the Sanitarium, made careful drawings of the cabinets, was taught how to use them, and returned to Vienna where he formed a company for their manufacture and sale. "The *Kellogischen Licht Bade* soon became fashionable," notes Schwartz, "and the cabinets were installed in the royal palaces of Great Britain, Germany, and Sweden. For years the electric light cabinet bath was popular in athletic clubs, where it frequently replaced the old Turkish steam baths."[30]

Over 1000 sauna cabinets were manufactured and installed in three years, in more than 300 Light Institutes in major cities. Among those whose health was restored were many of Europe's rich and famous: members of royalty, and "German medical men and financiers [who] soon recognized the value of the method," as Kellogg reported in his 1910 book *Light Therapeutics: A Practical Manual of Phototherapy for the Student and the Practitioner*. Once the *Kellogischen Licht Bade* became popular in Europe, more Americans traveled to Michigan to Kellogg's health spa—

including, it is said, Thomas Edison himself—to avail themselves of this unique treatment.

It seems clear that sauna therapy was not merely a fad. Otherwise, it would not have attracted such huge numbers of people, and often prominent ones. "King Edward of England was cured of a distressing gout at Hamburg by means of a series of light baths," wrote Kellogg. "He had the bath installed at Windsor and Buckingham palaces. Emperor William soon after followed his example, as did several other of the crowned heads and titled families of Europe."[31] Dr. Kellogg, eager to know how and why his invention was so effective in restoring health, conducted meticulous scientific tests on the effects of sauna therapy on various physiological functions in the body. In an 1894 meeting of the American Electrotherapeutic Association, he showed photographs of his electric light bath cabinets and read a detailed report on his experiments. His research will be described in more detail in Chapter 5.

The 20th Century After Kellogg

There are few places in the world where saunas are *not* found. "The beginning of the twentieth century saw a revival of the sauna," Virtanen writes, "as Norwegians became aware that certain contagious diseases could be prevented by proper bathing habits."[32] Thanks in part to the efforts of the Norwegian Medical Association, by 1922 various health groups, including the Sauna League, had been established in Norway. By 1956, public saunas in Norway numbered 959. Meanwhile, an athletic exchange between Finland and Sweden in the summer of 1939 motivated the Swedes to adopt Finnish specifications (regarding the quality of the rocks used for heating) in their sauna buildings. Research shows that in the mid-1950s there were many saunas in Russia made of lumber. In Siberia, saunas constructed of clay were reported. Body heating was also used in Estonia, Lithuania, and Latvia.

Virtanen mentions how even soldiers on the battlefield had their saunas.

> [During] the Winter War of 1939-1940…with the mercury dropping to 55-60 degrees [F] below zero [-48.3°C to -51.1°C]

and shortages of everything, [Finnish Field Marshal] Mannerheim never forgot his soldiers. He ordered the erection of saunas wherever soldiers quartered. They [saunas] were built in bunkers, dugouts, deserted buildings and sometimes even in tents. With the whistling sounds of shot, shell and shrapnel passing close overhead, the soldiers frequently prostrated themselves for protection, but never left for safety, as they thawed their frozen bodies in the 200 degree [F, or 93.3°C] heat of the sauna.[33]

Humans have not been the only ones to benefit from body heating. Virtanen remarks that the sauna is a current way of life in Canada

> not only for people but even for horses. At least one animal physical therapist has discovered that an extremely nervous horse calms down in a sauna. The therapist built a trailer and installed a heater in each of the side walls. Heavy planks were placed in front of the heaters to prevent the animal from touching the hot elements. At horse races, he uses the trailer sauna to calm down horses which are too nervous and would otherwise be eliminated from racing by the inspector. At first the horses are reluctant to enter the trailer sauna, but after one experience, they enter with eagerness.[34]

The above paragraph makes it clear that the horse sauna uses an electric heater (horses are deathly afraid of fire). Yet despite the favorable results with animals—or, for that matter, the medical success of Kellogg's electric light bath—some people feel resistant to the idea of using electricity to heat saunas. In his day, Dr. Kellogg was considered radical for installing electric light bulbs in his sauna cabinets. And today, purists still regard electricity in any form as an anomaly. They feel that saunas should be heated solely by hot rocks, or at the very least, fire. Most of the sauna connoisseurs I interviewed for this book who told me this are of Finnish descent. Bernhard Hillila, a university professor and college dean whose parents are both from Finland, raises his voice in protest in *The Sauna Is…*:

> With the American penchant for merchandising, there is…a danger that…the concept of sauna will be stretched badly out of shape to include sauna belts, sauna facial masks, sauna tubs, sauna cabinets, sauna tents, and steam rooms of all kinds! If the product involves heat, the ad man gets a sudden perspiration [pun intended] and says, "Let's call it sauna!"…[But the] term "sauna" is properly applied only to baths in which the

entire body receives dry heat and steam. It is to be hoped that the rapid spread and increased popularity will not lead to a changed, misdirected pattern.[35]

These strong sentiments are understandable, considering that the sauna was originally conceived not only as a place for physical healing, relaxation and socialization, but also spiritual communion and spiritual purification. The connection between physical and spiritual cleanliness has solid roots; fire and heat are seen as the means of purification for good reason. No wonder, then, that Navajo Indian Hoskie gave the following advice to a non-native regarding the proper conduct in a Native American sweat lodge: "Behave as you would in your white man's church."[36]

However—and I speak with great respect for traditional native ways—if our more modern methods heal, they are valid too. *Why not* call these newer methods "sauna therapy"? The premise is the same. Throughout human history, our therapies have changed as we have changed and evolved. Surely the modern, individual sauna cabinet must have its place, along with its electrical components. Perhaps it is our attitudes that need to be consistently realigned toward the sacred—for once this occurs, the materials of which a sauna is constructed may not matter as much.

Despite the changes that modern technology has brought to traditional practices—or perhaps because of them—body heating is becoming increasingly popular into this 21st century. According to a 1988 estimate reported by P. Valtakari in the *Annals of Clinical Research* (the entire issue was devoted to the sauna), in that year, the number of private saunas in Germany reached 400,000 (public saunas numbered 7000). This figure was an increase from 12,000 in 1970, according to other sources. By 1997, the number climbed to one million. Not only are saunas standard equipment in gyms, health spas, and hotels, but sauna therapy is regularly used at hospitals and university clinics. "Sauna bathing developed into a regular form of treatment complementing physical therapeutic measures as well as…the after-care of cardiac disorders and circulatory maladies," writes Valtakari. "Finns look askance at 'sauna bathing by prescription,' but in [what was then] East Germany physicians prescribe sauna baths, the expenses of which are at first wholly covered by health insurance."[37] In other parts of Europe—Austria, Switzerland, the Netherlands, France, Spain, and Italy—sauna use keeps growing. In Russia, the related *banya* or steam bath is as popular as ever.

As might be expected, the number of saunas is the highest in Finland. According to statistics cited by Hillila in his 1988 book, a staggering 80% of all rural families are estimated to have their own saunas. An editorial from about the same time in the *Annals of Clinical Research* provides a total number of 1.4 million saunas for Finland, or about one sauna for every three or four people. (However, the distribution is uneven, as some families own two or even three saunas—one for each of their homes—and this figure also includes the saunas in health clubs, hotels, apartment buildings, hospitals, and factories.) No wonder Hillila writes, "Finland is the only nation in the world with more saunas than cars."[38] The author presents an amusing anecdote of how much sauna is a part of the Finnish culture.

> Possibly the sauna strategy has also aided the government of Finland in its basic deliberations. It has been the custom of the Finnish cabinet to gather at 4 PM on Wednesday at Kesäranta, the official residence of the Prime Minister. The first item on the agenda is the sauna. After an hour and a half of steam cleaning, the cabinet members move on to formal deliberations. The parboiled officials are perhaps a little less brittle after the bath. Even inflation doesn't seem as ominous after one has endured 200° of heat.[39]

The Finns are so serious about their saunas, that their Olympic team carries a sauna with them whenever they travel. One of the first documented cases occurred in 1924, when the Finns had a sauna built for them during the Paris games. In August of 2001, my search of "sauna" in Medline's database yielded a surprising 404 entries, including an article on the secret of a good *löyly*! Clearly, the sauna revolution is here. In his article "Healthy and Unhealthy Sauna Bathing," Ilkka Vuori writes:

> As Finns we regard the sauna as essential to the survival of our nation through centuries of hardships caused by two powerful factors, an unfriendly environment and unfriendly fellowmen. For us sauna means health in the sense of good hygiene, relief of aches and pains, companionship, leisureliness, detachment from the everyday worries, physical and mental relaxation, good sleep, and thus general wellbeing.[40]

For some people, sauna bathing is a relaxing pastime. For others, ritual sweating means communing with the divine. For still others, having the regular use of a sauna is a life-saving necessity. Regardless of your reasons for using the sauna, it will be helpful to understand the mechanics of perspiring and why we sweat. That is the topic of the next chapter.

NOTES

1. John O. Virtanen, *The Finnish Sauna: Peace of Mind, Body and Soul* (Withee, Wisc.: O-W Enterprise, 1998), 2-3.

2. Finnish Sauna Society, "Development of the Finnish Sauna," http://www .sauna.fi/pages/develpt.htm (accessed March 3, 2003).

3. J. Peräsalo, "Traditional Use of the Sauna for Hygiene and Health in Finland," *Annals of Clinical Research* 20: 220.

4. Mikkel Aaland, *Sweat* (Santa Barbara: Capra Press, 1978), 15.

5. Egyptian Orthopedic Assocation, *The Edwin Smith Papyrus,* http://www.eoa .org.eg/oldest.htm (accessed October 3, 2002).

6. Ibid.

7. Virtanen, op. cit., 53.

8. Ibid., 54.

9. Ibid.

10. Sidney Licht, "History of Therapeutic Heat," in *Therapeutic Heat and Cold,* ed. Sidney Licht with Herman L. Kamenetz (New Haven: Elizabeth Licht, Publisher, 1972), 203.

11. Aaland, op. cit., 42.

12. Virtanen, op. cit., 59.

13. Aaland, op. cit., 178.

14. Virtanen, op. cit., 90.

15. Aaland, op. cit., 100.

16. Virtanen, op. cit., 179.

17. Aaland, op. cit., 137.

18. Ibid., 135.

19. Ibid., 50.

20. Paula Ford-Martin, "Hydrotherapy," in *Gale Encyclopedia of Alternative Medicine,* http://www.findarticles.com/cf_dls/g2603/0004/2603000437/p1/ article.jhtml (accessed November 21, 2002).

21. "Hydrotherapy," in *The Columbia Encyclopedia,* 6th ed., 2001, http://www .bartleby.com/65/hy/hydrothe.html (accessed November 21, 2002).

22. Ibid.

23. Kočka, Miloš. "Vinzenz Priessnitz, Founder of Modern Hydrotherapy" on <www.afx.cz/Priessnitz> (November 21, 2002).

24. Licht, op. cit., 208.

25. Ibid., 211.

26. Victor Horsley, "On Hydrophobia and Its 'Treatment': Especially by the Hot-air Bath, Commonly Termed the Bouisson Remedy," *British Medical Journal* (June 9, 1888), 1207.

27. Aaland, op. cit., 56.

28. George Knapp Abbott et al., *Physical Therapy in Nursing Care* (Washington, D.C.: Review and Herald Publishing Association, 1941), 22-23.

29. Licht, op. cit., 213.

30. Richard W. Schwartz, *John Harvey Kellogg, M.D.: Father of the Health Food Industry* (Berrien Springs, Mich.: Andrews University Press, 1970), 125.

31. John Harvey Kellogg, *Light Therapeutics: A Practical Manual of Phototherapy for the Student and the Practitioner,* rev. ed. (Battle Creek, Mich.: The Good Health Publishing Co., 1910), 3-4.

32. Virtanen, op. cit., 72.

33. Ibid., 125.

34. Ibid., 179.

35. Bernhard Hillila, *The Sauna Is...* (Iowa City: Penfield Press, 1988), 17.

36. Aaland, op. cit., 149.

37. P. Valtakari, "The Sauna and Bathing in Different Countries" *Annals of Clinical Research* 20: 232.

38. Hillila, op. cit., 18.

39. Ibid., 37-38.

40. Ilkka Vuori, "Healthy and Unhealthy Sauna Bathing," *Annals of Clinical Research* 20: 217.

CHAPTER 2

How and Why We Sweat

Sweat is the cologne of accomplishment.

HEYWOOD HALE BROUN, SPORTS COMMENTATOR
SPEAKING ABOUT RODEOS, CBS-TV, JULY 21, 1973

Have you ever heard the popular expression, "Don't sweat it"? It means *don't fret, because whatever your concern, it isn't worth worrying about.* According to this model, perspiring is not a good thing. Yet sweating is essential to maintain proper health. In fact, if we were prevented from sweating, we would become ill and die! That is why this entire chapter is devoted to how we sweat, and the positive changes that occur in the body when we do it.

Sweating is sometimes also called hyperthermia, which means "unusually high fever." Technically speaking, sweating is not always due to hyperthermia—for instance, one can also sweat when simply overheated, or when frightened—but the two are related. This chapter, however, will mainly discuss the sweating that occurs as a result of body heating.

The act of perspiration performs several important functions. It is a means by which the body removes excess water. It helps the body rid itself of excess heat. And it is one of the main ways in which the body removes waste material.

It is obvious that sweating gets rid of body heat and water, but many people ordinarily don't regard waste removal as a major function of sweating. However, elimination through the skin is intricately tied to the functions of the lymph and circulatory systems, the respiratory and urinary tracts, and the liver. Understanding the liquid waste management processes of the body—as well as how various fluids (blood plasma, lymphatic fluid, and urine) travel throughout the system—will help us appreciate how sweating directly lessens the body's overall elimination burden. If the skin discharges even a small part of the liquid waste through sweating, other bodily systems are spared a considerable amount of the work involved in sorting, processing and eliminating waste. Therefore, I will first describe briefly how various systems in the body function. After giving an overall picture of certain physiological relationships, I will directly explore sweating.

THE MAJOR WASTE ELIMINATION ORGANS

The Kidneys

One of the major channels of elimination of water in the body is the kidneys, a pair of bean-shaped organs on either side of the spine in the lower back. It is the job of the kidneys to precisely regulate the balance and distribution of water, mineral salts, hormones, and chemicals. About 70 % of unusable water in the system is eliminated as urine. (A very small amount of fluid is excreted in the feces.) Some of the urine consists of toxins that the kidneys filter and excrete. However, contrary to popular belief, the majority of urine consists not of dirty water, but simply the nutrient-rich blood plasma that the body cannot use at the moment. It is considered waste because these products are not needed at the time the urine is being excreted.

The kidneys do a wonderful job of filtering and excreting toxins and beneficial substances from the blood. But these urinary system organs are also rather delicate. They can become overloaded, congested, inflamed—

and ultimately, even infected—if they are forced to process too much waste or toxic material at once. Perspiration, then, serves a very useful function, because during sweating, the skin assumes some of the waste removal duties that are normally performed by the kidneys. When we sweat, elimination by the kidneys is actively suppressed so that a greater than usual amount of fluid is eliminated by the sweat glands. This gives the kidneys a chance to rest.

The Liver

The liver is a spongy organ, just under the rib cage on the front right side. The largest organ inside the body, it weighs about five pounds and measures approximately 8 to 9 inches x 4 to 5 inches. Among its over 500 functions, the liver plays a major role in waste purification by producing enzymes that break down harmful chemicals into more benign and manageable substances that the body can either eliminate or reuse. Toxins are either fat-soluble or water-soluble—that is, they bond to fatty tissue or to water, according to their affinity. Toxins can range from biological waste materials (hormones, microbes) to synthetic chemicals (petroleum products) to heavy metals (lead, fluoride). The next chapter contains more detailed information on such toxins.

The liver is powerful and resilient. However, not enough nutritional support or too many toxins will eventually clog it to the point where it can no longer produce adequate enzymes to neutralize foreign pathogens and other noxious material. The healthier your liver is, the more toxins will be excreted in your sweat. And, the more you sweat, the less your liver and intestines will be burdened with eliminating waste. See Chapter 8 for more details on how the liver detoxifies, and what you can do to support its function.

The Lungs

The lungs are two large sac-like organs on either side of the heart, comprised of highly elastic tissue that is moistened by mucous membrane. The lungs do more than deliver oxygen to the bloodstream and expel carbon dioxide (a product of cell metabolism). They transform some toxic chemicals into water-soluble byproducts, which are then excreted by the urinary system. Some toxins, such as volatile organic compounds (VOCs), can also be exhaled. A surprising 20% of fluid in the body is emitted in the form of water vapor through the lungs. When the body becomes hot, either through exercise or sauna therapy, the oxygen needs of the body increase by about 20%. This raises the respiration rate. As the respiration increases, so does the amount of water vapor emitted through the lungs.

The Skin

The skin is the largest organ of the body, weighing about six pounds and averaging about 20 square feet in area. Most people do not think of the skin as an organ like the heart or liver—since unlike these internal organs, the tissue of the skin envelops the entire outside of the body, and its tightly packed cells are spread out like a thin blanket instead of bulging in clusters. However, what characterizes an organ is the ability to perform multiple tasks based on messages sent to, and received from, other parts of the body. The skin, therefore, is identified accurately; for it is wonderful at "multi-tasking," processing bodily materials based on the feedback it sends to and receives from other biological systems.

The skin contains nerve endings, blood vessels, pigments, hair follicles, keratin-containing cells that waterproof the body and prevent bacteria from entering, and oil and sweat glands. Normal skin is supple, clear, smooth, and able to withstand a fair amount of mechanical stress. Consisting of the same type of tissue that in the developing embryo forms the internal spinal cord and neurons, it is very much an external "nervous system"—sensitive to pressure, pain, heat and cold. Since the skin is the interface between the body and its environment, it is the body's front line of protection. There is an insulating layer of fat beneath the surface of the skin to help keep us warm, and the skin prevents many types of bacteria from entering the body. It appears that the skin protects us in other ways, too, according to an exciting article in the December 2001 issue of *Nature Immunology*. German researchers have discovered a protein secreted by the sweat glands that acts as an anti-microbial agent. Called *dermcidin* (from the words that mean "skin" and "to kill"), this substance destroys many bacteria including *E. coli*, *Enterococcus faecalis* and *Staphylococcus aureus*, and the fungus *Candida albicans*. It is quite possible that the skin also has other important functions that haven't been discovered yet.

One square inch of skin contains 90 oil glands, also known as *sebaceous glands*. These glands secrete an oil known as *sebum*, which coats the hair follicles as well as the skin. Sebum seals in much-needed moisture, making the hair and skin supple and preventing drying and cracking (skin) or breakage (hair). People may think that the fat-like, waxy sebum eliminated by the sebaceous glands is the same as the unwanted body fat or *lipid* that gives us our "spare tire." But they are different types of fat; we do not emit lipid from the sweat glands. Sometimes excreted with the sebum are harmful bacteria that could clog the glands. Although skin is waterproof, it does absorb fats and oils, provided the molecules of fat are small enough to penetrate its pores. Other materials can also penetrate the skin, such as

FIGURE I

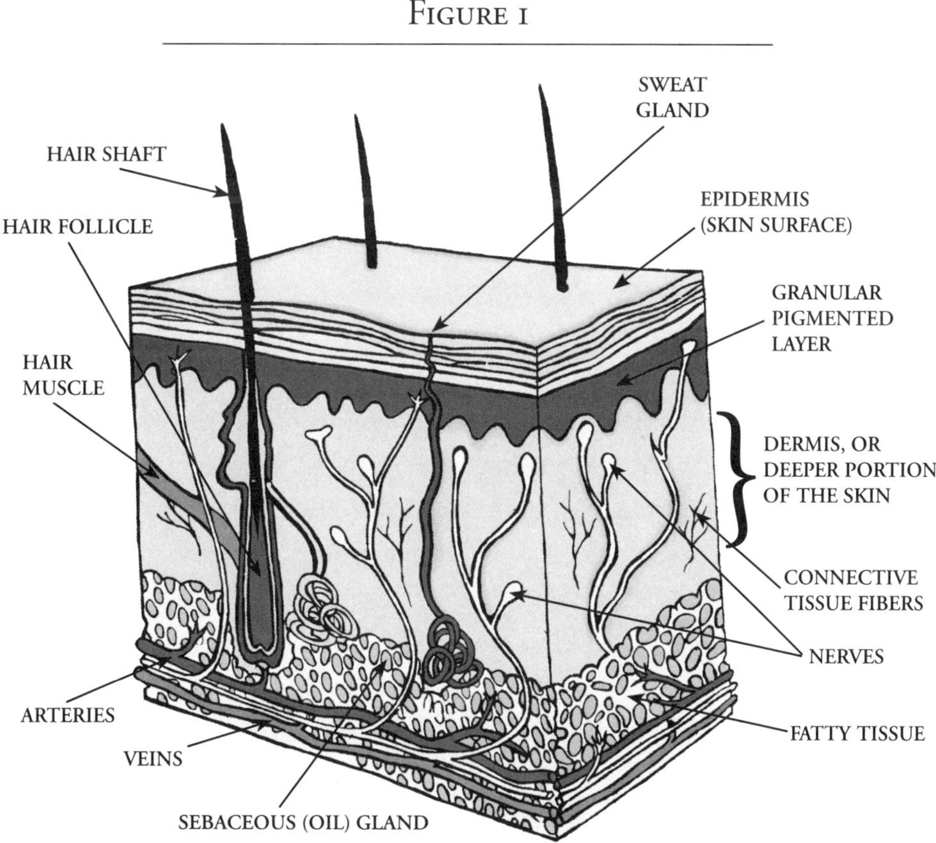

chemicals, heavy metals, some gases, and rays from the sun. (See Figure 1, a cross-section of skin containing sweat glands, on the previous page.)

The skin plays a major role in controlling body temperature through sweating. Although the skin is perceived as having different types of nerves—which respond accordingly to touch, pressure, temperature, and pain—their functions seem to overlap, as when the application of cold alleviates pain during tissue injury due to its numbing effect, or when the application of heat alleviates pain due to its relaxation of the tissues. (Heat has the effect of ultimately lessening the excitability of muscular tissue, thus calming the receptors for pain.) There are 625 sweat glands in an average square inch of skin, or approximately 2½ million sweat glands in the average person. Weighing approximately 100 grams (about three ounces), they are distributed throughout the entire body except for the nipples, external genitalia and lips. Along with nerves and hair follicles, sweat glands lie in the deepest part of skin tissue called the *dermis*, just above the fat. Sweat glands are long tubes that are coiled into a ball about one-third of the way up the skin, and which then straighten into single vertical channels called *ducts* that travel through the *epidermis* (the outermost layer of the skin).

There are two types of sweat glands. *Eccrine sweat glands* lead directly to the pores or openings of the skin and release the perspiration through the pores. They are especially plentiful on the hands, soles of the feet, and forehead, although they are present on the entire body. *Apocrine sweat glands* end in hair follicles and release the perspiration through the openings for the hair. (They also contain tiny muscles that rise when the person is cold, emotionally uneasy, or sexually aroused, a phenomenon known as "goose bumps.") These apocrine sweat glands are especially plentiful around the genitals and under the arms. Both types respond the same way to the body's signals to perspire. However, due to the different locations there are differences in the sweat. The sweat from apocrine glands contains proteins and fatty acids due to its sebum content. This makes the sweat thicker and more yellow, causing underarm stains on clothing. The odor that often accompanies sweat is not from the perspiration itself but from the bacteria on the skin and hair. Although women possess more sweat glands than men, men perspire more easily because they have a faster metabolic rate than women and generate more internal heat.

The body is always eliminating water through the skin. When the external temperature is comfortable, the fluid output called *insensible* sweat (meaning "not easily sensed") amounts to anywhere from one-and-one-half pints to a quart per day. Although not enough for us to notice, this small amount is very important since, along with the oil secretions, it helps to keep the skin moist and prevents drying and cracking. However, in this chapter and throughout the entire book, I will be focusing on the much larger quantity of visible sweat—called *sensible* (meaning "able to be sensed")—that is created by heat and muscle exertion. The body emits a number of different signals, and these signals reach a number of different bodily tissues before the sweat glands ultimately release the fluid we call sweat.

Nearly one-third of the perspiration emitted through the skin is discharged through the hands and feet. As stated in the *Edgar Cayce Handbook for Health Through Drugless Therapy*:

> Elimination through the skin is very important, for the skin normally does about one-twentieth of the work of the kidneys. When the skin elimination is speeded up, it can take care of practically one-tenth of the work that the kidneys usually do for the body. Therefore, stimulation through the skin is important for elimination...for it can help kidney function and prevent kidneys from becoming overloaded.[1]

Thus, with the kidneys, bowel, and lungs eliminating most of the body's water, the remaining 10% is normally emitted as perspiration through the skin. However, given the opportunity, the body can eliminate up to 30% of all waste through sweating. For this reason, the skin is sometimes called "the third kidney." As I will discuss shortly, the skin is given the opportunity to exercise its "third kidney" function during sauna therapy.

The Circulatory and Lymphatic Systems

When I began the research for this book, my very first question was "Where does sweat come from?" Once you appreciate how the circulatory and lymphatic systems work, it is easier to understand how the bodily fluid from both of these systems actually becomes what we call sweat.

The circulatory system is responsible primarily for supplying nourishment to the cells and transporting wastes to other systems in the body that are designed to eliminate them. Blood is comprised of *red blood cells, white blood cells* (which as a major part of the immune function of the body provide protection against pathogenic microbes and toxic chemicals), and some other materials, which float in a colorless liquid called *plasma.* The lymph system, although connected to nutrient distribution on a limited basis, plays a major role in the body's fluid regulation, immune response (the ability to protect itself against microbes, chemicals, and other harmful foreign agents), and waste removal. The *lymphatic fluid,* almost identical in composition to blood plasma, also contains a white blood cell called a *lymphocyte,* which is manufactured by the lymph tissue.

Lymphatic fluid is very thick and viscous. Compared to blood, which is about one-thirteenth of the body's weight, lymph accounts for a quarter to a third of the total body weight. Unlike the circulatory system, which has a heart to pump blood through its blood vessels, the lymph system doesn't have the equivalent of a heart to move the lymph through its channels. Instead, it must rely on mechanical pressure (such as the movement from physical exercise) to move the dense fluid. Thus, the lymph channels can become congested rather easily. That is why exercise (movement from within) and lymphatic massage (movement from without) are so important to help it move. For people who cannot exercise or receive a massage—or whose lymphatic systems are especially sluggish—sauna therapy no longer seems like a luxury but a necessity. Body heating causes both the lymphatic and the cardiovascular vessels to dilate, thus allowing the fluids from both systems to move more rapidly.

Due to the structures of the circulatory and lymph systems, the body's nourishment and waste collection cycles are intimately connected. In the cycle of blood circulation, the heart first pumps blood directly to the lungs, where the blood picks up fresh oxygen. Newly oxygenated blood immediately returns to the heart to be distributed throughout the body via blood vessels called *arteries.* The iron-rich hemoglobin in the red blood cells combines temporarily with the oxygen, giving these round cells their bright red color. (At the point when the red blood cells lose their oxygen and pick up carbon dioxide, they become darker red, traveling through the blood vessels called *veins,* which return to the heart.) The largest artery in the body, highly elastic to accommodate the pressure of a huge volume of blood, exits the heart. It is the *arterial capillaries*, however, that supply tissue cells with nutrients, since the capillaries are the only blood vessels small enough to fit in between each individual cell. It's important to recognize that our circulatory system is a single continuous network of many different types of blood vessels that are given a variety of names—arteries, veins, arterial capillaries and venous capillaries—according to their size and where they are located in the body.

Generally, all blood traveling away from the heart, filled with new oxygen from the lungs to deliver to the tissue, is either in arteries or arterial capillaries; and all blood traveling back to the heart, filled with carbon dioxide it has picked up from the tissue cells to deliver to the lungs to be expelled, is either in veins or venous capillaries. (The one exception to these rules is that the newly oxygenated blood travels first to the heart to refresh it.) Arterial vessels of all sizes are involved with nourishing the body cells. Venous vessels of all sizes are involved with waste removal from the body cells. It is the veins and venous capillaries, and not the arteries and arterial capillaries, that are closest to the surface of the skin.

The lymphatic system is a vast network of porous vessels and nodes, or gland-like clusters, that contain the lymph fluid. Some lymph clusters are in the throat (where they are called tonsils), the neck (noticed when we get swollen glands), the armpit, and the groin area. The lymphatic network roughly parallels the vessels in the circulatory system. However, since the lymph system deals so heavily with waste removal, its channels parallel *only* the veins and venous capillaries.

Toxin removal takes place during an exchange between the venous capillaries and the lymphatic vessels. A capillary is so tiny that red blood cells must pass through single file. At the point where the blood reaches a capillary, there is so much pressure and so little room in the channel, that some of the thin plasma fluid is squeezed from the capillary. This nutrient-rich, watery fluid that now bathes each cell is called *interstitial fluid*. After the cells take their nutrition from this interstitial fluid, they discharge waste products, which are a normal product of cell metabolism (the chemical reactions by which the cell sustains itself). Now it is time for the lymph vessels to play their sizeable role in waste management. Unlike the blood capillaries, which by design do not allow particulate matter to enter, lymph vessels are permeable. The waste-filled interstitial fluid gravitates to the nearest tiny *lymph capillary*. Once the liquid is drawn into the lymph capillary, it is called *lymphatic fluid*. This fluid travels to larger and larger lymph vessels, eventually arriving at the lymph nodes where it is cleaned by the lymphocytes and other immune cells. Lymphatic fluid can contain dead, treated microbial waste, heavy metals, and chemicals. After the lymph nodes neutralize and transform the toxic material, the treated waste trickles back into the venous bloodstream.

The cleaned, excess water that is now in the venous bloodstream must be eliminated by the body. When the fluid reaches the kidneys, the kidneys recycle back into the body those nutrients that can be used, and send the remaining liquid to the bladder for excretion.

THE FUNCTIONS AND BENEFITS OF SWEATING

Now we are ready to discuss sweat. What role does sweat play in the above picture?

As we saw before, sweat is classified as *insensible* and *sensible*. Insensible perspiration is excreted by the skin in such small amounts throughout the day that it is unnoticeable. It is believed to come solely from the spaces between the tissue cells, or in other words the interstitial fluid. Sensible perspiration, on the other hand, is the plentiful, running-down-your-face kind of sweat that occurs during body heating. During sensible perspiration, a much more complex process takes place. The sweat glands, responding to many different signals and needs of the body, are required to excrete much more fluid than the interstitial spaces can immediately provide. Therefore, the plasma from the capillaries flows into the interstitial spaces to replace what is being sweated out. After the capillaries release fluid into the interstitial spaces, the adjoining sweat glands then absorb that plasma fluid. Special cells within the sweat glands transform the fluid into its final form of sweat. What is now sweat travels through the sweat ducts to be excreted through the pores of the skin. (It is interesting that, depending on its function and location in the body, the fluid is called either blood plasma, interstitial fluid, lymphatic fluid, urine, or sweat. Except for the presence or absence of some proteins and mineral salts and maybe some toxins, it is basically the same liquid.)

Cooling the Body

The skin's role in removing wastes from the body is intimately connected to its role in regulating temperature. "Most of the heat produced in the body is generated in the deep organs, especially in the liver, brain, and heart, and in the skeletal muscles during exercise," write Arthur C. Guyton and John E. Hall, authors of the popular *Textbook of Medical Physiology*. "Then this heat is transferred from the deeper organs and tissues to the skin, where it is lost to the air and other surroundings."[2] It is the skin temperature that rises and falls along with the temperature of the environment. However, heat and cold management in human beings is designed so that in a healthy body, the deep tissues or core remain fairly constant.

Measured orally, body temperature ranges from a little less than 97°F (36.1°C) to 99.5°F (37.5°C). It can temporarily rise during strenuous exercise, sometimes to as high as 104°F (40°C); and it can fall during extreme cold, sometimes lower than 96°F (35.6°C). However, although the core temperature can vary a little, remaining within what are considered "normal" limits, it should not vary too much. Fever, produced for a specific reason by people who are ill, is another matter entirely, which I'll discuss shortly.

The *hypothalamus* of the brain contains a biological thermostat that is always alert for temperature changes in the body. The need for temperature regulation is signaled by nerves from inside the body and by nerves in the skin (which are in contact with, and always reacting to, the external environment). Once the hypothalamus decides what is needed to correct the body temperature, it sends signals to many different organs, glands and systems in the body. These signals first travel through the spinal cord, and then through certain nerves in the sympathetic part of the *autonomic nervous system*. (The autonomic nervous system functions automatically—that is, we do not have any conscious control over it—and *sympathetic* refers to the part of the autonomic nervous system that responds to alarm signals, as opposed to the need for relaxation.) Cooling of the body occurs in almost the exact inverse of how the body heats. The heart rate slows, pores close, and dilated blood vessels contract as body temperature returns to normal. Since the skin is no longer releasing copious amounts of fluid, more water is now sent to the kidneys—which is why one may feel a desire to urinate when the body is cooled after being overheated.

Different processes occur in the body, depending on whether it needs to be cooled or heated. If the person is cold, an automatic response of shivering will occur to produce more heat. Blood vessels in the skin will also contract to restrict blood flow to the body's core, thus preserving heat where it is needed the most. That is why extremities such as the hands and feet are the most in danger of freezing in bitter cold. If the person is overheated, the process is almost the opposite. Blood vessels in the skin dilate and the arterial capillaries force plasma into the spaces between each tissue cell, where the fluid is now called interstitial fluid. (The red and white blood cells and various proteins that were originally in the plasma remain in the blood vessels.) Then, the fluid migrates to the sweat glands through osmosis and hydrostatic pressure. *Osmosis* is the tendency of a liquid to flow from where there is more water to where there is less. *Hydrostatic pressure* means that as the fluid is pushed into the spaces between the cells, the pressure increases because there is less space between the cells. Since water cannot compress under pressure, hydrostatic pressure is even more of a factor than is osmosis in driving the fluid into the interstitial spaces.

Once the fluid reaches the coiled glands in the skin, it quickly fills the sweat ducts and flows out of the pores, where it is known as sweat. Since evaporating water cools whatever it leaves, the evaporation of perspiration will cool the body as long as the sweat leaves faster than it can be produced.

Perspiring, incidentally, makes the skin itself less sensitive to heat. This is convenient and appropriate, considering that people perspire *because* and *when* it is hot. If heat is supplied to the system faster than it is lost, the body temperature can safely rise by about six degrees Fahrenheit (a little more than three degrees Celsius).

Relieving Congestion

While the capillaries at the skin's surface are releasing their fluid into the sweat glands (via the interstitial spaces) to cool the body, they are also directly eliminating excess heat through the skin into the air. This is a direct result of their being dilated—which also accounts for the flushing, in varying degrees of redness, experienced by people who exercise, take saunas, or suffer from fever or sunstroke. When the capillaries are fully dilated, the rate of heat transfer from the core to the skin can increase by *eight times.*

The dilation of the capillaries makes a big difference in the quantity of blood they can hold. Normally, at a room temperature of about 70° F (21.1° C) with a resting heart rate, the amount of blood at the surface of the skin is about five to ten percent of the total blood supply. During intense heating of the body (say, if the person remains in a sauna for at least 20 minutes with sufficient penetration of heat into the tissues), the blood flow to the skin can increase *50% or more.* Dr. Kellogg, who in the late 1800s conducted some breakthrough experiments with many types of sauna cabinets, reported that when the blood vessels at the surface of the skin are fully distended, the skin can hold one-half to two-thirds of all the blood in the body. (This increase in blood flow to the skin does not increase blood pressure, however, because during body heating, all of the vessels in the cardiovascular system are stretched, and the internal vessels contain less blood.)

The dilation of blood vessels close to the skin does much more than simply dissipate heat—although that is of course an important function. Kellogg wrote in his 1910 book *Light Therapeutics*:

> Careful study of the blood supply of internal organs in relation to the skin shows that the blood vessels of every important internal organ are very directly connected with the vessels of the skin, through arteries or veins, or both....[When the blood flow to the skin's surface substantially increases] we possess in artificial congestion of the skin a method whereby we may quickly withdraw from the great vascular organs of the trunk from one-fourth to one-half of their total contents, thus affording almost instant relief to a congested liver, engorged spleen, hyperemic [containing too much blood] lungs, inflamed stomach or intestines, or congested spinal cord.
>
> ...This chronic congestion of vital organs necessarily results in derangement of functions, and often in change of structure. Passive congestion or stagnation of the blood in a part necessarily involves diminished oxygenation and accumulation of CO_2 and other toxic substances in the tissues. The result is partial asphyxiation and autointoxication of the congested parts through the accumulation of tissue poisons. A congested liver cannot do its duty as a bile-making and toxin-destroying viscus.[3]

Kellogg's elaboration of what occurs in a congested body is worth quoting at length because he had such a cogent and accurate understanding that autointoxication, or toxic overload of the body, causes disease.

> The congested stomach first manufactures an excessive quantity of highly acid gastric juice, but with a deficiency of pepsin [one of the digestive enzymes]. Sooner or later even the acid glands are worn out and hypopepsia [impaired digestion due to an under-secretion of pepsin] and apepsia [no pepsin secretion at all] result. The stomach then becomes a culture chamber for microbes of various sorts. Under the influence of the toxins produced, glands degenerate, resistance is lowered, chronic gastric catarrh [inflammation of mucous membranes] develops, cancer and other neoplasms [abnormal tissue growth] appear; through absorption of the toxins formed, the resisting power of the blood is lowered; general autointoxication occurs and various cachexias [states of general ill health, malnutrition, and wasting] develop; skin diseases of various sorts and general and local nervous disorders appear, especially the various forms of neurasthenia [a depressed state characterized by weakness and exhaustion]. Even melancholia and paresis [partial paralysis] may be traced to the influence of toxins generated in the alimentary canal.
>
> Similar results may follow congestion of the intestines. The resulting catarrh [mucous membrane inflammation] of the duodenum [the part of the small intestine that connects to the stomach] may extend into the liver and gall bladder, giving rise to jaundice, gallstones, hepatic abscess, pancreatic disease, appendicitis, hemorrhoids, the various forms of colitis, mesenteric tuberculosis, tubercular peritonitis [inflammation of the membrane lining the abdominal cavity], cancer of the intestines and peritoneum, and other maladies which are the outgrowth of lowered general and local vital resistance and traceable to a blood supply which has deteriorated by long retention in over-dilated vessels [in the deep tissues and organs of the body].[4]

Other illnesses that can result from congested blood are anemia, many kinds of pain in the nerves, muscles and joints, exhaustion, and "an almost infinite variety of mental and general nervous symptoms" such as dizziness, mental confusion, and depression.[5] About 20 years after Kellogg invented his incandescent bulb sauna, he wrote, "During the time which has elapsed since its first employment, this bath has been used under the author's general supervision in more than fifty thousand cases, aggregating several hundred thousand applications"![6]

Kellogg's enlightened emphasis on the importance of eliminating blood congestion is strikingly similar to the recognition in Chinese medicine that stimulating stagnant blood will help eliminate sluggish or weak chi (life force). Like the Chinese, who knew that meridians or energy channels correspond to certain organs and systemic functions, Kellogg also observed that the skin contains certain reflex areas which, when heated, correspond to and relieve congestion in particular organs. (We now know that these meridians physically exist at the widest sections of the fascia, called the fascial planes.) Not only is congestion of the inner organs almost always present in chronic disease, Kellogg advised, but pale skin is related to too much internal blood flow. (This is partly why the skin reddens and shines when people perspire: the blood is moving from the interior to the surface of the skin.) He also attributed the pallor of skin to a state of chronic spasm in the blood vessels just at the surface of the body.

Alkalizing the System

Kellogg was also aware that sweating helps induce an increased (desirable) alkalization of the system. (Although the liver and kidneys play a major role in regulating the acid-alkaline balance of the body, frequent intense perspiring can profoundly assist the process.) Toxins—whether acidic or alkaline themselves—have an acidifying effect on the body because they impair the energy metabolism of the cells and prevent biological wastes from being properly excreted. Over a relatively short time, these acid wastes produced by the body accumulate in the tissues.

A very interesting book by medical doctor Richard Kovács called *Electrotherapy and Light Therapy with Essentials of Hydrotherapy and Mechanotherapy* (published in 1949) demonstrates both Kellogg's legacy and the extent to which heat and light were routinely used as legitimate therapies by the medical community until the discovery of antibiotics. When a person perspires, Kovács wrote, "there is a loss of water, salt, urea and other nitrogenous substances, with a relative excess of alkali remaining in the blood and in the tissues" (presumably because so many acidic wastes were removed).[7] However, what was to Kovács in his day a "relative excess of alkali" may no longer apply in our current age, since so many people suffer from excessive systemic acidity that can result from illness, exposure to toxic chemicals, and an acid-forming diet consisting of sugar, too much grain and animal protein, and not enough vegetables.

Negative stress, with its acidifying stress hormones, also creates acidic wastes in the body. (*Stress* can be defined as the body's response to challenges created by internal and external input. If the body's resources are depleted or drained as a result of dealing with the input, the stress is negative. If the body responds to the input as a stimulating challenge so that growth and beneficial adaptation result, then the stress is positive.) Since a high level of systemic acids can augment any disease or unhealthful condition that already exists—as well as create new ones—I want to spend a bit of time discussing the acid-alkaline balance of the body, also known as the *pH*.

Simplistically put, pH is a term designating a mathematical formula that computes the acidity or alkalinity of the body. The following is excerpted from my recently published book, *The Handbook of Rife Frequency Healing*.

> The optimal pH levels for the blood, urine and various bodily tissues differ slightly from one another. However, in order for the person to maintain absolute health, the one body area whose pH *must* stay within a very narrow range of alkalinity is the arterial blood plasma. Depending on which authority is being cited, the ideal pH range for the blood plasma is from about 7.35 to 7.45 or 7.5. If the blood deviates too much from its ideal pH for too long a period of time, the person becomes sick and eventually dies....
>
> The body is basically internally alkaline by design (the skin is naturally acidic). How, then, does it become acid? Acidic waste products are constantly being created during the course of normal everyday metabolic processes. If these acidic wastes are not expelled, they end up poisoning the system. It is the job of the respiratory tract, the chemical and physiological buffering system (which includes the liver), and the urinary tract to regulate the acid-alkaline levels. The respiratory tract

alters the rate of carbon dioxide ventilation from the bodily fluids. This in turn changes the ion concentration through a series of biochemical processes. The chemical and physiological buffering system of the body goes through a number of different steps to produce extra chemicals, which also counteract the acidic pH imbalance in the blood plasma. It is the urinary tract network, however, that is by far the most efficient method the body has for getting rid of acids. The kidneys play a prominent role in excreting acid through the urine—although even this method has its limitations. The blood transports excess acid to the kidneys only a little bit at a time, and slowly. No matter how hard the kidneys are forced to work (assuming they don't become overloaded), there is only so much acidity that they can excrete. Eventually, when the kidneys have done all they can, and there are still excess corrosive acids and acid-forming substances that threaten to damage the bloodstream, the acids are simply relocated elsewhere in the body to protect the blood. The wastes get stored in the extra-cellular fluids (fluids surrounding the cells), the connective tissue, the joints and even the organs. This is how a chain reaction of deterioration in bodily functions starts to occur. It is this autointoxication, in which one is poisoned by one's own toxic wastes, that lays the foundation for degenerative diseases which include arthritis, allergies, fibromyalgia, diabetes, cardiovascular problems, kidney stones, bone loss and cancer.

The body's finely tuned needs clearly show that storing overly acid *or* alkaline wastes in the tissues to get them out of the bloodstream—while a necessary short-term emergency intervention by the body—is hardly the ideal solution to a pH imbalance. Bone loss is a good example of a highly unbalanced, overly acid system. It also graphically illustrates a malabsorption or shortage of calcium and other minerals, which are key factors in maintaining the proper pH. Most of the calcium we ingest is not used for bone construction, but instead freely circulates in the body to be utilized in different metabolic processes, including the neutralization of systemic acid. The pH balance of the blood is so crucial that when no more calcium is available in the system, the body leaches it from the bones.[8]

This unfortunate scenario is all too common. Too many acids in the body cause more than bone degeneration, however. As if degenerative conditions weren't bad enough, most bacteria, viruses, parasites, and fungi love a mild degree of acidity. (They do die in terrain of very high acidity as well as very high alkalinity; but at those extremes, you can't survive either.) The same unbalanced pH level that causes a deterioration of the body's tissue also allows these microorganisms to proliferate. And when they do, they excrete acidic wastes into the bloodstream, creating a vicious cycle of more acidity, and hence more microbes—and more infectious diseases. In case there are any remaining doubts that sweating alkalizes the system, consider that the pH of perspiration is acidic. It can be somewhat acidic at 6.8 (7.0 is neutral), or extremely so at 4. This scale acquires greater meaning when you realize that the numbers on the acidity/alkalinity scale do *not* represent equal divisions. Each number higher than the one before it represents an *exponential* increase: 1 is ten times greater than 0, 2 is 100 times greater than 0, 3 is 1,000 times greater than 0, and so on. This means that even a small change in pH levels makes an enormous difference.

In *Reverse Aging*, Sang Whang addresses both the problem of stagnant blood and excess acidity: "Acid coagulates blood, thus causing poor blood circulation around the places where the acids are accumulated. This in turn causes some organs to act sluggish and we start to see the symptomatic signs of aging."[9] The poorest circulation is often at the capillaries, through which red blood cells can pass only one at a time. Even if a person's diet and health improve enough to make the system generally more alkaline, the tiny capillaries won't benefit from this change as long as they remain clogged, surrounded by the acid wastes that have accumulated deep in the tissues. Body heating, however, expands the capillaries enough to loosen and break up or dissolve the toxins, which can then exit the body through urine and sweat.

Of course, it is possible that someone's system might be too alkaline (although according to microbiologist Robert O. Young, excessive alkalinity is always the result of the system's attempts to compensate for an over-acid condition). Neither extreme is healthy. But sweating helps the body clear out all debris, acidic and alkaline, allowing the tissues to be restored to their original pristine state.

Circulatory and Respiratory Changes

The circulation of blood in the lungs is closely related to cardiac output. During exercise, Guyton and Hall write, "both oxygen consumption and total pulmonary ventilation increase about 20-fold between the resting state and maximal intensity of exercise *in the well-trained athlete*."[10] [emphasis theirs] This figure may be the origin of claims by some sauna therapy proponents that during body heating, the oxygen needs of the body increase by about 20%. However, it's important to remember that sauna therapy isn't exercise. As I will discuss later in this chapter, there are some important differences between the two. People who are *not* well-trained athletes, who are sitting passively inside a sauna rather than jogging or rowing, may find that their oxygen consumption and total pulmonary ventilation do not conform to the above.

Nevertheless, the circulatory system does undergo many changes when a person sweats. The heart may beat up to 160 beats per minute, due to the increase of blood to the skin to reduce temperature and the corresponding increase in metabolic rate. With blood circulating so much faster, the amount of blood that can be pumped may be twice the amount that is pumped during normal rest. This allows a more rapid delivery of nutrients to body tissues as well as improved waste removal. Kovács recognized that the increase in circulation from body heating causes a "rise of the pulse-rate in the ratio of about 10 beats for each degree Fahrenheit, just as it does in fever."[11]

Body Heating and Weight Loss

Sauna manufacturers and dealers frequently claim that sweating causes weight loss. The promotional material from various companies ranges from modest to extravagant. The most conservative estimate states that a 20-minute to 30-minute sauna session—providing the person perspires consistently—yields a loss of 200 to 300 calories, an energy expenditure roughly equivalent to running two or three miles. The most extraordinary claim gives a 2000 calorie loss, roughly equivalent to the energy expended by someone in superb physical shape rowing or jogging for 30 minutes.

Some medical doctors scoff at even the more conservative figure. They declare that all weight lost during a sauna session is from water rather than fat, and that once the bodily fluids are replenished, the weight will immediately return. It is understandable that one might be skeptical of manufacturers' claims—especially if they sound extravagant. But at the same time, assertions from uninformed doctors who are antagonistic to the mere mention of sauna therapy are not reliable, either. Thus, we need to piece together the truths in these two contrasting views to determine whether or not people really lose weight from doing sauna therapy.

Perhaps the most concise claim as to why one loses weight in the sauna is from Major Ward Dean in his letter to the editor in the August 7, 1981 issue of the *Journal of the American Medical Association*. Many sauna manufacturers cite this issue of the journal when referring to the number of calories expended in the sauna.

> The fact overlooked by most people who attempt to debunk saunas and other devices that cause enhanced sweating is that the water does not just "leak out" of the body. Sweating is a part of the complex thermoregulatory process of the body involving substantial increases in heart rate, cardiac output, and metabolic rate, and consumes considerable energy. In a sauna...the only means of maintaining body temperatures in the normal range is by evaporation of sweat, a process that consumes approximately 0.586 kcal per gram of water lost. A moderately conditioned person can easily "sweat off" 500 g[rams] in a sauna, consuming nearly 300 kcal [calories]—the equivalent of running 2 to 3 miles. A heat-conditioned person can easily sweat off 600 to 800 kcal with no adverse effects. *While the weight of the water lost can be regained by rehydration with water, the calories consumed will not be....*Regular use of a sauna may impart a similar stress on the cardiovascular system [as running]—and its regular use may well be as effective a means of cardiovascular conditioning and burning of calories as regular exercise.[12] [emphasis added] [For the sources of the information on cardiac output, the writer cites T.H. Benzinger, "Heat regulation: Homeostasis of Central Temperature in Man" in the *Physiology Review* 49 (1969): 671-759 and J.R. Brobeck, editor, *Best & Taylor's Physiological Basis of Medical Practice, 9th Ed*, 1973, p. 133. For the sources of information on metabolic rate, the writer cites G.T. Koroxenidis, J.T. Shepherd, and R.J. Marshall, "Cardiovascular Response to Acute Heat Stress" in *Journal of Applied Physiology* 16: 869-872 and L.B. Rowell, G.L. Brengelmann, J.A. Murray, et al., "Cardiovascular Responses to Sustained High Skin Temperature in Resting Man" in *Journal*

of Applied Physiology 27:673-680. For the source of information on calories lost during body heating, the writer cites Guyton's *Textbook of Medical Physiology, 4th Edition*, 1971, pp. 833-834.]

If an increase in metabolism can augment the amount of body heat that is produced, then conversely, given enough heat, the body can—and does—increase its speed of metabolism. Thermal and chemical messages in the body are intertwined in a process called *chemical thermogenesis*; and these processes are supported by the laws of thermodynamics. The following data, from a very interesting British textbook with the deceptively bland title of *Clayton's Electrotherapy 10E*, explain why. (The numerous contributors to this book explain cellular function on many levels—physiological, biochemical, electromagnetic—to provide an understanding of the success of different non-invasive treatments, including heat, laser therapy, ultraviolet and far infrared therapies, electrical stimulation, and ultrasound.)

"When heat is added to matter," writes Kenneth Collins, "a number of physical phenomena result from increasing the kinetic energy of its microstructure. [Kinetic energy is energy in motion.] These may be summarized as follows:"

1. Rise in temperature: The average kinetic energy of constituent molecules increases.

2. Expansion of the material: Increased kinetic energy produces a greater vibration of molecules which move further apart and expand the material....

3. Change in physical state: Changing a substance from one physical state (phase) to another requires a specific amount of heat energy....

4. Acceleration of chemical reactions: Van't Hoff's Law states that "any chemical reaction capable of being accelerated, is accelerated by a rise in temperature...."[13]

These natural laws point to the changes in body chemistry and the expansion of blood vessels that induce other changes that occur during fever, exercise, or saunas. Some increase in metabolism does occur in the body when it is subjected to high heat. We already know that the metabolic rate rises about six percent for every degree Fahrenheit rise in the body temperature. With the adipose (fat) cells heated at high enough rates to cause substantial molecular friction, the enzymes and hormones will break them down and transport them through the bloodstream for the body to use as energy. The more energy burned, the more weight the person loses.

Despite the above data, it must be emphasized that *the results of heating the body from an external source are not identical to results from an internally generated fever*. In fact, the two modalities might be seen to operate on opposing principles. Dr. William MacKay, Associate Professor in the Department of Physiology at the University of Toronto, explains:

> During fever, the hypothalamus deliberately elevates the core body temperature and keeps it there. In the sauna, where the body temperature is elevated by external heat application, the hypothalamus is unwilling to allow a significant rise in core body temperature. As body temperature rises in the sauna, thermoreceptors in the hypothalamus detect the rise in temperature. In response, the hypothalamus activates mechanisms to cool the body—that is, keep the body temperature at its normal level. These mechanisms include skin vasodilation and sweating, of course, *but also a reduction in secretion of hormones that increase metabolic rate*.[14]

This reduction in metabolic hormones, including thyroxin from the thyroid, helps clarify why people *might not necessarily* lose weight from sauna therapy. "However, one also has to contend with the fact that all metabolic reactions are sensitive to temperature," MacKay points out. "The higher the temperature, the faster *all* metabolic reactions proceed. So just by temperature effects alone, metabolic rate will be elevated; although because of that the endocrine system will be trying hard to slow metabolism down. It is classic homeostasis at work."[15] As I will discuss later in this chapter, according to Dr. MacKay, during a fever, the body can switch from burning glucose to burning fat for energy. Although one probable reason for this is the starvation of microbes (most of which feed on glucose), conceivably one might also lose that extra abdominal bulge. But there is no guarantee that this will happen. This points to the wisdom of doing some form of aerobic exercise shortly before entering the sauna.

Despite the above, there is a very interesting study called "Repeated Thermal Therapy Improves Impaired Vascular Endothelial [lining of the blood vessels] Function in Patients with Coronary Risk Factors," which strongly supports weight loss during sauna bathing (without exercise). Authors M. Imamura and colleagues were not exploring weight loss per se, but instead wanted to find out whether sauna therapy helps repair the cells lining the major blood vessels of the heart (it does). However, they also incidentally discovered that after 15 minutes of sauna therapy every day for two weeks, their subjects not only had a *significant* decrease of body weight, but their fasting blood sugar levels *also* decreased significantly. A lower fasting blood sugar level means that when the person awakens, the level of glucose in his or her blood is lower than usual. I attribute this lower reading to the increase in metabolism. The body burns fuel more quickly, which depletes some of the glucose that normally circulates through the blood to feed the tissues. (The heat source in this sauna used far infrared heating, which will be discussed in detail in Chapter 4.) Since the authors were not biased toward reporting weight loss but instead were looking for something else entirely, their finding assumes even more significance.

How much cold is applied after the body is heated, and even the degree of chill, may also affect weight loss. In an article called "How the Sauna Affects the Endocrine System," K. Kukkonen-Harjula and K. Kauppinen studied the effects of sauna bathing on the increase of thyroxin (the thyroid hormone which increases the body's metabolic rate) and TSH (thyroid-stimulating hormone, which the pituitary gland secretes to induce the thyroid gland to secrete more thyroxin). The authors write that if one gradually cools at room temperature following a sauna, there is no increase in these hormones. However, they write, "If the sauna is followed by cold exposure (a shower or a swim), the concentration of TSH is increased."[16] (Please note that *this procedure is not safe for everyone, especially for those with a heart condition.* Read Chapters 6, 7, and 8, and check with your doctor, before undergoing sudden extremes of heat and cold.)

"There is no question that cold-sensitive thermoreceptors are much more powerfully stimulated by rapid cooling than gradual cooling," concurs MacKay. "The stronger sensory signal would then elicit a more vigorous response from the hypothalamus to activate the thyroid. So I would agree that the net stimulus to the thyroid is more powerful with rapid cooling. Indeed, one might conjecture that this aspect of sauna therapy may be the most important for aiding weight loss." [17]

A final explanation for weight loss during body heating may be due to the beneficial heating of a critical enzyme called 5'-deiodinase. The thyroid gland is responsible for regulating the body's metabolism through its output of thyroxin (also known as T4). However, it is not T4 that is actually absorbed and utilized by the cells, but the physiologically more active hormone called liothyronine (or T3). The body uses the 5'-deiodinase enzyme to convert T4 to T3. Metabolic processes occur correctly only when this conversion takes place.

Significantly, though, T4 cannot be converted into T3 if the body temperature is too much below normal (98.6°F or 37°C). The shape of an enzyme depends on its temperature: too much *continual* heat makes the enzyme too tight, and too much *continual* cold makes the enzyme too loose. Due to chemical insult, dietary indiscretions, emotional trauma, or other stress, some people's body temperature—and hence enzyme temperature—becomes too low to convert the thyroxin to liothyronine. (This condition is called Wilson's Thyroid Syndrome, named after the doctor who discovered it.) People with Wilson's Thyroid Syndrome are in a vicious cycle. If the body temperature is too low, the enzyme becomes too loose and the body cannot readily convert T4 to T3. This can make the body temperature even lower, which in turn makes the enzyme even more misshapen and more unable to perform the proper conversion of T4 to T3! One can have an adequately functioning thyroid gland, with lab tests that show sufficient T4 in the bloodstream—yet have low thyroid *activity* in the *cells* (indicated by tests for T3 levels), which is a truer indicator of metabolic function. Low T3 levels indicate low thyroid *system* (as opposed to low thyroid *gland*) function. A person can experience clinical symptoms of hypothyroidism due to low performance of either the thyroid gland, or of the thyroid system.

The treatment of choice for Wilson's Thyroid Syndrome consists of a drug containing *only* T3 (rather than T4, or a combination of T3 and T4). Once the extra T3 in the body starts increasing the temperature, the 5'-deiodinase enzyme resumes more of its proper shape and starts converting more T4 into T3. With the resulting higher body temperature, the enzyme functions even more efficiently and a normal temperature is eventually reached—

at which point (according to Wilson's findings) the person no longer needs T3 medication. Since Wilson's Thyroid Syndrome is a temperature-related condition, it seems clear that in addition to the effects of the (necessary) exogenously administered T3, heat from a sauna might conceivably warm the 5'-deiodinase enzyme enough to raise the metabolism at least a bit (which would assist with weight loss). A far infrared sauna is best for this function, for reasons that will be explained throughout this book.

Thus, many factors are involved in weight loss during body heating. Clearly, the weight loss discussion is complex and unresolved. It does not appear that there is any simple "yes" or "no" answer.

Toxin Elimination

There is a charge—mostly voiced by the conventional (allopathic) medical community—that sweating does not substantially eliminate toxins from the system. This claim simply is not true. First, interstitial fluid is a component of sweat. Since waste products of cellular metabolism are contained in interstitial fluid, it seems obvious that sweating does indeed help the body get rid of toxins. Second, fat stores are universally recognized as depositories of toxins that are not easily metabolized. Even though certain heavy metals gravitate toward bone, these and environmental poisons (such as many pesticides) often are found in fat cells because by nature, lipids surround poisons to prevent them from contaminating the rest of the body. When the metabolism speeds up, the body breaks down the fatty tissue and digests it for energy. At this point, poisons that were held by the fat cells get dumped into the bloodstream, to be broken down by the liver and then removed with perspiration. Details on the toxins found in sweat, and some of the issues surrounding chemical poisoning, will be discussed detail in the next chapter. For specific detoxification programs, see Chapter 8.

It must be noted that Dr. Kellogg himself did not believe that many toxins were eliminated through perspiration. He felt, rather, that the real value of sweating lay in its alleviation of the congestion of the inner organs. However, in Kellogg's time, many of the chemical poisons that surround us and which we take for granted as a part of modern daily life had not yet been invented, so they could not have been excreted. Given the fivefold increase in degenerative diseases today, which are certainly related to poor quality food, environmental contaminants and so on, I believe that the good doctor would have found many more poisons excreted in his clients' sweat had he conducted tests in the 21ˢᵗ century. Kellogg's comparisons of sweat from various types of saunas are described in Chapter 4.

THE PURPOSE AND EFFECTS OF FEVER

The elevated body temperature that we call *fever* is a different phenomenon from the elevated temperature that occurs during sauna therapy. However, there are many similarities between the two. Also, medically induced high fevers are often induced with special heat cabinets or used as a treatment along with regular sauna therapy. Therefore, I want to discuss what happens in the body during normally occurring fever and medically induced fever.

Fever is a condition in humans and all warm-blood animals that naturally occurs during illness, when the temperature rises as part of the body's immune response. As mentioned earlier, a generally safe zone of temperature increase is considered to be about six degrees Fahrenheit (a little more than three degrees Celsius). However, during serious illness, the body temperature may rise by as much as eight degrees Fahrenheit (about four degrees Celsius). Such high temperatures constitute a medical emergency.

One major purpose of fever, as described by Stephen E. Langer and James F. Scheer in *Solved: The Riddle of Illness*, is that it "encourages quick inflammation in the immediate area of an infection and keeps it from spreading."[18] I will address this phenomenon in the next chapter in my discussion of endogenous biological materials.

Another purpose of fever is the production of heat. First, the *macrophages* (immune cells that destroy microbes) send a hormone-like biochemical message to the brain that a fever is needed in the body. Then the brain signals the *thyroid* and *adrenal glands* to work together to speed up the body's metabolic rate so that extreme heat is produced. All of this raises the "set point" of the body's temperature. Raising the set point means that the baseline for the minimal amount of heat required by the body rises, just as when you turn up the thermostat on the heating system in your house. The *hypothalamic* portion of the brain, knowing that more internal heat is required, then sends a biochemical message in the form of a thyrotropin-releasing hormone to the *pituitary gland*. The pituitary, in turn, transmits thyroid-stimulating hormone (TSH) to the thyroid gland. In response, the thyroid secretes extra thyroxin, which increases the rate of cellular metabolism throughout the body. At the same time, the adrenal glands secrete epinephrine and norepinephrine. These hormones help increase the metabolism by stimulating activity in certain tissues such as heart and skeletal muscle, by dilating blood vessels, and by altering the blood flow. Part of this increase in metabolism stimulates the process of *perspiration*. Langer and Scheer write:

> Experiments by G.W. Duff and S.K. Durum showed that at two degrees centigrade [3.6 degrees Fahrenheit] of fever, certain immune system defenders—T-cells and antibodies—increased by 2000 percent over their number at normal body temperature. Similar findings were reported by another research team. Antibody production in the spleen cells has been found to increase dramatically during a fever. Scientists have concluded that the hormone-like substances, called interleukin-1, set off body defense cells to fight infection and also send the brain signals to increase body temperature to provide an ideal climate for the multiplication of defense cells. Many physiologists believe that human beings are equipped with a temperature regulation system which puts a ceiling on fever at approximately 41.11 degrees centigrade (106 degrees Fahrenheit).[19]

In addition to the above research, a 1937 study by a Mayo Clinic doctor on "The blood picture before and after fever therapy by physical means" (using the hot air Kettering hypertherm sauna) found a 58% increase in white blood cell count after fevers of 104° to 106.8°F (40° to 41.6°C) were induced in subjects. Moreover, the white blood cell increase remained several hours after the fevers were induced.

Not only are the body's immune defenses marshaled through fever, but many pathogenic microbes cannot survive in temperatures above, say, about 105°F (40.6°C). For instance, the growth rate of the polio virus is reduced up to 250 times at 104°F (40°C). The Lyme disease spirochete (a dangerous corkscrew-shaped bacterium) dies at the same temperature. Temperatures of about 106°F (41.1°C) cause the death of the *Streptococcus pneumoniae* bacterium, which causes pneumonia, middle ear infections, arthritis, and inflammation of the heart, brain, intestinal, and spinal cord membranes.

High heat also kills tumors: cancer cells die at temperatures from about 104°F to 107°F (40°C to 41.7°C). Dr. Jeffrey Freeman, founder of the Europa Institute of Integrated Medicine, explains the mechanism of this process:

> Researchers have found that the blood vessels in normal tissue actually open up (to dilate) when heat is applied, in an effort to flush out the heat and cool the cell environment down. Because a tumor is a more tightly packed group of cells, blood circulation is restrictive and sluggish. When heat is applied to the tumor...temperature continues to rise to destructive levels. This process continues over a period of time even after the treatment....The tumor cells are now extremely susceptible to destruction by radiation or by additional heating.[20]

Artificially induced *hyperthermia* (an abnormally high body temperature, or fever) can be created when heat is applied either to the entire body, or to individual areas when the cancerous tissue is local and circumscribed. Sometimes, minute amounts of mistletoe (mistletoe is lethal in large doses) are injected to produce heat. Or, the doctor can inject other herbs or drugs, or use hot water, far infrared, or some other heat-generating method. After the client's temperature is raised to that of a high fever, ice or cold water are carefully applied and the temperature returns to normal. This takes place in a highly controlled environment with various life support monitoring equipment, where blood glucose, electrolytes, and other vital sign levels are very carefully watched. Freeman notes that many types of cancer respond well to hyperthermia: cancer of the bladder, bowels, breast, liver, lung, lymph, prostate, stomach, and uterus. "Cancer patients whose previous treatments have proven unsuccessful may benefit from hyperthermia," he writes. "Most patients receiving hyperthermia find it very tolerable....There is no danger" as long as the person is monitored by the physician. The machines used for the therapy are water-cooled, thus maintaining a constant temperature. Those receiving allopathic care such as radiation or chemical treatments "are able to reduce the dosage....This results in far less [overall] toxicity [to the body]."[21]

In all high-temperature treatments for illness, the microbe-killing capacity of fever is augmented by the body's increased production of white blood cells as part of a heightened immune response. That is why a hot bath, exercise or a sauna at the beginning of a cold or flu can prevent it from escalating, or stop it entirely.

People do not need to be technologically advanced to understand the benefits of hyperthermia. In the West Indies, natives suffering from syphilis or cancer have cured themselves by deliberately subjecting themselves to infections from such high fever diseases as malaria and typhoid. And the survival function of high temperatures is so important that animals whose bodies are unable to generate a fever by themselves will purposely manipulate their environment to create one. Langer and Sheer report:

> [R]esearcher M.J. Kluger and his associates [made] a stunning discovery on infected lizards. Lizards do not have a built-in fever-generating system such as ours and must find fever-inducing sources on the outside. The Kluger team learned that sick lizards have an instinct which makes them seek hot environments in order to raise their body temperatures to fever level when they are sick. Infected fish, too, swim to warmer water to raise their temperatures and combat illness.[22]

When one is ill, microbes are destroyed by more than the direct "cooking" effect of high heat. They are further disabled because, during fever, the body uses a different kind of fuel for energy than when it is experiencing normal temperatures. Ordinarily, the body takes *glycogen* (a long chain sugar molecule) that is stored in the liver and breaks it down into *glucose* (a simpler form of sugar), which then circulates through the bloodstream to supply energy to the body cells. The drawback is that pathogenic microbes as well as the body's tissues use glucose for energy. However, at high enough temperatures, the body metabolizes fat (and in extreme conditions, protein) in addition to glucose to meet its increased energy needs. "By switching to energy sources other than glucose, the body lowers its glucose levels in the blood plasma," explains Dr. MacKay. "The reduction of plasma glucose helps curtail the possible proliferation of bacteria." [23]

Nature is elegant; it always has more than one purpose for any function. In a striking synchronous chain of events, while the body is generating a fever it also produces extra enzymes, which immune cells require in order to break down toxins and foreign particles. MacKay notes that since high heat destroys enzymes, the body will create heat shock proteins if the fever continues. These proteins bond to, or "chaperone," the enzymes to protect them from the high temperatures. Fever also produces changes in the blood's concentration of neurotransmitters and peptides (made from amino acids, the building blocks of protein). These affect the brain by inducing relaxation (which is why sick people want to rest), thus allowing the body to focus solely on healing.

The feverish body also secretes certain hormones such as beta-endorphin, norepinephrine and possibly even growth hormone. Beta-endorphin is an endogenous (meaning "produced by the body") painkiller, similar in chemical composition to synthetic morphine. As you might imagine, the alleviation of pain is an indispensable function for people who are injured or ill, which is why heating pads, sweating, sauna bathing, and other ways of increasing body heat relieve pain. Norepinephrine dilates the blood vessels and changes the blood flow in the body. Growth hormone promotes lipolysis, or a breakdown of fat stores as an energy supply (a convenient function, since the body is quite busy and needs fuel)—although different studies have yielded somewhat contradictory data about whether or not body heating causes a significant increase of growth hormone. One 1980 study shows an increase in growth hormone resulting from a session of body heating. Kukkonen-Harjula and Kauppinen write that "usually" there is an increase of growth hormone, although individual differences are "considerable" and younger people have a greater increase than the elderly. But they cite another finding, that though there is a substantial increase of growth hormone at first, as sauna bathing continues the levels decline.[24] Medical doctor William Rea, who specializes in environmental illness, writes in *Chemical Sensitivity*: "The different results of these studies [about the changes in growth hormone levels] may be due to variations of total body pollutant load in the researchers' respective patient populations."[25] Therefore, whether sauna therapy increases the production of growth hormone is apparently dependent on several factors. (Conceivably, if the body could safely be brought to high enough temperatures in the sauna—especially if the sauna uses far infrared radiation (FIR) as its heat source—a fair approximation of a fever condition, as well as increased amounts of growth hormone, might be produced. Why FIR could make a difference will be discussed in Chapter 4.)

The Body's Heat Adaptation Mechanisms

I should mention at least briefly some of the mechanisms the body develops to adapt to continuous heat, whether it's from living in a tropical climate or taking lengthy daily saunas. When someone is regularly exposed to heat for about four to six weeks, the body increases its sweat output, usually from about one to three quarts per hour. As the periods of sweating become more numerous, the loss of salt—which at the beginning is a substantial 15 to 30 grams a day—decreases over time, usually diminishing to 3 to 5 grams a day. This is because the cortex of the adrenal glands secretes more of the hormone *aldosterone*, which causes the sweat glands to reabsorb sodium from the kidneys before the sweat is released through the skin. However, the potassium salts in the body still tend to be excreted. Since the body requires a precise balance of sodium and potassium, the potassium must be replenished, either through supplements or potassium-rich foods such as bananas. As the person becomes even more experienced at sweating, still less salt is excreted, and even the potassium does not have to be replaced as much.

Another adaptation of the body to sustained heating, worth mentioning again, is the continued production of "heat shock" proteins. These protect the enzymes so necessary for thousands of chemical reactions in the body.

Despite the body's adaptability to heat, however, it cannot adapt well indefinitely to very high temperatures. Dr. Kellogg was aware that although applications of heat can be stimulating and refreshing, there is a point at which heat is no longer beneficial. An overheated body becomes exhausted and no longer responds as it should. The augmented enzyme output suffers, because some of the proteins that comprise the enzymes are heat sensitive and are destroyed above a certain heat threshold. The skin can become burned. In addition, continual body heating without any respite actually causes a *decrease* in the body's ability to perspire, since in an overwhelmed system the brain overheats and the hypothalamus shuts down, no longer able to perform its temperature-regulating function. Under such conditions, where the heat remains too high with no relief, heatstroke can result. It generally begins with fatigue and dizziness or light-headedness, and if not treated can end in unconsciousness and even death. The differences between simple heat exhaustion and the medical emergency of heatstroke, along with their respective treatments, are discussed in detail in Chapter 7.

The type of sauna one uses, and the application of cold after the heat, may determine how much benefit one derives from sauna therapy. Of course, there is obviously a difference between being in a very hot room for 15 minutes, as opposed to an hour, or being in 180°F (82.2°C) for half an hour, as opposed to 80°F (26.7°C) for half an hour. Your own sensations are a valuable guide in showing you how much heat is too much.

For these reasons, Dr. Kellogg did not leave people in his light cabinets for too long. He also gave his clients sponge baths or immersed them in cold water before re-introducing them to the light cabinet. In addition, he installed fans in his later model saunas so that the perspiration would be whisked away immediately. Leaving sweat on the skin for prolonged periods can cause unhealthful conditions such as prickly heat rash. People unused to sweating should be acclimatized to sauna therapy slowly and remain comfortable. Also, plenty of mineralized water should be available to replace the fluids and electrolytes lost through perspiration. (Electrolytes are minerals in a particular form. They are discussed in more detail in Chapter 3.) Kellogg wrote:

> For producing the [desired] effects, long applications are not necessary. Three to six minutes [in the light cabinet] are ordinarily sufficient. The duration of the [sauna] bath need be only enough to produce moistening of the skin from perspiration. In certain classes of cases, [however,] longer baths are needed. This is especially true of obesity, rheumatism, gout, and in diabetics who are strong and not emaciated. In these cases it is necessary to continue the bath sufficiently long to produce an elevation of temperature, so as to stimulate oxidation of the protein wastes. For this purpose the duration of the bath should be fifteen to thirty minutes, or until the temperature taken in the mouth reaches 100° to 100.5°F [37.8° to 40.6°C].[26]

Kellogg is an invaluable resource, integrating serious and meticulous medical research with a well-rounded holistic approach. No one today could find legitimate fault with his methodology, despite the fact that his book is almost 100 years old. Most of what he wrote is as applicable today as it was a century ago. Those portions that are no longer pertinent say more about how much sicker people are today, than they do about the quality of Kellogg's work.

SUMMARY

Briefly, the documented physiological effects of heating the body above normal temperatures are as follows:

- accelerated heart rate, causing increased cardiovascular circulation, especially at the surface of the skin
- enhanced lymphatic circulation
- increased production of hormones, including beta-endorphin, nor-epinephrine, and (depending on conditions, such as the application of cold afterward) thyroxin
- increased production of white blood cells
- increased production of enzymes
- relaxation of the muscles
- selective stimulation of the parasympathetic nervous system (responsible for the relaxation response)
- the killing or disabling of microbes

These effects in turn lead to the following benefits:

- the elimination of stagnant blood and the decongestion of organs, which in turn stimulates better organ function
- faster metabolism (the rate at which nutrients are assimilated and toxins are removed)
- increase in systemic alkalization
- decrease or total elimination of pain in the nerves, muscles and joints in the majority of cases
- reduction or elimination of disease

Once the physiology and biochemistry of sweating are clear, it is easy to understand why so many seemingly miraculous assertions are made about sauna therapy. These claims of better health are not inflated. Virtually every condition of ill health can either be eliminated or substantially improved by improving organ function and the better distribution and assimilation of nutrients. These processes augment toxin removal, kill microbes (that were not initially affected by the high heat), and help balance the pH of the body (which generally means an increase in systemic alkalinity). As

I discuss in Chapter 6, the ability of the body to repair itself under optimal circumstances either influences, or directly causes, a complete or partial reversal of infectious diseases and degenerative conditions.

That said, there is one caveat to the general principles I have just outlined. People are very different, each with their own unique physiology and biochemistry. Kukkonen-Harjula and Kauppinen write, about their own research:

> Some of the information available on the effects of sauna baths on the endocrine system is inconsistent. This is probably because the bathing arrangements in the experimental situations may have varied and the subjects have not always been accustomed to the sauna. The diurnal changes of hormone secretion, meals and physical exercise preceding the sauna exposure, or individual characteristics (age, sex, health, amount of adipose tissue) should be considered….Only a few studies have compared different ways of taking sauna baths and consequent physiological effects. In our study the changes in the concentrations of hormones in blood in young men were small in a sauna of 80°C [176°F] (dry heat) and somewhat greater in a sauna of 100°C [212°F] (dry heat). The greatest hormonal responses were obtained in a sauna of 80°C [176°F] with added steam ("löyly") … Some of the changes in hormonal secretions in the sauna are similar to those that occur during physical exercise, but some [are] unique to the sauna.[27]

Despite the dissimilar characteristics of the test subjects, the differences in saunas used in body heating studies, and even the sometimes contradictory research results, I think that there is enough positive and convincing data about sauna therapy to make it worth trying. The next chapter, which discusses the increased toxic load that we all carry, may help convince you even more.

Notes

1. Harold J. Reilly and Ruth Hagy Brod, *The Edgar Cayce Handbook for Health Through Drugless Therapy* (New York: Berkeley Publishing Group, 1986), 72.

2. Arthur C. Guyton and John E. Hall, *Textbook of Medical Physiology, Tenth Edition* (Philadelphia: W.B. Saunders Company, 2000), 822.

3. John Harvey Kellogg, *Light Therapeutics: A Practical Manual of Phototherapy for the Student and the Practitioner, Revised Edition* (Battle Creek: The Good Health Publishing Co., 1910), 44, 48.

4. Ibid., 48-49.

5. Ibid., 49.

6. Ibid., 51.

7. Richard Kovács, *Electrotherapy and Light Therapy with Essentials of Hydrotherapy and Mechanotherapy* (Philadelphia: Lea & Febiger, 1949), 328.

8. Nina Silver, *The Handbook of Rife Frequency Healing: Holistic Technology for Cancer and Other Diseases* (Stone Ridge, NY: The Center for Frequency Education, 2001), 27-28.

9. Sang Whang, *Reverse Aging* (Miami: JSP Publishing, 1999), 114-115.

10. Guyton and Hall, op. cit., 973.

11. Kovács, op. cit.

12. Ward Dean, letters to the editor, *Journal of the American Medical Association* 246 (August 7, 1981), 623.

13. Kenneth Collins, "Thermal Effects," in *Clayton's Electrotherapy 10E,* ed. Sheila Kitchen and Sarah Bazin (London: WB Saunders Company Ltd., 1996), 95-96.

14. William A. MacKay, personal communication, December 3, 2002.

15. Ibid.

16. Kukkonen-Harjula, "How the Sauna Affects the Endocrine System," *Annals of Clinical Research* 20: 264.

17. MacKay, op. cit.

18. Stephen E. Langer and James F. Scheer, *Solved: The Riddle of Illness* (New

Canaan, CT: Keats Publishing, Inc., 1984), 37.

19. Ibid., 37-38.

20. Jeffrey Freeman, "Why We Use Hyperthermia" (handout, Europa Institute of Integrated Medicine, 1999), 1.

21. Ibid., 2.

22. Langer, op. cit.

23. MacKay, op. cit., September 3, 2001.

24. K. Kukkonen-Harjula, and K. Kauppinen, op. cit.

25. William J. Rea, *Chemical Sensitivity, Volume 4: Tools of Diagnosis and Methods of Treatment* (Boca Raton: Lewis Publishers, 1997), 2445.

26. Kellogg, op. cit., 53.

27. Kukkonen-Harjula, op. cit., 264-265.

Chapter 3

What We Sweat, and Why We Need to Get Rid of It

Better keep yourself clean and bright;
you are the window through which you must see the world.

GEORGE BERNARD SHAW,
IRISH DRAMATIST AND LITERARY CRITIC (1856-1950)

In America, billions of dollars are spent each year to make us smell as though we don't sweat. Advertisers would have us believe that human beings should emit the aroma of jasmine or musk—or better yet, not have any body odor at all. But it is normal for any biological material, including human skin, to emit a scent. There is really no reason to hide one's normal chemical signature, other than bondage to custom and fear or disgust of normal bodily functions.

On the other hand, a downright stinky or pungent body odor indicates that poisonous materials (such as bacteria) have accumulated in the system or on the skin faster than they can be expelled; and to eliminate the odor, the person's health must be improved. In this case, it is normal to have a negative response to noxious odors because molecules of the unhealthy material are physically entering your system through the air you're breathing. But the breath fresheners, colognes, and deodorants that all promise to make us sweeter-smelling merely mask odors by numbing the nasal passages—they do nothing to address the cause of the odor. To make things worse, most of the personal care items used for cleansing the body and face, or covering up foul scents, are themselves loaded with harmful chemicals that don't belong in the body. This will become evident as I continue.

The following pages provide a brief overview of some of the chemicals in our environment, how ubiquitous they are, and why it's important to eliminate them. Sherry Rogers, a doctor specializing in environmental medicine, bluntly states: "Toxicity is a one-way street leading to disease; the key to healing the impossible is to reverse the toxicity."[1] She feels so strongly about this, her book is called *Detoxify or Die*. Once you realize the effect of toxins on your health, sauna therapy may seem more indispensable than ever.

THE BURDENED BODY

Numbers vary as to how many new chemicals and chemical compounds are created weekly, monthly or yearly—but it is certain that as the perceived need for chemicals increases, so does the number of chemicals. Of those chemicals that become new products and are added to our food, water or soil, less than half have been approved by our government agencies. Consider the following data from a 1982 article, "Evaluation of a Detoxification Regimen for Fat Stored Xenobiotics."

> Over four million distinct chemical compounds have been reported in the literature since 1965, with 6,000 new compounds added to the list each week....More than 3,000 chemicals are deliberately added to food and over 700 have been identified in drinking water....Over 400 chemicals have been identified in human tissues, with some 48 found in adipose [fat], 40 in [breast] milk, 73 in the liver, and over 250 in blood plasma. The characters of chemicals found in adipose tissue are diverse, but tend to reflect biologically persistent or often used materials such as DDT, PCB, dioxin, nalkanes, PCP and THC.

Chemicals stored in adipose and other tissues pose a continuing physiological and psychological threat to human health. Dioxin has been associated with ischemic vascular disease and with other physiological as well as psychological effects as long as ten years after initial exposure. Oncological studies have shown a significant association between PCB and DDE levels in fat and increased cancer incidence. In addition, PCB exposures have resulted in increased plasma triglycerides, even in the absence of overt symptoms of PCB toxification. PCBs in monkeys not only resulted in increased blood lipids, but negatively affected the ability to maintain pregnancy. Further, they have been related to personality and cognitive functioning of persons unexpectedly exposed.[2]

A study appearing in the 1995 *Proceedings of the American Public Health Association* states:

> The EPA reports that literally every American has accumulated measurable levels of some thirty different toxic chemicals in their tissues. More recent reports set the tally at one hundred and seventy-seven. Every woman's breast milk boasts pesticides, [and other pesticides such as] lindane, chlordane, [and] dieldrin and sixty-five isomers of PCBs and dioxins. The average man's semen has thirty-five different forms of PCBs. The human body has become the final repository, the final toxic waste dump. Increasing toxic body burdens have been associated in the literature with increased risks, health effects, and symptomatology. It is not surprising this chemical plethora is having an adverse effect on the population at large.[3]

Leaping ahead about five years, in a Public Broadcast Service special on the chemical industry's suppression of evidence that their own products cause cancer, televised in the spring of 2001, newsman Bill Moyers had his blood drawn and analyzed. Out of 150 common industrial chemicals, Moyers' blood contained *over 80*. Among them were alcohols, solvents, pesticides, petroleum-based synthetics, PCBs, and persistent organic pollutants (POPs). Moyers is in his 60s. It took years for these chemicals to build up to their present levels in his bloodstream; and 50 years ago, there were far fewer chemicals than there are today. If Moyers has these levels of contaminants in his body now, what must it be like for a young child or infant—who must deal with even more chemicals, but whose immune system is not as fully developed as that of an adult? Mr. Moyers is not unique in where or how he lives; most people are as toxic as he. DDT, a pesticide that does not biodegrade well and has been banned since the 1960s for that reason, has even been found in the fat of polar bears in the Arctic!

Everything that we eat, drink, inhale, and in many cases touch, goes right into the body. The chemicals can be stored anywhere—in the organs, glands, muscles, even the bones—but one place where toxins are concentrated is the fatty tissue. Fat is present not only beneath the skin, but surrounds the organs. The brain and nervous system are predominantly comprised of certain types of fat (the brain is 65% to 70% fat), which is why chemicals can be so dangerous and produce so many and varied effects, ranging from motor impairment to mental confusion. In fact, some doctors believe that especially in people who are sensitive to chemicals (such as those having a formal diagnosis of multiple chemical sensitivity or environmental illness), the inhalation of chemicals injures the hippocampus and limbic areas of the brain, thereby accounting for the symptoms of emotional distress, learning disabilities, memory loss, and other cognitive impairments.

"If storage of chemicals and drugs in adipose tissue was a static phenomenon, or if these chemicals caused no harm, further research might be unjustified," states an article from the Foundation for Advancements in Science and Education. But these chemicals are highly active. Human exposure to one type of pesticide leads to a

> lifetime adipose tissue burden of DDT. Chemicals which store in fat do not remain there indefinitely, nor are they pharmacologically benign....Once these lipophilic [fat-loving] chemicals move from the fat to the blood, they are carried to every organ in the body, including the target organs for which they pose a threat. The result is a significant risk of adverse health effects, both chronic and acute.[4]

"Our bodies act like sponges, absorbing the chemicals to which we are exposed," write Jacqueline Krohn and Frances Taylor in *Natural Detoxification*.

> Water-soluble chemicals are absorbed and then excreted. However, fat-soluble chemicals accumulate in our fat cells and cell

membranes....When the body is under stress [as during illness, emotional anguish, or nutritional deprivation], it releases these chemicals from the fat to circulate in the bloodstream.
Later, these chemicals will return to the fat cells and cell membranes, to be released another time. The release and return cycle of these chemicals continues indefinitely unless we help our
bodies rid themselves of toxins.[5]

Thus, any toxin not excreted by the body can be recycled continually
into the bloodstream, re-exposing the system again and again. Since every
cell in the body contains some fat—even if it's a very small amount—the
toxins can actually lodge anywhere.

It should be noted that women have more problems with toxins than
do men because, with a higher percentage of fat in their bodies, they have
more places to store the poisons. As Krohn and Taylor point out, women's
smaller size in general also causes them to become ill from chemicals more
quickly than their male counterparts. Also, women's higher levels of estro-
gen and progesterone can interfere with the efficiency of some enzymes
utilized in the detoxification process. Finally, due to lower levels of the enzyme called *alcohol dehydrogenase*, women are less able to detoxify alcohol.
This includes the alcohols in solvents as well as the kind that you drink.

Given the pervasiveness and danger of common chemicals, it is no surprise that David Steinman provides figures of "Typical Background levels
of Pesticides and Industrial Chemicals in the Blood" in *Diet For A Poisoned
Planet*. What might appear to be insignificant amounts can in fact be lethal
because the chemicals are so dangerous: it does not take much to poison
a human being. Moreover, the levels that exist in a person's blood and fatty tissue are now higher than they were in 1990, when the book was published. It is horrifying to think that tables such as Steinman's even have to
exist as we humans continue to poison ourselves and our environment.[6]

The United States Environmental Protection Agency agrees. Its chill-
ing 1982 *National Human Adipose Tissue Survey*, on the amounts of poisons taken from the fat cells of surgery patients and cadavers, reports PCBs
in 86%, four out of five dioxins in more than 90%, eight of the nine benzene–related volatile organic compounds in more than 90%, benzene in
96%, and 1,4-dichlorobenzene found in all. And the December 1986

Type of Chemical	Specific Chemical	Amount in Parts Per Billion (ppb)
Aromatic Solvents in Blood	Benzene	less than 1 ppb
	Ethylbenzene	less than .5 ppb
	Styrene	less than 1 ppb
	Toluene	.6 ppb
	Xylene	1.5 ppb
Halogenated Volatile Hydrocarbons	Chloroform	less than 1 ppb
	Dichlorobenzene	less than 1 ppb
	Dichloromethane	less than 1 ppb
	Perchloroethylene	1.1 ppb
	1,1,1 trichloroethane	1.6 ppb
	Trichloroethylene (TCE)	less than .5 ppb
Chlorinated Hydrocarbon Pesticides and Industrial Pollutants	Benzene hexachloride	.3 ppb
	Chlordane	.8 ppb
	DDT	1 to 5 ppb
	Dieldrin	less than .3 ppb
	Heptachlor	.3 ppb
	Hexachlorobenzene	less than .3 ppb
	Lindane	less than .3 ppb
	Pentachlorophenol (penta)	12 ppb
	PCBs	1 to 2 ppb
Ketone Solvents in Blood	Methyl ethyl ketone (MEK)	less than 20 ppb
	Methyl isobutyl ketone (MIBK)	less than 20 ppb
	Methyl n-butyl ketone (MBK)	less than 20 ppb

National Human Adipose Tissue Survey reports that 100% of fat samples from Americans contain chlorinated solvents and heavy metals, including aluminum, beryllium, cadmium, lead, and mercury.

There is no way to completely avoid dangerous chemicals (although you can certainly take steps to minimize exposure). Even if you think you're healthy now, remember that the effects of chemicals are cumulative. By the time symptoms of chemical toxicity manifest, the body is already seriously impaired.

Toxins and Their Effects

Different Types and Danger Levels of Toxins

Toxin literally means "poison." Any substance that is irritating or harmful to the body, has a negative effect on cell structure and function, stresses biochemical and organ functions, or undermines health, can be considered a poison. An article called "Detoxification Biochemistry" states:

> Toxins may be of external origin (also referred to as xenobiotics or exogenous toxins), such as chemicals in the air, water, food additives, or drugs. They may also be generated internally (also referred to as endogenous toxins) as the end-products form the metabolism of hormones, bacterial byproducts, and other complex molecules.[7]

Toxins can also come from radiation, harmful electromagnetic fields, and even emotions. Negative emotions such as frustration, sorrow and rage create acidic wastes in the body.

Of all the different kinds of toxins, biological materials are the most benign. Chemicals not indigenous to the human body—both organic chemicals and heavy metals—are often found in the same manufactured items. (In this context, the word *organic* simply means any compound containing at least one carbon atom.) Foreign chemicals especially can cause moderate to severe health problems and even death. First I will discuss endogenous biological materials, and then the many types of exogenous toxins.

Endogenous Toxins: Biological Materials

This category consists of waste produced by the body in the course of normal metabolic functioning and also pathogens and the waste they excrete. Some of the bodily substances that migrate out through sweat are intrinsically beneficial. They are considered waste only because the body cannot utilize them at the time they are being eliminated. Guyton and Hall note some constituents: lactic acid, potassium, sodium, urea, aldosterone from the adrenal glands. According to Martha M. Christy, author of *Your Own Perfect Medicine*, other ingredients may include minute traces of biological materials such as certain amino acids (arginine, lysine, ornithine and tryptophan);

vitamins including ascorbic acid, biotin, folic acid, inositol, and riboflavin; minerals including calcium, iodine, iron, magnesium, phosphorus, potassium, and zinc; other nutrients including glucose; and hormones including aldosterone, dopamine, estradiol, and epinephrine.[8] However, although one's own bodily products are usually unneeded rather than harmful (poisonous), this is not always the case. "The improper formation or metabolism of normal body chemicals, such as hormones and neurotransmitters, can cause a harmful imbalance," write Krohn and Taylor.

> Internal toxins also include substances that our bodies create in response to various conditions, and which become toxic in excess amounts. For example injury, anesthesia, and pollution cause the body to produce free radicals that are toxic to all tissues. Exercise can cause an excess of lactic acid in the muscles, resulting in stiffness and pain in people who cannot properly process it.[9]

Emotional and physical trauma, and negative stress—feelings of being overwhelmed rather than challenged—can also generate internal toxins. It is possible that, if left in the system to re-circulate, the stress hormones could reattach to the receptor sites of cells and evoke uneasy emotional and physiological responses similar to those elicited at the time they were generated.

The excreted waste (or mycotoxins) from pathogens—viruses, bacteria, fungi, and parasites—are also biological materials. Mycotoxins can cause inflammation and infection—which, although related, are different from each other. A picture of the interplay between the two will help us to better understand how the body deals with some of its internal toxins.

Inflammation is the body's way of dealing with irritation—regardless of whether the irritation is caused by microbes (infection), chemicals, friction, heat, or toxins. During inflammation, various scavenger cells gather at the problem site to ingest dead and damaged tissue. The scavenger cells also act as a cushion or barrier between the local damaged tissue and the surrounding healthy areas. In addition, an increased supply of blood is generated by the immune response to bring extra nutrients, oxygen, and hormones to the repair site.

Infection, on the other hand, is a pathological, diseased state of the tissues involving microbes. The microbes force their way into various cells in the body and, as a byproduct of their own metabolic and survival functions, introduce waste materials into the tissues that don't belong there. (The speed at which microbes proliferate depends on the body's pH, the amount of oxygen in the system, and glucose levels, among other factors.) The body reacts to this biological assault by feeling pain (the nerves are being chemically irritated), malfunction (microbial toxins unfavorably alter the body's pH, poison the system, and hamper waste removal), and/or swelling.

This is the point at which infection and inflammation overlap. The body responds to localized microbial infection through swelling to contain the infection and protect the surrounding tissues from being inundated by pathogens. But inflammation itself can cause infection. For example, during a non-microbial swelling such as an injury, if the scavenger cells cannot break down and digest the damaged tissue quickly enough, the injured cells in the area will putrefy. Then, an infection due to microbial contamination and/or endogenous toxins will result. Unfortunately, on those occasions when the body's inflammatory response lingers past the point of usefulness, the swelling continues for too long, slowing down the circulation in the area and thus preventing healing. (At this point, many people try to eliminate the swelling with the opposite effects of heat and cold, through the alternating application of ice packs and sauna, or cold and hot water.)

It's important to remember that any debris—no matter what its cause—that remains in the system without being cleared, can cause inflammation and eventually infection.

Exogenous Toxins: Organic Chemicals and Heavy Metals

Toxins that are not produced by the body itself can enter the system through the skin, respiratory tract, and gastrointestinal tract. As we progress further into the 21st century, it begins to appear that any condition in the body can be directly caused, or exacerbated, by synthetic chemicals.

The organic culprits include pesticides, fertilizers, and volatile organic compounds (VOCs)—among which are formaldehyde, toluene, benzene, and styrene. These are found in antifreeze, carpet, disinfectant, laundry detergent, polishes and varnish, shampoo, even packaged foods. Heavy metals (also known as toxic metals) also find their way into the body.

Cadmium, lead, mercury and zinc are found in cleaners, cosmetics, paint, solvents, vaccinations, and thousands of other items.

It is almost impossible to avoid chemicals. Detergents, heavy metals and solvents abound in cleaners, soaps and personal care products. Hydrocarbons and sulfur dioxide are in automobile, bus and airplane exhaust. Carpet contains acetone, benzene and ethylbenzene, formaldehyde, phthalate, styrene, toluene and xylene, in addition to heavy metals that give them their bright color. Clothing is treated with fire retardant and fabric softener. Computers, telephones, electronic devices, and thousands of other things outgas molecules of plastic. Deodorizers and mothballs are made from dangerous petrochemicals. Fertilizers also contain petrochemicals. Furniture, glue and adhesives contain solvents. Pesticides, insecticides, fumigants, and fungicides, purposely made to be deadly, are registered poisons with the United States government. They are sprayed onto our crops and now are embedded in cooking utensils and children's toys. Shoe polish is comprised of dyes synthesized from coal tar, which in turn is derived from petroleum. Second hand cigarette smoke alone contains (among other chemicals) acetone, acetylene, ammonia, benzene, carbon monoxide, DDT, formaldehyde, heavy metals, hydrogen cyanide, methane, methyl alcohol, nickel compounds, nicotine, and propane.

The list is endless. Medical doctor Doris Rapp, who devotes an entire chapter to chemical pollution in *Is This Your Child? Discovering and Treating Unrecognized Allergies in Children and Adults,* itemizes the presence of various compounds in detail. Information on the sources of formaldehyde alone fills nearly two pages. Readers might be most familiar with formaldehyde's use as an embalming agent for corpses. But formaldehyde also can be found in adhesives and glues, antifreeze, beer and wine, detergents, carpet; polyester clothing, fabric and fabric dyes; furniture and wood items; ink, rat poison, newsprint, many types of paint; personal care items such as cosmetics, deodorants, mouthwash, nail polish, shampoos, and toothpaste. Air fresheners, pharmaceuticals, photography supplies, plastics, tissues and toilet paper, upholstery foam, wallpaper, even pharmaceuticals and some vitamin supplements house formaldehyde as well.[10] Dr. Rapp discusses in detail the wide range of symptoms in children and adults that are caused by toxic chemicals, as well as the many measures involved in reclaiming health.

The problems caused by these poisonous chemicals are virtually unlimited. For those who think in terms of specific *diseases* (which are collections of symptom-pictures to which medical personnel have given specific names), many medical sources conclude that toxic chemicals can either cause or contribute to, among other conditions, asthma, autism, cancer, environmental illness, epilepsy, multiple sclerosis, and Parkinson's disease. For those who relate more to *symptoms* (which describe how different areas of the body are affected), toxic overload can manifest as body odor and bad breath, brittle nails and hair, burning eyes, cardiac problems, coated tongue, constipation, diarrhea, gastrointestinal cramping, headaches, hemorrhoids and ulcers, irritability, pain in muscles or joints, ringing in the ears, sinus infections, sneezing, wheezing and other respiratory problems, and all sorts of skin problems such as boils and rashes. Emotional symptoms include anxiety, irritability, depression, and outright panic attacks. Exposure to just polychlorinated biphenyls (PCBs) causes cancer, fatigue, headaches, high blood pressure, impaired balance, liver malfunction, limb pain, muscle weakness; and impaired mental function such as inability to concentrate, memory loss, mental confusion, and insomnia. As already discussed with the chart on page 66, only 1 PPB to 2 PPB are required for symptoms to appear.

"Heavy metals" is a category of toxins whose name can be confusing, because some of these metals, such as zinc, sound just like the minerals we need in our diet. But the form in which a mineral appears can determine whether it is beneficial or dangerous. With the exception of ionic minerals (also called electrolytes)—which are beneficial minerals carrying an electrical charge, and tiny enough in structure to pass across a cell membrane— the minerals that nourish us are *compounds*, combined with one or more other elements. So the "calcium" that we ask for in the health food store, even though the single name suggests the presence of only one element, is actually a *compound* (calcium carbonate, calcium lactate, calcium citrate, and so on). This helps explain how zinc can be either helpful or harmful. If the zinc is bound to another element and thus assimilable by the body (such as zinc gluconate), it's a nutrient. If it's *unbound,* it is highly poisonous. The phrase "heavy metals" or "toxic metals" pertains not only to some unbound minerals, but also to minerals that, no matter what their form, can never be nutrients and are always lethal to the body. These include aluminum, cadmium, lead, and mercury. (For more information, see *The Handbook of Rife Frequency Healing.*)

The symptoms and diseased states that result from heavy metal poisoning alone keep growing. Dr. Sherry Rogers writes that heavy metals are most insidious because

> they can mimic any symptom, like perplexing peripheral neuropathy (strange numbness and tingling, loss of sensation, loss of nerve control, unusual pain) in arms or legs. The brain is a frequent target organ and certainly our epidemic of depression, mood swings, brain fog with inability to concentrate, learning disorders, attention deficit disorder, memory loss, lowered I.Q., irritability and aggression are all manifestations at least in part of the onslaught of heavy metals in our air, food and water.... [They also] usually present as the most incurable and hopeless [conditions] like multiple sclerosis, manic depression, lupus, or chronic fatigue.[11]

Countless numbers of researchers are investigating the effects of heavy metals. The following list summarizing the major toxic metals, their health effects, and what items contain them, is derived from the work of four sources: medical doctor Stephen Edelson, naturopath-osteopath Ross Trattler, medical doctor Lawrence Wilson, and the Environmental Defense website. Dr. Edelson—who specializes in programs that detoxify heavy metals and poisonous chemicals from the system—feels that many serious conditions are actually autoimmune disorders. This category includes Type I diabetes, chronic fatigue, Crohn's disease and ulcerative colitis, autoimmune hepatitis, some kidney disorders, lupus, multiple sclerosis, myasthenia gravis, polymyositis, rheumatoid arthritis, scleroderma, numerous thyroid problems, and vasculitis. "I believe that heavy metal and/or chemical toxicity is a causative factor in nearly every autoimmune disorder, if not all," he declares. In his experience, "the heavy metals most often found at unacceptable levels in the body are aluminum, arsenic, cadmium, lead, mercury, nickel, and tin."[12] Other practitioners find many problems with copper toxicity as well.

Some of the symptoms caused by cumulative doses of various metals (depending on the degree of exposure) are listed below:[13]

Metal	Found in	May cause
Aluminum	Antiperspirant and deodorant; antacids, laxatives and other over-the-counter medications; baking powder; beverage cans; cigarette filters; cookware; dental amalgams; some foods such processed cheese and salt; tobacco smoke; toothpaste	Brain degeneration, leading to Alzheimer's disease, dementia and memory impairment; digestive disorders such as colic and gas; nerve damage leading to motor and behavioral dysfunction; seizures; skin rash
Arsenic	Automobile exhaust; beer; cigarettes; paints; processed salt; herbicides and insecticides; wood preservatives	Diarrhea; headaches; liver and kidney damage; muscle spasms; weakness
Cadmium	Auto exhaust; cigarette and marijuana smoke; evaporated milk and other refined foods; fertilizer; paint pigments; silver polish; fertilizers; fungicides; rubber; rubber carpet backing	Acne; arthritis; back pain; cancer; emotional disturbances including a tendency toward violence; emphysema; heart disease including arteriosclerosis and high blood pressure; infections of various kinds; kidney and liver damage; nausea and vomiting
Copper	Alcoholic beverages from copper brewery equipment; meats (copper sulfate is given as a growth enhancer) and other foods; pesticides, insecticides and fungicides; water from the plumbing pipes	Anemia; arthritis; autism, schizophrenia and stuttering; hypertension; liver enlargement and inflammation; myocardial infarction; nausea and vomiting; postpartum psychosis; Wilson's Syndrome (thyroid malfunction); toxemia of pregnancy
Lead	Automobile exhaust; canned food with lead seams; cigarettes; leaded gasoline fumes; some glazed dishware; hair dye; ink; paint; pesticides; solder	Anemia; arthritis; bone disease; cataracts; degeneration of motor neurons; constipation and diarrhea; nausea and vomiting; mental retardation in children, and lowered intelligence and emotional instability in both children and adults; gout; hypertension; impotence and sterility; kidney, liver, pituitary and thyroid damage; muscle aches; seizures; vertigo

Metal	Found in	May cause
Mercury	Adhesives; batteries with mercury cells; cosmetics such as mascara (especially waterproof); dental fillings (so-called "silver" amalgam fillings); drugs and over-the-counter medications such as calamine lotion; paint; personal care items such as contact lens solution; pesticides and fungicides; fabric softener; tuna and swordfish; vaccines (the mercury derivative thimerosal is even deadlier than mercury and is used as a preservative)	Birth defects and chromosome damage; emotional disturbance; gingivitis and tooth loss; headaches; hearing loss; insanity; learning disabilities and mental retardation; nerve impairment and tremors; gastrointestinal problems including abdominal cramping, nausea and vomiting; skin eruptions; thyroid disorders; vertigo; vision loss; yeast infections
Nickel	Batteries; cigarette smoke; various foods such as hydrogenated vegetable oils, margarine, peanut butter, herring, oysters, and tea	Allergies; birth defects; central nervous system disorders including brain damage, loss of sensation and motor control, and tremors; cancer; cardiovascular diseases including arteriosclerosis, high blood pressure and irregular heartbeat; infertility and miscarriage; kidney damage; muscle weakness; respiratory disorders including asthma, bronchitis and emphysema; skin disorders including dermatitis and photosensitivity
Tin	Air pollution and industrial waste; coated food cans and processed foods	Central nervous system disorders including brain damage, loss of sensation and motor control, and tremors; muscle weakness; respiratory disorders including asthma, bronchitis and emphysema

Dr. Edelson notes a 1997 National Resources Defense Council report where 845 million pounds of poisonous chemicals were applied to American crops. Here are "just a few" of the toxic chemicals (including pesticides) he lists in his book, to which people are exposed each day.

- Benzene: Found in cigarette smoke, gasoline, inks, oils, paints, plastics, rubber, detergents, explosives, pharmaceuticals, and dyes. One study estimates that 45% of our exposure to benzene comes from cigarettes, especially if you smoke or are exposed to second-hand smoke.

- Chloroform: Found in cleaning solvents, floor polishes, insecticides, artificial silk, and lacquers.
- Dichlorobenzene: Found in deodorants, insecticides, metal polishes, moth proofing, lacquers, and paints.
- DDT (dichlorodiphenyl-trichloroethane): This pesticide, which was outlawed in the United States in 1972 because it is extremely toxic, can still be found in soil and other substances, including—according to a study done by the Southwest Research Institute in the 1990s—carpeting. The Institute discovered that 90 of 362 Midwestern homes examined by their investigators had DDT in the carpeting, likely brought into the homes on the soles of people's shoes.
- Formaldehyde: Found in nearly all indoor environments. Foam insulation, particle board, pressed wood products, grocery bags, waxed papers, facial tissues, paper towels, wrinkle resisters, adhesive binders in floor coverings, backings on carpet, and cigarette smoke contain formaldehyde.
- Hexane/Heptane/Pentanes: Found in glue, cement, adhesives, paint thinner, plastics, gasoline, ink.
- Toluene: Found in petroleum products, carpets, carpet glue, copy paper, paint.
- Trichloroethylene (TCE): Your dry-cleaned clothes may be making you ill: more than 90% of the TCE produced is used in dry cleaning products and metal degreasing. TCE is also used in printing inks, lacquers, varnishes, adhesives, and paints. The National Cancer Institute lists TCE as a liver carcinogen.
- Xylene: Found in rubber, paint, ink, photo processing, plastics, insecticides, petroleum products.[14]

This chapter can only summarize the dangers of chemicals and heavy metals and their effects on human beings. There are excellent books on the market that explain in detail how toxins harm the body and how you can recover from them. However, even the above summary should give you an idea of how severely toxins can effect us.

Studies of Toxins Released through Sweating

Do heavy metals actually exit the body during sweating? Mikkel Aaland asserts that during a brief 15-minute sauna, the skin through sweating can eliminate the same amount of heavy metals as would require 24 hours for the kidneys to excrete. The journal articles and research studies corroborating this are impressive. A study called "The excretion of trace metals in human sweat" has found that the average concentrations of nickel and cadmium are higher in sweat than in urine. Mercury is also eliminated by sweating, according to another research article. H.B. Lovejoy and colleagues write:

> The most recent article to suggest that mercury losses by sweating may be substantial appeared in the National Geographic Magazine. In the mining of cinnabar ore in Spain [the ore naturally contains high levels of mercury], miners with clinical signs of mercurialism were placed in a hot environment where forced sweating occurred. This sweating procedure constituted treatment for the removal of mercury from the body....sweating may be a significant avenue for the elimination of absorbed mercury.[15]

Next, the authors cite a study in which supervised sweating affected the excretion of mercury in industrial workers who manufactured chlorine using the mercury cell process, and thus were heavily toxified.

> The concentration of mercury in the sweat was considerably higher than that in the urine on a comparable volume. The quantity of mercury eliminated in sweat within the 1½ hour period represented from 50% to almost 200% of that contained in the 16-hour composite urine sample for the mercury cell circuit participants. The individual with the highest sweat rate also had the highest mercury concentration in his sweat.
>
> The mercury concentration in the sweat of the controls was very low and approached the [very low, close to non-existent levels of mercury]....The elimination of mercury via sweat has been shown to constitute a significant route for the removal of mercury from the body (bloodstream). Information from this small study group tends to support the concept that "sweating them out" reportedly used in mercurialism cases among cinnabar miners may be a valid treatment for rapid removal of absorbed mercury. Since the mechanism involved in sweat bypasses the kidney's role in the elimination of mercury...sweating should be the initial and preferred treatment of patients with elevated mercury urine levels.

The authors conclude by commenting on difficulties some researchers have had in "establishing a relationship between mercury exposures and urine mercury levels," since other data showed smaller levels of mercury in the urine than one might expect from the degree of mercury exposure. Until the above study, researchers had not considered "sweating as a possible significant route for the elimination of mercury from the body."[16] Now, it is well known among clinicians that high levels of mercury can be, and are, emitted through intensive perspiration.

What about pesticides and organic compounds? Are they excreted through sauna therapy as well? An article by Zane R. Guard and Erma J. Brown in the *Townsend Letter for Doctors & Patients* posts some before-sauna and after-sauna test results for six people with peripheral neuropathy and/or multiple sclerosis suspected to be linked to chemical exposure. The results of three out of six people whose levels of chemical exposure were measured before and after the sauna therapy are excerpted on the next page.[17] Of the other three not shown, one had between a 90% and 99% reduction of symptoms, the second had a 99% reduction of symptoms, and the third (who had been exposed to Agent Orange) had a 50% reduction of symptoms.

It is impressive to see the reduction in the amounts of chemicals, and the percentage of improvement in symptoms, after a medically supervised program of sweating. Significantly, Gard and Brown write:

> In the literature we found many reports of cases in which the onset of multiple sclerosis appeared to be precipitated by widely differing conditions: trauma, diet, pregnancy, emotional stress, exertion and fatigue, changes in temperature, tobacco, urban-rural, geographic and climactic aspects, heavy metals, dental caries, organophosphates, and organic solvents.
>
> In the United States, there appears to be a concentration of MS north of the 37th parallel latitude, which coincides with geographic areas relying heavily upon petroleum products. This correlates throughout the world, except in an area of Florida and in some South Sea islands. This strange exception is thought due to the high use of pesticides. A higher incidence is found in cities where there is a greater amount of automobile exhaust... Also we must consider the higher incidence occurring in the wheat belt, fruit growing and dairy farming

Exposure Source	Number of Days on Program	Medical Complaints	Toxicants	Pre-Program Results (ppb)	Post-Program (ppb)	Symptom Reduction
Pesticides: Flea bombs; exposed to powder in yard	50 days	Central Nervous System Depression; Peripheral Neuropathy; Musculo-Skeletal Disorders.	DDT	0.8	.0	99%
			DDE	3.4	1.1	
			Chlordane	12.5	.0	
			Heptachlor	.9	1.0	
			Hept. Epoxide	.6	.3	
			TransNonachlor	1.6	.0	
			Endosulfan	11.6	.0	
			Benzene	2.0	.0	
			Toluene	1.5	.0	
			Tri Methylbenzene	.6	.0	
			Xylene	1.2	.3	
			Dichloremethane	4.8	.0	
			Chloroform	4.5	.5	
			TetraCE	5.5	.0	
			Dichlorobenzene	2.8	.0	
Pesticide sprays in home and garden, all her life.	Two courses of treatment: 1-28 days 1-12 days	Extreme fatigue, Muscles weak; Occasional seizure-like activity. Paralysis of legs intermittently.	DDE	4.0	.0	99%
			Isocy.	8.00		
			AntiParietal	Positive		
			AntiBrush B.	Positive		
Volatile Hydrocarbons	25 days	Central Nervous System Depression; Peripheral Neuropathy foot drop.	Benzene	2.3	2.1	75%—and temporary, because subject was re-exposed and then had relapse.
			Toluene	1.0	1.0	
			Ethylbenzene	.5	<.5	
			Styrene	.7	<.5	
			111, TCA	6.8	0.9	
			TCE	.9	<.5	
			Tetra CE	3.4	.8	

industries. Their practices with respect to mercurial dusts and sprays, lead-arsenate, and management of livestock afflicted with parasites may be in question.

An extensive literature search, coupled with clinical observations within the past five years, indicates a strong correlation between the appearance of inflammatory disease of the central nervous system and exposure to organic solvents.[18]

In addition to heavy metals, pesticides, petrochemicals, and other organic chemicals, drugs are excreted through sweat. A 20-year-old review of the scientific literature by D.W. Schnare and colleagues relates to substances found in sweat. "A variety of chemicals have been identified in sweat, including n-alkanes, paraffinic hydrocarbons, methadone, amphetamines, antiepileptics and morphine.... The effectiveness of this pathway [perspiration] is significant, with as much material excreted through the sweat as through the urine."[19]

It is valuable to hear from the subjects themselves what they experience during sauna therapy. The following accounts from narcotics officers who unwillingly absorbed PCP while doing their job are from an article called "Chemical Hazards in Law Enforcement."

> "As I was sitting in the sauna I suddenly felt like I was floating," stated Michael Del Puppo, a narcotics officer who had liquid PCP deliberately thrown into his face four years ago (a favorite practice of illicit laboratory operators seeking to disable and escape from officers). "The walls were moving in on me. When the horribly bitter taste of PCP started coming out in my mouth again I felt sure that the [sweating] program was actually getting the stuff out of my body. No other treatment had done that."
>
> ...Leonard Villahermosa, after completing the [sauna therapy] program in August 1983, said: "While I was in the sauna I actually began to taste the PCP in my mouth. I could also smell it about my body. After about a week things started to change; it caught me by surprise. I had been having headaches every day for a very long time and suddenly one day I realized that I didn't have a headache anymore. After that I just kept getting better and better. Toward the end of the program I felt great.
>
> "After completing the program I took another series of tests. The personality test score, IQ test score, and reaction time test score all showed my improvement. After talking with a cousin,

he said, 'You sure do sound different. You must feel pretty good.'
Everyone, since that time, has said the same thing and they still
are saying it."[20]

Gard and Brown describe a 32-year-old women who underwent detoxification therapy using a sauna. She had been diagnosed with systemic lupus erythematosus since the age of 15, and among other health problems
suffered from blurred vision, chemical sensitivity, ear infections, fatigue,
muscle spasms and weakness, nosebleeds, and sinusitis.

> A fat-biopsy revealed levels of chlorinated pesticides…Her
> headaches soon disappeared, but her joint pain would flare then
> subside during sauna sessions. After 30 days…she began to
> hallucinate as a response to the release of fat-stored anesthetics,
> accompanied by a distinct anesthetic odor. The hallucinations
> were usually followed by a response similar to that of a patient
> in a recovery room. [There is a] 90% improvement of her lupus
> condition, without the use of medication. She continues to [use
> the] sauna following [pesticide] exposure to prevent the symp-
> toms… [Interestingly, her brother] also has lupus and original-
> ly was in better health than his sister. Now she feels she is 100%
> better than her brother who is on conventional therapy."[21]

THE NEED FOR PREVENTION

In the summer of 1973, the Michigan Chemical Corporation substituted a flame retardant it manufactures for a dairy cattle magnesium oxide supplement, which it also manufactures, and distributed it as feed.
According to Mary S. Wolff and colleagues, the chemical used as flame
retardant—PBB (polybrominated biphenyl)—

> has been found to be hepatoxic [poisonous to the liver], neuro-
> toxic [poisonous to the nervous system], immunotoxic [poison-
> ous to the immune system], and carcinogenic…Such compounds
> are…poorly metabolized, if at all. This, with their low volatili-
> ty and lipid solubility, leads to accumulation and long-term stor-
> age in the body….Pronounced effects on dairy cattle followed, in-
> cluding marked decrease in milk production, aborted pregnancies,
> hyperkeratosis [abnormal thickening of the skin], lameness, and
> abnormal growth of the hooves.[22]

The repercussions of this event affected the entire state of Michigan. As one might imagine, the people who ate the widely distributed meat, milk, cheese and butter from these cows—not to mention the farmers themselves—became moderately to severely ill, as did the animals, with liver, with neurological, and with immune disorders. More than 200 farms were quarantined during 1974 to 1976, since, according to the authors, "they had been found to have more than 0.3 ppm [parts per million] of PBB in livestock, milk, or poultry." Five years after the event, "PBB was widely found as a residual tissue contaminant in the population of Michigan....approximately 97% of the residents of the state had measurable amounts of PBB" in both the bloodstream and body fat.[23]

The residents of Michigan had no control over what they ingested in that case, but in general, consumers can avoid dangerous chemicals by reading the labels of the most common household products. The scope and breadth of what we are putting into our bodies is almost unbelievable. I will give examples of two common ingredients.

The first, aluminum, is a toxic metal commonly found in antiperspirants. Like all heavy metals, aluminum was never meant to be inside the body. Aluminum is absorbed directly through the skin into the lymph nodes of the armpit. Ironically, when the body tries to excrete the chemicals by sweating, people apply even more aluminum-filled antiperspirant to keep themselves dry! Evidence suggests that this vicious cycle can eventually lead to cancer—and that many more women than men get breast cancer not necessarily because of a sex-linked genetic disposition, but because women shave their armpits and then apply antiperspirant and deodorant directly onto their bare skin. Without the hair to block the chemicals from seeping into the skin, the chemicals migrate to the lymph nodes. Either these chemicals are inherently very poisonous at minute amounts—sometimes at as little as 1 ppm—or the levels are much too high for the body to break them down efficiently. Once the lymphatic vessels get clogged with chemicals, we're in serious trouble, for *lymphocytes* (white blood cells produced by the lymph glands, and which devour microbes and systemic toxins) are the first line of defense in a healthy body. As I mentioned in Chapter 2, the lymphatic system relies on mechanical pressure (such as exercise, movement, and massage) to pump the fluid through the vessels; it does not have the equivalent of a heart. With the lymph vessels sluggish and clogged, the waste materials remain to poison the surrounding tissues.

The second example of a very common toxic chemical is sodium laurel sulfate (SLS). Sodium laurel sulfate and its derivatives are popular detergents present in almost every brand of shampoo, soap, body lotion and cream, and even toothpaste. Sodium laurel sulfate is commonly used by manufacturers because it creates luxurious foam and also very effectively homogenizes (mixes together) the ingredients in a preparation by increasing a substance's permeability. However, SLS not only efficiently penetrates the skin, but even passes through the blood-brain barrier where it can affect brain tissue. When put into a concoction such as toothpaste that contains fluoride—or anti-bacterial soap (which by law must contain registered pesticides as a legal requirement of being "anti-bacterial")—SLS becomes a *carrier* for other, often more dangerous chemicals. Sodium laurel sulfate by itself dries the skin, can cause severe eye and skin inflammation, and can even interfere with vision. But furthermore, according to Judi Vance, author of *Beauty To Die For*, some Japanese studies indicate that SLS damages the DNA in our cells. Whether or not the Japanese studies are correct, the fact remains that the most commonly used product in soaps and other personal care products, SLS, causes other poisons to be more efficiently absorbed into the system.

With the hundreds of chemicals that can course through our bodies daily, perhaps the most concise—and the strongest—summary on the benefits of sweating is made by medical personnel David E. Root, David B. Katzin, and David W. Schnare. In a paper presented at the National Conference on Hazardous Wastes and Environmental Emergencies in May of 1985, they categorically state: "A considerable portion (10-15%) of the toxic materials excreted through the body will come out through the sebaceous sweat."[24] For poisonous materials where less than .5 PPB can make a huge difference in how one feels, this is a strong recommendation for sauna therapy.

It should be clear from the studies cited in this chapter that body heating is highly beneficial for people with serious health problems. However, using a sauna on a regular basis to detoxify will prevent the problems before they start. Given the prevalence of toxic chemicals in our lives, the frequent use of a sauna would seem to be a necessity rather than a luxury. In the next chapter I discuss the different types of heat used in various saunas, so you will be able to choose the kind that can help you the most.

NOTES

1. Sherry A. Rogers, *Detoxify or Die* (Sarasota, Fl.: Sand Key Company, Inc., 2002), 179.

2. D.W. Schnare et al., "Evaluation of a Detoxification Regimen for Fat Stored Xenobiotics," *Medical Hypotheses* 9 (1982): 265-282.

3. R. Michael Wisner et al., "Treatment of Children with the Detoxification Method Developed by Hubbard," *Proceedings of the American Public Health Association: National Conference, San Diego, 1995*, reprint, unpaginated.

4. Foundation for Advancements in Science and Education Research Bulletin, *Fate and Distribution of Cocaine, Diazepam, Phencyclidine (PCP) and THC (Marijuana): A Technical Review* (August 1985), 1.

5. Jacqueline Krohn and Frances Taylor, *Natural Detoxification, A Practical Encyclopedia: The Complete Guide to Clearing Your Body of Toxins,* 2nd ed., rev. and exp. (Port Roberts, Wash.: Hartley & Marks Publishers, Inc., 2000), 5-6.

6. David Steinman, *Diet for a Poisoned Planet* (New York: Harmony Books, 1990), 302-303.

7. HealthComm International, Inc., "Detoxification Biochemistry," *Technical Bulletin* (2000), unpaginated.

8. Martha M. Christy, *Your Own Perfect Medicine* (Scottsdale, Ariz.: Self Healing Press, 1994), 116-117.

9. Krohn, op. cit., 6.

10. Doris Rapp, *Is This Your Child? Discovering and Treating Unrecognized Allergies in Children and Adults* (New York: William Morrow, 1991), 286-287.

11. Sherry A. Rogers, *Total Wellness* Newsletter (May 2000), 3.

12. Stephen Edelson and Deborah Mitchell, *What Your Doctor Won't Tell You about Autoimmune Disease* (New York: Warner Books, 2003).

13. Data compiled from Edelson, op. cit.; Environmental Defense website at http://www.scorecard.org (accessed November 18, 2002); Ross Trattler, *Better Health Through Natural Healing: How to Get Well Without Drugs or Surgery* (New York: McGraw-Hill Book Company, 1985), 330-334; and Lawrence Wilson, personal communication.

14. Edelson, op. cit.

15. H.B. Lovejoy et al., "Mercury Exposure Evaluations and Their Correlation with Urine Mercury Excretions: 4. Elimination of Mercury by Sweating," *Journal of Occupational Medicine* 15 (7), 590.

16 . Ibid., 591.

17. Zane R. Gard and Erma J. Brown, "Literature Review and Comparison Studies of Sauna/Hyperthermia in Detoxification," *Townsend Letter for Doctors & Patients* (August/September 1999), 78.

18. Ibid., 76.

19. Schnare, op. cit.

20. Robert B. Amidon, "Chemical Hazards in Law Enforcement," *Journal of California Law Enforcement* 18 (3), 29.

21. Gard, op. cit., 79.

22. Mary S. Wolff, PhD, et al., "Human Tissue Burdens of Halogenated Aromatic Chemicals in Michigan," *Journal of the American Medical Association* 247 (15), 2112.

23. Ibid., 2114-2115.

24. David E. Root et al., "Diagnosis and Treatment of Patients Presenting Subclinical Signs and Symptoms of Exposure to Chemicals Which Bioaccumulate in Human Tissue," *Proceedings of the National Conference on Hazardous Wastes and Environmental Emergencies* (Cincinnati, Ohio, May 14-16, 1985), 152.

The Three Types of Heat

The idea is not to have the best sauna on the block,
but to get the entire block into the sauna.

HAROLD TIER
PRESIDENT, FINNISH SAUNA SOCIETY

To paraphrase the writer Gertrude Stein, a sauna is a sauna is a sauna. But is it? It *is* true that in different saunas, if the temperatures are optimal; if the heat penetrates deeply, evenly, and consistently into the body; and if the moisture content of the air in each unit is the same, sweating will yield equally good results. Yet there are many factors, more than you might think, that determine temperature, heat penetration, moisture content, and so on. Each method of inducing perspiration has its own advantages and disadvantages. Since the heating method used by a particular type of sauna will, to a large extent, determine its effects on the body, this chapter is devoted to the physics of heat and how heat travels, and how the science of heat applies to sauna therapy. Readers who are not technically-minded or not interested in the mechanics of heat transfer, might be tempted to skip this chapter. However, perhaps you are dealing with a serious illness and are thinking of buying your own sauna. Or perhaps you had a disappointing experience in someone else's sauna, and are not sure whether it was due to an inferior unit or to an incompatibility between the unit's method of heat transfer and your unique needs. In either case, understanding the principles of heat transmission can help you choose the sauna and the heating source that are right for you.

Heat Transmission

Throughout the ages, the chambers used for body heating have been as diverse as the cultures that practiced it. But regardless of whether the chamber was a pit in the ground, wooden cabinet, marble alcove, clay room, or cloth tent, with the exception of a sand bath (as we'll see in Chapter 5) there were basically two circumstances under which heat was administered: the person was either immersed in water, or surrounded by air. I will not be discussing immersion in water since a sauna is not a water bath. Therefore, in our discussion of heat treatment, we are referring to the body surrounded by air, with the air holding varying degrees of moisture ranging from relatively none, to light mist, to heavy steam.

To begin, I want to define heat. According to *Fundamentals of Heat and Mass Transfer*, "Heat is energy in transit due to a temperature difference."[1] The molecules of a substance are literally vibrating, which produces *energy in motion*.

Regardless of the way in which heat is transmitted, according to the Laws of Thermodynamics:

- Molecules at a higher temperature move faster than molecules at a lower temperature.
- Heating a substance generally causes it to expand. (Since the molecules are moving faster, they tend to bump into each other more; so the collision makes them ricochet out and take up more space.)
- Heat travels from the object or area that is hot to the object or area that is cold.

As you read the descriptions below of the three types of *heat transfer*—conduction, convection and radiation—be aware that the three methods can overlap: anything with a temperature emits radiation (or radiant heat), no matter how the heat is *initially* transmitted. And once a solid body is heated, it eventually transfers that heat to its other parts through conduction. However, it is still useful to understand these three categories. Later, you will see how they relate to sauna therapy, and how you can use your knowledge of heat to decide what type of sauna to use or buy.

Conduction

Conduction is the transmission of heat by direct physical contact of two bodies of different temperatures, or within a single body whose parts are at different temperatures. If your hand is cold and my hand is warm, and I hold your hand to warm it, the heat (following a basic Law of Thermodynamics) will flow from my warm hand to your cold one. If you used a hot water bottle to warm your hand, the same principle would apply.

Conductive heat is so much a part of our everyday lives, many of us are familiar with the process without being aware of the term. When you stir honey into your hot tea and forget to take out the metal spoon, the water may heat the spoon so much that you no longer can comfortably hold the spoon. If the bulb in your lamp burns out, before replacing the bulb you wait for it to cool to avoid getting burned. And when your car starts to overheat, you pull off the road, open the hood and check the engine with a cloth protecting your hand, because the metal parts are too hot to touch with your bare skin.

Conductive heat also plays a prominent role in healing. As reported in *Therapeutic Heat and Cold*:

> Almost as soon as man [sic] learned to build fires, he noted that stones in or near them maintained their heat for a long time. He soon learned to place the heated stone against a painful part....[However, t]he oldest form of conductive heating was contact with the waters of thermal springs [among other sources]....Hot water is perhaps the most widely applied agent of conductive heating, whether it be a local soak or compress or a full tub. Many variations have been used and many special containers and appliances have been tried. Water has been poured, thrown or rubbed on the body. Pools, tanks and other containers [such as animal skins and hollow dried gourds] have been devised especially for therapeutic heat.[2]

Here is a more detailed, technical explanation of conductive heat. Heat always travels from the hotter toward the colder part due to the nature of how molecules travel and collide. Molecules that are hot are faster-moving than molecules that are cold; so as heat molecules vibrate and move, they bump into the colder ones. This molecular collision in turn causes *those* molecules to move faster (which also makes them hotter); and then *they* bump into *their* neighbors (which move faster and become hotter), which in turn bump into *their* neighbors, and so on—just like the successive fall of tiles in a game of dominoes.

Thus, when I want to apply a warm pack to skin, the heat travels from the warm to the cold area. Conversely, if I want to cool my skin, when a cold pack is applied the warmth travels *from* the warmer skin *to* the cold pack. In *Clayton's Electrotherapy 10E*, Kenneth Collins writes: "The rate of heat transfer depends on the difference in temperature between the regions in contact, the surface area of contact at the boundary, and the thermal conductivity of the materials in contact."[3] For instance, water is a much better conductor of heat than air, and metals are much better conductors of heat than wood.

As I will discuss shortly in the section on the electromagnetic spectrum, anything with a temperature above absolute zero is also *radiating* heat. Radiation is direct heat. However, when any other modality of heat transference is added, such as conduction, you have an indirect heating method as well. *Conduction is the end result of all other heating processes.*

Convection

Convection heat is another familiar method of heating. Early in their schooling, children are taught the truism, "Hot air rises." They see that when they are in a hot shower, steam rises to the ceiling. The family dog likes jumping on the couch during a cold season because the floor is cold, and the air on the couch (which is higher than the floor) is warmer. And when repeating a recipe, a good baker always puts the cake into the oven on the same rack because there can be enough temperature variation in the upper and lower portions of the oven to significantly affect how the recipe turns out.

Convection, then, is the dispersion of heat from one point in space to another due to the circulation of a fluid such as water or air. Here, the molecules of a *fluid*, rather than a solid, are responsible for the transport of heat. (Note that I said *transport* of heat. Once the heated molecules touch the cooler ones, the eventual *transfer* of heat is by conduction.)

A fluid can be either a liquid or a gas. However, since with liquids the distinction between convection and conduction can be ambiguous, it is much easier to explain convection heating in terms of air. When air comes into contact with a heated object or body, its temperature rises. The molecules in the vicinity of the hot object move faster and further apart, and this region of air becomes less dense than the air surrounding it. So the hot air rises and is replaced by cooler air, which in turn becomes heated. This is how currents are formed through convection. The same process occurs with wind.

You may have heard of a convection oven. Electric heating coils are at the top and bottom of an enclosed metal box. Fans are placed in the oven to increase the air movement beyond naturally occurring convection. The fan moves the air, the hottest air rises, and there is a continuous cycle of moving air. This process decreases cooking time by about one-third.

Don't forget that even though the heat is *dispersed* primarily by displacement of the fluid—in other words, through the *currents that convection creates*—ultimately, the heating of an object occurs through *conduction*. Once the molecules of water or air collide, Collins writes, there is an "immediate process of energy transfer from one fluid particle to another."[4]

Again, all objects with a temperature above absolute zero are *radiating* heat; and radiation is direct heat. However, convection as a method of heat transference provides an indirect heating method as well.

Radiation

In this nuclear age, when one hears the word "radiation" it's easy to think of a dangerous nuclear powered reactor. But radiation simply means the emanations of energy that are emitted by a source, whether that source is a nuclear power plant, a radiator that's used to heat your house, or the sun. Radiation can be harmful or beneficial.

The Electromagnetic Spectrum

The electromagnetic energy that travels through space or air and is emitted by the sun is the most common form of radiation. As I explain in *The Handbook of Rife Frequency Healing*, the electromagnetic spectrum consists of many different lengths of energy oscillations that comprise our universe:

> Most of the waves on the electromagnetic spectrum are invisible to the human eye except for the small band of visible light, which we see as colors. The most important thing to remember about electromagnetic waves is this: *even though we cannot see most of the frequencies themselves, we can nonetheless utilize the electromagnetic waves, as well as visually see, thermodynamically sense (temperature-wise), or perceive in some other way, the byproducts or effects of the electromagnetic waves that manifest as physical phenomenon.* For instance, radio waves and x-rays are part of the electromagnetic spectrum. Radio waves are rather long and x-rays are much shorter. We cannot "see" these frequencies in the usual sense, but inventions make it possible to harness them for the purposes of radio broadcasts and taking pictures of the inside of the body.
>
> … What some people think of as distinct energies or energy phenomenon—electric waves, radio waves, microwaves, infrared light, visible light, ultraviolet, x-rays, gamma rays—are all oscillations on the electromagnetic spectrum, progressively ranging from very low to exceedingly high. *We tend to think of this continuum of cycles per second as separate phenomena or unrelated energies because we perceive them differently with our senses (and often perceive them not at all).* For instance, we cannot see radio waves, microwaves or infrared, but between infrared and ultraviolet radiation, a brief section of the electromagnetic spectrum *is* visible to us visually. We call this "visible light." But it is important to remember that on one level, visible light is not something radically unconnected to, for instance, microwaves or gamma rays. All are lower or higher frequencies that simply *have different manifestations* and uses for us on the physical plane at this time.[5]

All wavelengths on the electromagnetic spectrum oscillate, or possess a back-and-forth movement. These wavelengths travel at 186,000 miles per second in a vacuum, otherwise known as the speed of light. As you can see from the diagram on page 94, the electromagnetic spectrum spans a continuum of energies. These energies are characterized by either their frequencies (the *number* of *cycles per second*, or CPS, at which they vibrate), or their wavelengths (the *distance* of *one complete cycle*). At the beginning of the chart (the bottom) are the largest wave forms. They are literally miles in length: 100 megameters is 62,137 miles, at 3 CPS. As the oscillations *increase* in number *per second*, by definition the *size* of the oscillations becomes smaller. "It is evident that the shorter waves must vibrate at a greater frequency and vice versa," wrote Kovács in *Electrotherapy and Light Therapy with Essentials of Hydrotherapy and Mechanotherapy.* "A homely comparison to visualize this may be a motley army of giants and dwarfs, all under orders to reach the same goal simultaneously; in order to do so the giants step out leisurely, while the dwarfs run and take hundreds of steps for each one of the giants."[6] Depending on the wavelength (size) of the particular electromagnetic wave, electromagnetic energy may be reflected away from the surface of the object or body, may pass right through, or may be absorbed by it.

Electromagnetic wavelengths, measured from the longest to the shortest, are: the extremely low frequency waves (ELF) we use for power and telephone (measured in megameters), radio waves (meters and kilometers), and microwaves (measured in centimeters and meters). Next comes infrared radiation (IR)—near (NIR), middle (MIR), and far infrared (FIR) radiation (all measured in microns)—followed by visible light (measured in microns), ultraviolet radiation (called ultraviolet light, measured in angstroms), x-rays (also measured in angstroms), gamma rays (measured in milliangstroms), and finally, cosmic rays.

Infrared Radiation (IR)

Of the various types of radiation that the sun emits, several are capable of producing heat in body tissue: microwaves, high-frequency radio waves, and infrared radiation (IR). Some microwaves and high-frequency radio waves can produce tissue damage. Fortunately, most of the time there are not enough traveling through the atmosphere to cause any problems.

Infrared radiation, on the other hand, comprises a full 80% of the sun's

THE ELECTROMAGNETIC SPECTRUM

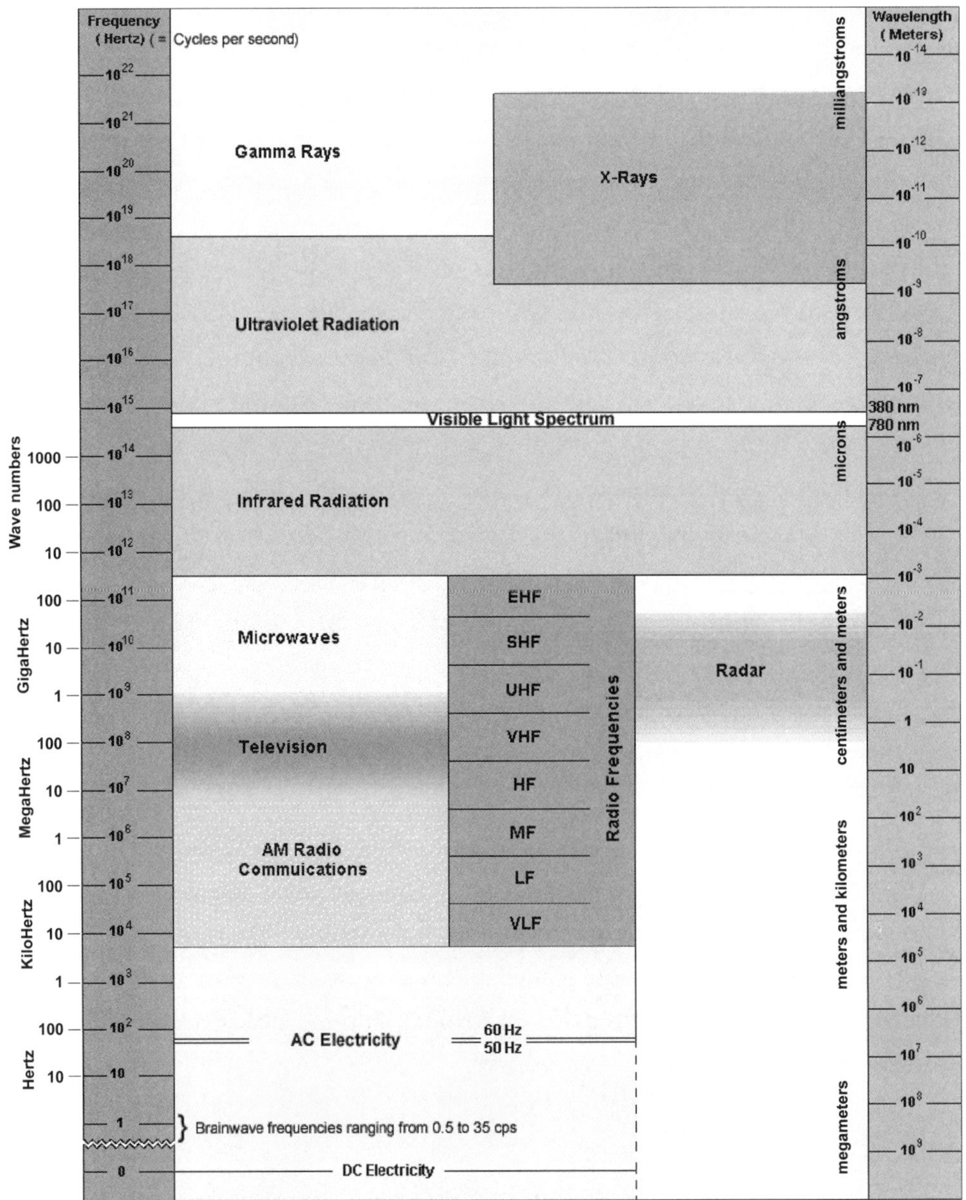

Items on the left side of this chart are measured in frequency; items on the right are measured in wavelength. As you can see, there is often an overlap between various categories—X-rays, for example, exist within the gamma ray and ultraviolet regions of the EM spectrum, just as radar exists within the microwave and television band. (In fact, the word "radar" is shorthand for the phrase "Radio Detection and Ranging.")

emissions—and is also what gives us our heat and promotes life. It is this healing IR bandwidth that interests us for the purposes of sauna therapy.

Infrared radiation exists on the electromagnetic spectrum just below the frequencies for visible light, so it is not visible to the eye. How then do we know that it exists? The discovery of radiation in the infrared spectrum was made by Sir Frederick William Herschel, a German musician and astronomer who was well-known in his time. After Herschel moved to England in 1757, he and his sister Caroline built telescopes that they used to locate and catalogue double stars and nebulae, and which Herschel used to discover the planet Uranus in 1781. It wasn't until 1800, though, that the astronomer conducted his celebrated experiment that established infrared

Close-up of the Infrared Spectrum

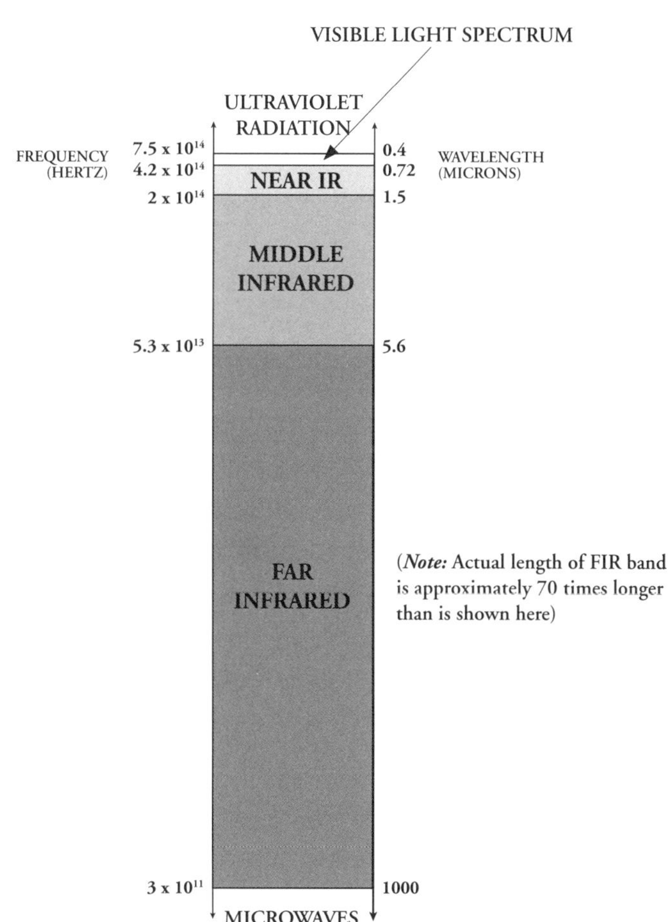

radiation as part of the scientific record. Herschel never intended to discover infrared wavelengths; he was trying to ascertain the temperature of each band (color) of visible light. First he separated sunlight into its seven colors by shining it through a prism. Next he placed a thermometer within each color to take its temperature. Then he provided "controls" by placing one thermometer each just beyond the red and violet portions of the visible light. A control in an experiment is used to provide a comparison against whatever is being tested or measured. In this case, Herschel assumed that these regions of invisible radiation would not register any appreciable temperature, which made them an ideal backdrop against which he could measure what he was *really* testing for, the temperatures of visible colors. But the scientist made a surprising, accidental discovery. Violet registered the coolest temperature, and red the hottest, in the visible light spectrum—but the region just below the visible red wavelengths had an even higher temperature than visible light! This region was later named infrared. "Infra" means "below," to indicate its position relative to visible red light—"below red" on the spectrum, as it is slower moving in frequency. (Similarly, "ultra violet" means "above violet," as it is a higher frequency than violet.)

Infrared radiation is emitted by many different sources: the sun, planets, animals, plants, humans, and inanimate objects such as fire, sand, a warm sidewalk, a desk, even an ice cube. Any object that emits any amount of heat at all—that is, a temperature above absolute zero (-459.67°F, -73.15°C, or 0° Kelvin)—radiates IR. The specific wavelength that an object most strongly radiates is determined by its temperature. Or, put another way, the temperature of an object correlates to the electromagnetic frequencies it emits in the infrared range. Also, the relationship between temperature and wavelength is inverse: higher temperature means shorter wavelengths, and lower temperature means longer wavelengths. Wavelengths in the IR range are measured in microns (one micron equals one-millionth of a meter). Temperatures on the infrared band range between absolute zero (at the longest wavelength of 1000 microns) to 6782°F or 3750°C (at the shortest wavelength of .72 microns). As with visible light, IR is either reflected (bounced off the object that it hits, basically in a straight line), refracted (scattered or bent, since it changes direction), or absorbed when it hits an object, depending on the kind of material of which the object is composed.

Although IR is invisible to the human eye, some animals and insects can "see" in the infrared range—for instance, a rattlesnake can perceive warm-blooded prey in a dark cave. (These animals and insects are able to translate the infrared heat radiated by objects and other living bodies into an image that is not exactly visual in the way we think of the term, but which is based on a separate sensory system.) Humans have learned to mimic the visual acuity of animals by inventing machines that detect even slight differences in the heat that emanates from a source. Since infrared radiation has longer wavelengths than visible light, it cannot be detected by ordinary photographic plates; but specially built electronic sensors do the job. The IR that is invisible to us under ordinary circumstances is captured on special film and translated into colors on the visible spectrum that we *are* able to see. The coldest IR spots appear as purple, slightly warmer areas are visible as green, and extremely hot regions are seen as red. Images of ordinary objects taken with IR cameras may be unusually colored, but it is clear what these objects are. This kind of "super-vision" is used in many arenas.

The ways in which infrared can be used are almost limitless. Thermography devices detect abnormalities in body systems, since warmer or colder areas of the body can indicate everything from tumors to degenerating tissue to unusual brainwave activity. Security cameras used by police and the military can detect people inside buildings due to the heat they emit in comparison to their surroundings. Infrared satellites monitor weather in the sky, note changes in the deepest ocean currents, and can even find planets in outer space. Today, infrared radiation technology is so much a part of our everyday lives that it's even in our living rooms: the remote control for the television set emits an invisible electromagnetic beam in the IR range, and a special heat-sensitive mechanism on the TV responds. But even more amazing is the healing relationship between certain wavelengths in the IR range and human beings. This relationship directly pertains to sauna therapy and will unfold throughout this chapter.

The frequencies that all lie within the category of infrared radiation are subdivided into three smaller categories, each possessing a slightly different quality. The numerical boundaries between the categories can seem somewhat arbitrary, since, depending on what source you read, the wavelength sizes of each infrared category vary slightly. However, Linda Hermans-Killam—the author of an extensive NASA-related website explaining how infrared radiation is used in astronomy—suggests a reasonable guideline: "The main factor that determines which wavelengths are included in each of these three infrared regions is the type of detector technology used for gathering infrared light."[7] Therefore, according to this formula, far infrared has the longest wavelengths, ranging from about 5.6 to 1000 microns; middle infrared has medium long wavelengths, ranging from about 1.5 to 5.6 microns; and near infrared has the shortest wavelengths, ranging from about .72 to 1.5 microns. (See the diagram on page 95.) The temperature ranges of near, middle, and far infrared differ, since an object's temperature corresponds to the wavelengths that it emits.

Far Infrared Radiation (FIR)

The part of the infrared radiation spectrum that we are interested in as it relates to sauna therapy is a tiny portion of the FIR range: those wavelengths that range from about 7.0 microns to 9.0 microns in length and which radiate heat from (respectively) approximately 285° to 122°F (140.6° to 50.0°C). (Don't forget, the shorter wavelengths are hotter and faster-moving.) Human beings normally emit a temperature of 98.6°F (37°C), which falls into the far infrared range of about 9.35 microns. In Chapter 2, I discussed the effects of temperatures at or slightly above 98.6°F (37°C) on human tissue. Simply put, warmth not only feels good, but it stimulates life processes. Feeling good from being comfortably warm, and the growth of plant or animal biological tissues, are synonymous. Nature has evolved us to create and respond to particular electromagnetic wavelengths that not only radiate the precise amount of heat we need to feel comfortable, but give us life. (We naturally equate far infrared radiation with heat. However, although heat is an important benefit, and one we can easily perceive, it is also possible that heat is only one of the manifestations of those particular wavelengths on the electromagnetic spectrum that we call FIR.) "The development and reproduction of all life forms on Earth depend upon Far Infrared Rays in sunlight," writes author Zhang

Jian Dong in an interesting (if somewhat crudely translated) book from Malaysia.

> After laying their eggs, all insects depend on sunlight to hatch them and propagate. This is all done by Far Infrared Rays. Sea turtles lay their eggs on the sandy beaches and bury them in the sand. Under the heat of the sun, especially the effects of Far Infrared Rays acting on the eggs for a period of time, tiny turtles appear. This is one of the life forms which Far Infrared Rays have contributed. If there were no sunlight, all these would not have taken place. As such, we call Far Infrared Rays in sunlight the "Light of Life."
>
> Our bodies too can produce Far Infrared Rays. The intensity of Far Infrared Rays produced by the human body is ever-changing. When its intensity is high, we will feel healthy and will be able to overcome ailments. However, when it begins to decline, the human body will be subjected to attacks by ailments and disease, age quickly and there will be a decline in the state of health. And when we are about to face death, Far Infrared radiation of the human body will be near zero....the human body requires a continuous supply of Far Infrared Rays from Mother Nature to boost the powers of the Far Infrared Rays found in our bodies.
>
> ...Just as Far Infrared Rays are able to cause the albumen and egg yolk to develop into various organs...[and] hatch the eggs of insects, sea turtles, chickens and other animals, causing them to develop blood vessels, nerves, skeletons, skin and feathers, it can similar cause changes to the human body...[it can] activate, revitalize, reactivate, develop and strengthen the various organs in our bodies when it is absorbed....[8]

In an article called "Biological Activities Caused by Far-infrared Radiation," the authors review the existing scientific literature on the effects of FIR. They conclude that the effects of FIR on human and other living systems are "biologically active."

> Recently much attention has been paid to health-improving or food-preserving activities of far-infrared rays, especially among the people of Japan....Pioneering attempts to experimentally analyze an effect of acute and chronic radiation of far-infrared rays on living organisms have detected a growth-promoting effect in growing rats, a sleep-modulatory effect in freely

behaving rats and an insomniac patient, and a blood circulation-enhancing effect in human skin.[9]

Most infrared radiation (far, middle, and near) from the sun is filtered by the gases in the atmosphere, but enough reaches the earth to cause some dramatic effects. The FIR travels in straight lines through the air directly into the body, since the oxygen and nitrogen molecules of air are unable to block FIR waves. Although a small amount of the radiant heat is lost to the atmosphere—enough to raise the air temperature slightly—most of the rays must reach a solid body that then converts the rays to heat. This helps explain why the air temperature can noticeably drop during the summer when clouds cover the sun. Once in the skin, the rays are absorbed and then reflected into deeper layers of tissue.

Although heat-producing wavelengths are all called "infrared," the three bandwidths have different qualities from each other. And within a single bandwidth, different rays—even ones that are close to one another in wavelength—can produce very different effects. For example, in the late 1940s, 50s and early 60s, infrared cookers were popular. But the word "infrared" covers a broad range of frequencies. Unless the frequencies from the cookers were specified by the manufacturer, the consumer had no idea what these appliances were emitting. In a 1999 issue of *Journal of Food Engineering*, the authors compare hamburger patties cooked by middle infrared and far infrared. The experiments they report showed great differences in how the two batches of meat were heated. FIR yielded closely matched temperatures between the surface and the inside of the hamburger. For the same core temperature to be reached in each batch, the MIR-cooked hamburgers required a much higher surface temperature than did the FIR-cooked meat. But this meant that there was more drying and charring on the surface of the meat cooked with middle infrared. The far infrared-cooked meat required a shorter cooking time, and its energy consumption was almost half of that of the MIR-cooked meat.

Similarly, near infrared heats very differently than far infrared. An article on FIR appearing in *Complementary Healing* points out that "When near infrared (NIR) waves heat organic substances the surface gets hotter than the interior, and the interior gets heated by conduction from the surface. By contrast, far-infrared penetrates deeply with a very uniform warming effect."[10] FIR directly goes into the body about 1½ inches—sometimes a bit more or less, depending on the fat and water content of the body, and the ratio of fat to muscle. The skin's thickness and amount of pigmentation, the blood supply to the area, and the degree to which the skin microstructure scatters the wavelengths, also affect penetration. Short wavelengths are scattered to a greater extent than long.

The water molecule is a very efficient absorber and emitter of FIR, notably in the range of about 9 microns, because it *intrinsically resonates* within these particular wavelengths. This characteristic is called *resonant absorption*. Whereas other wavelengths on the electromagnetic spectrum (for instance, in the much longer radio frequency range) pass through water, a 9.4 micron far infrared wavelength will be absorbed by the water itself and cause its temperature to rise. In *Energy Medicine: The Scientific Basis*, James L. Oschman describes resonant frequency in detail.

> Any object has a certain natural or resonant frequency. Strike it, bump it, pluck it, or heat it, and it will tend to vibrate at a specific frequency. This applies to a bone, a piece of wood, a molecule, an electron, or a musical instrument....In the living body, each electron, atom, chemical bond, molecule, cell, tissue, organ (and the body as a whole) has its own vibratory character [as well]....In terms of vibrations, the human body can be compared to a symphony orchestra. Each molecule corresponds to a particular instrument. Each bend, rotation, or stretch of a chemical bond has a certain resonant frequency, and will give off certain "notes" if it is energized. Since molecules, water, and dissolved ions are constantly bumping into each other at body temperature, all parts are constantly jiggling and absorbing and emitting energy.
>
> ...When two objects have similar natural frequencies, they can interact without touching; their vibrations can become coupled or entrained. For electromagnetic interactions between molecules, the word "resonance" is used more often than entrainment. In the older literature you will find the term "sympathetic vibrations."[11]

The amount of far infrared radiation emitted by a body or object is part of its electromagnetic signature. The movement of atoms and their constituent particles—as well as the movement of the chemical bonds between molecules—change direction, rotation and orbit, thus creating important changes in their electrical and magnetic fields. "Vibrations are a fundamental part of physics," writes Oschman. "There is a wide spectrum of electromagnetic vibratory frequencies, covering some 90 octaves. Any therapeutic interaction, whether it uses sound, heat, laser beams, herbs, aromas, or movements, involves one or more portions of this energy spectrum."[12]

People's ability to absorb and emit FIR is related to the ability of water to absorb and emit FIR. Since the human body is comprised of almost 70% water, this helps to explain why people respond in such a positive way to FIR, particularly in the ranges of roughly between 6 to 14 microns. Further, as Inoué and Kabaya point out:

> [I]t must be mentioned here that the molecular structure of water is greatly modified by far-infrared radiation. NMR [Nuclear Magnetic Resonance] studies have recently revealed that *water clusters become much smaller in size after an exposure to far-infrared rays....Such a change means that the motility of water molecules is highly activated by the far-infrared radiation. Hence, it might be speculated that far-infrared radiation stimulates the penetration of water molecules into various sites inside the body tissue* and also modulates dynamic functions of humoral factors in the body fluid.[13] [emphasis added]

This exciting discovery has some far-reaching implications. It makes sense that if water acquires a smaller molecular structure (also referred to as becoming "wetter"), living tissue absorbs it more easily. This means that the body becomes better hydrated, allowing for a more efficient transport of minerals into the cells as well as a more efficient expulsion of waste materials from the cells. That FIR induces this effect makes further sense when we consider the benefits that sweating has on the body. This information also helps explain the recent popularity of so-called "clustered" ("wetter") water, and other similar waters.

But far infrared radiation affects water in another unusual way, too. Serge Jurasunas writes:

> ...[W]e know that the functional mechanism of electromagnetic far-infrared rays is their ability to shorten the cluster (chain) of polluted water. By shortening the long chain of water, gaseous polluting substances such as C_{12} [carbon-12], Co [cobalt], CO_2

[carbon dioxide], SO_2 [sulfur dioxide], contained in the long chain of water, are expelled into air, while heavy metals such as Hg [mercury], Cd [cadmium], etc. precipitate to the bottom.[14]

Thus with far infrared radiation, there is a mechanical cleavage, and therefore a beneficial chemical separation, of the polluting substances from the water contained in the cells. Once dissociated from the water, the chemicals are managed more easily by the body for removal. An extra benefit is the "wetter" water's ability to adhere to the cell surfaces and act as a medium for various biological processes within the cells. Although in the above paragraph Jurasunas is discussing *tenko-seki*—the native Japanese SGES, or "super-growth ray-emitting stone" that has slightly higher FIR-emitting properties than other minerals such as granite or tourmaline—similar (though perhaps not quite as dramatic) results can also be applied to far infrared radiation that is emitted from other sources. Here is yet one more reason why so many people in far infrared saunas get such good results in eliminating heavy metals from their bodies.

For many reasons, then, FIR may be viewed as a nutrient. A living human sends and receives FIR on a regular basis. James Oschman, Richard H. Lee, and other authors have written about the unusually high levels of different electromagnetic rays (especially FIR) that are emitted by practitioners of numerous healing modalities like massage, Therapeutic Touch, and the Chinese healing art Qigong (pronounced "chee gung"). This is why almost all healers characteristically have warm or even hot hands (the palms generally emit energy between 8 and 14 microns). Another example of extra high FIR emission occurs during fever, a strategy that the body uses to heal itself. Thus a certain narrow band of FIR that is bio-regenerative has important ramifications if it is the primary or only wavelength used as the heat source for a sauna.

As you become familiar with the three ways in which heat travels, you realize that the method of heat transport—radiation, conduction, convection, or a combination of these methods—can make a huge difference not only in how much you perspire, but also in your subjective experience of sweating. The type of heat transfer you prefer determines the heat source that you'll want to use. And the heat source you use will determine the construction materials you'll want for your sauna. This is the subject of the next chapter.

NOTES

1. Frank P. Incropera and David P. DeWitt, *Fundamentals of Heat and Mass Transfer,* 4th ed. (New York: John Wiley and Sons, 1996), 2.

2. Sidney Licht, "History of Therapeutic Heat," *Therapeutic Heat and Cold* ed. Sidney Licht with Herman L. Kamenetz (New Haven: Elizabeth Licht, Publisher, 1972), 204-205.

3. Kenneth Collins, "Thermal Effects," *Clayton's Electrotherapy 10E,* ed. Sheila Kitchen and Sarah Bazin (London: WB Saunders Company Ltd., 1996), 96.

4. Ibid.

5. Nina Silver, *The Handbook of Rife Frequency Healing: Holistic Technology for Cancer and Other Diseases* (Stone Ridge, N.Y.: The Center for Frequency Education, 2001), 39, 121-122.

6. Richard Kovács, *Electrotherapy and Light Therapy with Essentials of Hydrotherapy and Mechanotherapy* (Philadelphia: Lea & Febiger, 1949), 310-311.

7. Linda Hermans-Killam, "Infrared Astronomy: Near, Mid and Far Infrared," Infrared Processing and Analysis Center (NASA's infrared astrophysics data center, operated by CalTech), http://www.ipac.caltech.edu/Outreach/Edu/Regions/irregions.html (accessed Aug. 12, 2003).

8. Zhang Jian Dong, *Conybio F.I.R.: Health Knowledge* (Luala Lumpur, Malaysia: Conybio, undated), 126-128.

9. Shojiro Inoué and Morihiro Kabaya, "Biological Activities Caused by Far-Infrared Radiation," *International Journal of Biometeorology* 33: 145.

10. Valerie H. Free, "Far-Infrared: Technologies that Harness the Sun," *Complementary Healing* (1998), 7.

11. James L. Oschman, *Energy Medicine: The Scientific Basis* (Edinburgh: Churchill Livingstone, 2000), 121, 123.

12. Ibid., 122.

13. Inoué, op. cit., 150.

14. Serge Jurasunas, "A Far Infrared Ray Emitting Stone (SGES) to Treat Cancer and Degenerative Diseases," *Townsend Letter for Doctors & Patients* (June 2000), 124.

CHAPTER 5

Construction of the Sauna

Ah, to build, to build!
That is the noblest art of all the arts.

HENRY WADSWORTH LONGFELLOW,
U.S. POET (1807–1882)

In the last chapter, I discussed the three ways in which heat is transmitted. As a general rule, people have different responses to conduction, convection, and radiation heat—and to the media that convey them. Preference for a particular heat source will depend on the thickness of skin, the amount of water and fat in the body, constitution, diet, the climate in which the sauna is being used, the amounts and types of toxins in the person's body, the state of wellness and illness, and so on. As we shall see, there are many factors to consider—heater design, construction materials, and more—in answer to the question, "What type of sauna should I use?"

DIFFERENT HEAT SOURCES FOR DIFFERENT SAUNAS

There are several natural heat sources possible for a sauna: sun, heated sand, fire (totally or partially enclosed, or in a completely open area), and stones that have been previously heated before being brought inside the chamber. Each of these methods has advantages and disadvantages. Electricity, a heat source that is not naturally-occurring, will be discussed throughout this chapter and in much greater detail later in its own section, "Challenges of Radiant Electric Heat."

The Sun

The sun, as the sustainer of all life on this planet, was the original radiant heat sauna. It is hard to imagine a better natural source. For back-to-nature purists, sunbathing (often nude) is the simplest form of hot air therapy, although indoor hot air solariums were built by many cultures from the ancient Greeks to early 20th century Germans in the blossoming Natural Hygiene movement. Unfortunately, holes in the ozone layer caused by pollutants and hydrocarbon exhaust from autos and planes have allowed a more than usual amount of destructive ultraviolet wavelengths to reach us, so this has made sunbathing a less pleasant and safe experience in the past 50 years. Also, the success of sunbathing depends on the angle and intensity of the sun's rays. The earth is slightly tilted on its axis, and earth's orbit follows a slight ellipsis (elongated circle). Consequently, the angles of the sun's rays change as the seasons change, especially as one travels farther away from the equator. In semi-tropical and tropical climates, sunning must be limited for safety. The best way to utilize sunlight in these regions may be to build enclosures of special glass that blocks out all or most of the harsh wavelengths in the electromagnetic spectrum but allows the desired wavelengths to shine through.

One might assume that an hour in the sun would produce a similar effect as being inside a sauna. In fact, under optimal circumstances, the sun is the ideal healer—as it is meant to be; after all, humans evolved under sunlight. For some people, sunbathing works even better than a sauna, because in addition to life-promoting far infrared wavelengths, the sun contains the heavily germicidal ultraviolet wavelengths. However, Kellogg and other scientists recognized that a narrow, focused band of infrared radiation in the FIR range—minus all the other wavelengths, especially one of the three UV bands which is harmful to the skin and not particularly germicidal—could generate certain responses in the body that full-spectrum sunlight might not achieve, especially if people wished to heat their bodies for extended periods of time. Many ill people do not have the stamina or biological efficiency to extract and amplify the benefits of specific wavelengths. Under these circumstances, it makes sense that isolating and extracting the desired wavelength, to help conserve the resources of an already weakened system, may be much more helpful than the sun's complete range of electromagnetic rays. Currently, the easiest way to accomplish this narrow-spectrum approach is by using electricity.

Hot Sand

Hardly anyone thinks of a sauna in relation to immersion in sand, but in some parts of the world this method is still popular. The bather is surrounded by sun-heated sand and left for a period of time. Once warmed, the silica (the chief ingredient of sand) holds the heat for hours. Some cultures that used solariums also placed sand onto the floor to heighten the effects of the sun. Again, such a heating arrangement would only work in those parts of the world where the sun is hot and one can rely on the presence of certain wavelengths year-round. Sand bathing uses a combination of radiant and conductive heat. It's important to remember that any time conduction is used as a prime heating method, the assimilation of heat into the body tissues slows down.

A modern version of the sand bath uses the FIR-emitting *"tenko-seki"* stone discovered in a mine on Kyushu Island, Japan. (The benefits of this rock were discussed in more detail in the previous chapter.) Granite and tourmaline emit almost as much FIR as does *tenko-seki*. Theoretically, any FIR-emitting mineral, if there was enough of it, could be used as a "bath" with good results.

Fire

Heating a sauna with fire is the most popular method around the world, except in highly industrialized urban areas whose method of choice is electricity. There is something friendly and even magical about a fire: one is treated to a light show as the fuel burns and the perspiration starts to drip. There are several types of fire-fueled saunas, due to the different kinds of fuel and the varied methods of containing the fire.

To many rural people, the only real sauna is one that uses a wood-burning fire. This is understandable, as fire has been the main heating method for saunas throughout humankind's history. Wood is usually readily available and works well—although it does have to be replaced, and if the fire is not maintained constantly it will flicker out. Fire has a romantic and earthy appeal, although some people do not like to be around open fire, since it can pollute, and the smoke can contain irritants and allergens. (There are conflicting studies as to whether particles from wood fires are carcinogenic.) Coal, although used occasionally in some parts of the world, is generally not even regarded as a sauna fuel, since it is highly toxic when burned and can be quite dangerous to people with sensitive lungs.

Fire can be contained in a clay oven or metal stove, or burn in a partially or completely open pit in the room itself. Fire that is enclosed in a clay oven or metal stove gives off mostly radiant heat. If the fire is in a partially or completely open pit, a fair number of convective air currents may be produced. But regardless of whether the fire is in an open or enclosed space, the pleasantness and safety of the sauna experience is still determined by how efficiently the fire burns, and even the type of wood used.

Heated Stones

People familiar with Native American sweat lodges know that properly treated stones can be a wonderful heat source. Some sweat lodges are heated by wood-burning fires, but most use large igneous rocks, which hold warmth for a long time. First the rocks are heated outdoors to immensely high temperatures in a wood fire. The rocks are then placed into a pit at the center of an enclosed lodge. The lodge is a low, dome-shaped structure made of long curved branches covered with animal skins, blankets or canvas. The heat is primarily radiant, although, since heat rises, the larger the area the more convective air currents are produced. In *Sweat*, Mikkel Aaland describes in great detail how to test the stones to make sure they are suitable for a sauna. The stones must be the right size, packed neither too loosely nor too tightly, and they must not explode or crumble into powder when heated. Although Aaland is discussing the smaller rocks used in a Finnish-style sauna onto which water is poured to make steam, it is reasonable to assume that the selection of very large rocks for a sweat lodge must be made with equal care.

Strictly speaking, a Native American sweat lodge is not a sauna but a revered holy ritual used by numerous native tribes for centuries. Although sweat lodges provide the physical benefits of a sauna, the purification is also intended to occur on emotional, mental, and spiritual levels. In most sweat lodges, depending on the tradition, various herbs for purification (such as chapparel) as well as water are tossed onto the rocks. When herbs vaporize on hot rocks, this creates lots of smoke, which can make it difficult to breathe and offset the benefits of the volatile oils released from the herbs. (I will discuss the effects of steam shortly.) The air can be so thick, Aaland reports, that some natives used to bring homemade respirators with them into their lodges so they could withstand the huge amounts of hot smoke and steam. People with sensitive lungs might not want to visit a sweat lodge unless they know beforehand how much water and herbs will be poured onto the stones. The quality of the air can vary greatly, depending on who is facilitating the sweat ceremony. My first sweat lodge experience was delightful; but the second time, I had to leave because I couldn't breathe through the dense smoke and scorching steam. The medicine man in charge of the fire felt that in order for it to be a "real" sweat, the fire should be as hot as possible and elicit the strongest possible physical and emotional responses, even if one responded negatively.

Building a sweat lodge is time consuming and you need the space for it. Unless you live in the country with a constant temperate climate, have access to the building materials, can leave the lodge standing all year round once you have built it, and are willing to spend about five hours preparing the fire and the rocks each time you want to sweat, don't consider this a substitute for a daily or even weekly sauna. However, if you have the opportunity to attend a traditional native sweat lodge as a special event, it can be a powerfully spiritual, positive transformative experience—provided the medicine man (or woman) doesn't exceed your limits of heat and smoke.

EFFECTS OF MOISTURE IN THE AIR

When I discuss "sauna" in these pages about moisture, I am referring solely to sauna rooms or chambers, since in a cabinet the head is exposed to fresh air.

The Production of Negative Ions

For many body heating aficionados, a sauna is not a real sauna without water. In fact, one sauna manufacturer told me, in Europe, a sauna is defined according to three criteria: it must be a wood-lined room; the heat source (which can be either electrical or a fire) must reach a minimal temperature of 140°F (60°C); and the unit must be outfitted with hot rocks upon which water can be thrown, in order to get a good *löyly*. It is illegal to call anything else a sauna.

For both the Finns and Native Americans, throwing water onto hot rocks to create a light vapor is an important ceremony. However, the presence of water vapor in either an electric-heated or fire-heated rock sauna goes beyond aesthetic appeal or even the quality of heat. Very light steam can make the difference between a feeling of well-being or the onset of illness. Western science has finally confirmed what native cultures have intuitively known for centuries: that the moving water is healing because it produces beneficial negative ions.

An *ion* is an atom or molecule with either a positive or a negative charge. Normally, the number of protons (which have a positive charge) and electrons (which have a negative charge) are equal. However, if an electron gets bumped off an atom, the atom assumes a positive charge. If a lone electron whirling around finds an atom and latches on to it, the atom then becomes negatively charged. An excess of positively charged ions is caused by electrical machinery, smog, and non-natural environments such as automobiles and building interiors that contain synthetic materials. Positively charged ions in the air make people feel fatigued and restless, partly because they attract carbon dioxide that displaces valuable oxygen when we breathe. The immune response can begin to falter, opening the door not only to insomnia, migraines and respiratory illnesses, but also to arthritis, allergies and other autoimmune conditions.

Negative ions are created by plants during photosynthesis, by fire, and by *moving water*—particularly if it falls through the air in a waterfall, ocean spray or shower, or is vaporized into steam when poured onto the hot rocks of a sauna. Large numbers of negatively charged ions in a room or in the environment energize, rejuvenate, and make people feel secure and calm. Research shows that these subjective good feelings are due in part to the relaxing alpha brain wave patterns that are induced. The healing effect of negative ions is so important that NASA provides a negative ion generator for astronauts after space flights. And many hospitals in Europe routinely place the units in sick people's rooms, where the negative ions enhance the healing from burns and even help people recover from some forms of cancer.

Aaland describes how the Finns—regarded as the world experts on saunas—responded to the introduction of electric heaters in saunas and the positive ions they produced.

> The effect of negative ions on sweat bathing was discovered when researchers were trying to account for the tremendous popularity of sauna wood burning stoves over electric stoves. Subjective reasons, such as the fragrance of burned wood, did not fully explain why Finns felt so refreshed after time in a wood heated sauna and quite dulled from certain electrically heated saunas. Tests showed that the practice of splashing water on super-heated rocks produced an abundance of negative ions. Many electric stoves, it turned out, were not getting the rocks hot enough and the glowing metal heating coils were spurting more positive ions in the air. Researchers learned that if the rocks were properly heated in electric stoves, the positive ions, being larger and less mobile [than negative ions], would ground out on the hot stones. The buying habits of the Finns, perhaps the most sophisticated of sweat bathers, has forced many Finnish electric stove companies to pay particular attention to their sauna stove design...it is likely [that] similar negative ion production occurs in any sweat bath that converts water to vapor quickly. The Native American Indian sweat lodge comes to mind.[1]

Most sauna designers and installers tell me that the best electric stoves allow the rocks to be placed directly among the electric heating coils instead of on top of a grill or in a tray. This requires an exceptionally well-made, insulated, safe stove—but the benefits seem to be worth the extra effort and price.

Moisture as a Lubricant

There is another, more obvious reason for wanting some water vapor in a sauna. Moisture lubricates the mucous membranes that line the respiratory passageway, helping them filter out dust and dirt from the air before it reaches the lungs. This gives the body some protection from pathogenic microbes. Moisture can also help to loosen and expel phlegm from the lungs and sinus cavities, which is why many people favor a steam bath when they have a cold or more severe respiratory infection. Finally, the proper amount of moisture in the air also allows the lungs to easily exchange carbon dioxide for fresh oxygen. Air that is too dry makes it difficult to breathe freely. If there is not enough moisture in the air, the mucous membranes dry out, and in extreme cases may even burn. (People from humid climates who visit dry desert regions sometimes need to spray salt water into the nose to prevent the formation of crusts and sores—at least until their bodies acclimate to the dryness.)

However, at the other extreme, clammy wet heat is usually not bearable either. It can be hard to breathe in air that is too humid. Excess humidity also holds heat—in the body and in air—in warm climates. This is because air that is already saturated with moisture does not absorb very much perspiration from the skin, so there is less evaporation. The perspiration then remains on the body, trapping dirt and heat in the pores of the skin. On the humid eastern coast of the United States, temperatures in even the mid-70s Fahrenheit (mid-20s Celsius)—which by itself is not uncomfortably hot—induce the majority of folks to turn on their air conditioners. In contrast, in desert climates, even when the temperature climbs into the 90s or 100s Fahrenheit (from around 32° to the low 40s Celsius), people may not feel a need for air conditioning if the air is dry. Dry air quickly absorbs perspiration, and the subjective cooling effect is immediate. The mechanics of hot, wet air—and the body's corresponding inability to cleanse and cool itself—explain why people living in warm humid climates may exude more unpleasant body odor, need more frequent showers, and even feel more clammy and cantankerous, than those in drier climates. Once when I was in Arizona, the temperature climbed to 110°F (43.3°C). Yet I was comfortable, and wore the same outfit for three consecutive days because even on the third day the garment was still as fresh as if it had just been pulled off a clothesline. This is very different from my experience on the Eastern United States seaboard: I find that a mere 70°F (21.1°C) is unpleasant if the air is humid. Clothing sticks to the skin and may need laundering after one day.

The science of water evaporation explains why the balance between beneficial amounts of water vapor and undesirable quantities of steam must be carefully negotiated in a sauna. John O. Virtanen, the Finnish-born author of *The Finnish Sauna*, writes:

> [W]e can employ a fairly accurate rule-of-thumb: if the *kiuas* [stove] is up to proper heat but the humidity is insufficient, there is generally an unpleasant "dry" smell in the room; if, on the other hand, a "steamy" smell is present, the humidity has risen above the accepted level and the *kiuas* may be underheated or undersized. Even in small saunas, the heater's *löyly* capacity should be such that it can convert at least one quart of water into *löyly* in 15 minutes with no resultant unpleasant odors when the water is thrown over the rocks at 3-minute intervals.[2]

The Electric Light Bath Compared to Russian and Turkish Steam Baths

Perspiration Levels

The slow or even total lack of sweat evaporation in humid climates helps explain Dr. Kellogg's discovery in 1894 that steamy Turkish or Russian baths and even hot water baths were not as effective as his dry electric light baths for inducing perspiration. In fact, the amount of perspiration produced in the electric light bath compared to the Turkish and Russian baths was almost double. Thick, continuous water vapor is steam—making the device no longer a sauna but a steam bath—but the comparison here is useful, since some people mistakenly call a steam bath a sauna. In such an environment what is sometimes perceived as perspiration is simply the water from the steam that remains on the skin. Both Turkish and Russian baths use liberal amounts of steam and heat primarily through convection (as well as radiation), which is the least efficient way of inducing a sweat. Kellogg's light bath heated primarily through radiation (significantly, the bulbs emitted quite a bit of heat in the far infrared range), and only secondarily (and very slightly) did the cabinet heat by means of convected air currents. Unfortunately, no tests were done with saunas that use wood burning fires. However, Kellogg's research is still very useful to us because each sauna that he tested used primarily one, and at the most two, methods of heat transfer.

The ways in which Kellogg determined which saunas induced the most perspiration were very elaborate, not only for his time but also by today's standards. "My earliest experiments in the use of the electric-light bath showed me that it was capable of producing very characteristic effects," he wrote. "This led me to undertake a series of physiologic experiments for the purpose of placing its therapeutic use upon a rational basis, and for the purpose of comparing the effects of the electric light, Turkish, and Russian baths." Three healthy young men stayed in each type of sauna for five, 10, 20, and 30 minutes, on different days, with diet and other conditions "being made as nearly alike as possible." Kellogg tested for carbon dioxide elimination, urinary secretion, perspiration, surface and internal temperature, numbers of both red and white blood cells, and levels of hemoglobin in the red blood cells. To determine carbon dioxide elimination, he designed a special, delicate air meter to measure "all the air expired during the ten minutes before the experiment, collecting an average sample of the air for analysis. During the bath the air was collected for the same length of time….the results obtained were corrected for barometric pressure and vapor tension so that the figures…[were] properly comparable."[3] At the end of the experiment, Dr. Kellogg found a significantly higher amount of various bodily secretions in the urine when the men took Russian and Turkish saunas than when they took electric-light baths. Kellogg summarized the results:

> The diminished amount of urea, total chlorides, and total solids present in the urine during the twenty-four hours in which the subject was subjected to the electric light bath, was evidently the result of increased elimination by the skin, showing that the electric light bath is much more powerful than either the Turkish or the Russian bath as a means of stimulating vicarious eliminative work upon the part of the skin.

> The amount of perspiration induced by the incandescent electric light bath was fully double than that induced by the Turkish bath in the same length of time.
>
> The amount of perspiration induced by the Russian bath was less than that induced by the electric light and the Turkish bath.[4]

Other researchers have also confirmed the effect of too much moisture in the air—though again, what is "too much" depends on the individual. Kellogg's teacher Dr. Wilhelm Winternitz, who popularized the electric light bath in Europe and thus boosted its prominence in the United States, is quoted by Kellogg as having said:

> Another advantage of the electric light bath is that it does not interfere with heat elimination. It in fact encourages heat elimination by encouraging free perspiration. Many other forms of hot applications, particularly hot-water baths and sweating packs, cause retention of bodily heat [due to the lack of evaporation of sweat from the skin]. In the electric light bath, the heat elimination and the excretion of effete matters which accompany vigorous perspiration proceed with increased activity at the same time the rays of radiant heat are penetrating the tissues, elevating the temperature of the blood, and quickening all the vital processes....Ordinarily a much higher temperature is necessary before symptoms of sweating occur in the vapor bath.[5]

The comment about the air temperature inside the sauna is important. The electric light bath read 81°F (27.2°C), the Turkish bath, 128.5°F (53.6°C), and the Russian bath, 101.8°F (38.8°C). The body temperature of the subjects (all taken when they had been in the sauna for the same period of time) was also different. The average temperature of the subjects who had been in the electric light bath was 99.6°F (37.6°C); and the temperatures of those in the Turkish bath averaged 98.7°F (37.1°C). No readings were taken for the Russian bath, but due to its similarity to the Turkish one might assume similar numbers.

The amount of time required for the subjects to begin sweating was less in the electric light bath. In Kellogg's cabinet, the subjects took an average of 3 minutes 32 seconds, compared to 5 minutes 35 seconds in the Turkish bath, and 6 minutes 45 seconds in the Russian bath.

Thus the large quantity of steam in Russian or Turkish baths can make it difficult to breathe easily or sweat copiously. Dr. Kellogg preferred radiant heat not because he made cabinets that used that principle; he made sauna cabinets employing radiant heat because they *worked*. Compared to conduction and convection (whether via hot water, hot air, or hot metal), radiant heat is a much more efficient way to heat the body. "The electric light bath," he concluded, "is incomparably superior to every other means yet devised for raising the temperature of the skin or of the body in general."[6]

Heat Penetration: Its Depth and Effects

In addition to the other benefits of radiant heat, Kellogg found that the "thermic heat rays" (as he called them) "have wonderful penetrating power and reach the deep-lying tissues fully two inches below the surface"—so that "even the brain, the spinal cord, the liver, the lungs, the heart, the lymphatic glands, the thyroid gland and other of the most important structures of the body" are "under the influence of thermic stimulation."[7] The doctor then compared radiant heat with conductive heat and convective heat, both dry and moist. He wrote:

> Convection heat has no power of penetration. It heats only the surface with which it comes in contact, although, of course, a solid body placed in a heated atmosphere gradually acquires the temperature of the medium with which it is surrounded through conduction of heat from the surface to deeper parts....It is important to note the radical difference in therapeutic power between thermic applications in the form of radiant energy and those procedures in which heat is applied by means of media, whether solid, liquid or gaseous. When heated objects such as the hot-water bag...are brought in contact with the skin, the superficial layers of the skin are heated, and then little by little the temperature of the deeper layers is gradually raised by conduction. The process is very slow, however, and as various investigators have shown...the deeper tissues are cooled off as rapidly as [they are] heated, the heat being conveyed away by the blood and lymph. A moist hot application...is a more effective heating procedure than a dry hot application, for the reason that the skin is saturated with water and thus

becomes a better conductor; but the difference in effect is not great.…A dry hot application, by inducing perspiration, after a time moistens the skin so that practically the effect of a moist application is obtained.[8]

The application of heated air or vapor to the surface of the body likewise produces its effects by heating the surface only, heat being slowly conducted to the underlying layers of tissue, and thus gradually raising the body temperature; but no marked effect is produced upon the deep-lying structures— nerve trunks, viscera, etc.—unless the procedure is continued for a sufficient length of time to raise the temperature of the blood. [At this point, the air must be extremely hot in order to produce a deep heating of the body.][9]

In the case of the electric-light bath, whether administered by means of the incandescent light or the arc light, the effect is very different indeed. When the light rays fall upon the skin, they penetrate the deeper structures to the extent of two inches or more. This effect is instantaneous, so that the thermic stimulation of the deeper structure begins with application and continues in full play to the end of the procedure….[10]

Kellogg then analyzed why radiant heat penetrates so thoroughly.

The highest degree of thermic stimulation through radiant heat may be produced upon the deeper structures of the body irrespective of the temperature of the skin surface or of the air surrounding the body. Prolonged applications to the skin are depressing through the reflex effects which they evoke, whereas thermic applications to the deeper lying structures are highly stimulating…a hot application to the cutaneous [skin] surface through reflex action lessens heat production, whereas heating of the muscular structures increases heat production by stimulation of the thermogenic tissues.[11]

Above, Dr. Kellogg was commenting on the tendency of the body to shut down its sweating apparatus with the continual application of heat. This point helps us understand why hot tubs and hot baths—taken alone, without alternate timed applications of cold—although relaxing, are generally not as healing as a sauna.

What if Kellogg had compared his own device to a relatively dry sauna heated by either a wood-burning stove, open fire or hot rocks? All saunas emit radiant heat (remember, anything that has a temperature radiates heat). But some saunas also emit a fair amount of heat via convection, depending on the size and shape of the room and ventilation—and especially if heated by an open fire. This decreases the benefits that can be obtained only from radiant heat. And although fire radiates, it also creates convection currents (updrafts) as hot air rises. If the fire is totally enclosed in a stove or oven, there is much less chance of updrafts, but now the room can become too hot to withstand for long periods, as some of the heat lies outside the beneficial FIR band.

Challenges of Radiant Electric Heat

The use of electricity as a heating source is a very recent phenomenon in the history of body heating. This section, then, is devoted to the special problems and challenges of electric heaters.

Eliminating Burning

Compared to fire, light bulbs are obviously easier to manage and maintain, and they cannot become as hot. However, this does not mean that Kellogg's electric light bath would be the best sauna today. At the Battle Creek Sanitarium, clients were warned not to go too near the bulbs in the light cabinet, since the bulbs (there were 32 of them) eventually did get too hot to touch. A friend of mine, who had worked at Battle Creek Equipment Company decades ago developing exercise equipment (including steam cabinets), regularly took saunas in Dr. Kellogg's original electric light baths. "I really enjoyed it," he reminisced, "but I didn't like those bulbs that stuck out all over the place. It was too easy to get burned." (He was thus inspired to later invent a FIR sauna cabinet of his own.) Today at the Battle Creek Lifestyle Health Center, a descendent of Kellogg's spa, old working models of the electric light bath are in perfect condition and still used. But they have not been altered in any way; the light bulbs are not covered with screens or mesh to prevent burns.

An upgrade, then, of the electric light bath, would be an electric heater enclosed in a protective covering. Most modern radiant heaters for saunas consist of metal coils or quartz heated by electrical power, or (this is less common) gas powered heaters that are ignited either electrically or by a match. Depending on the size of the room and the air flow, there will be considerable amounts of convective heat transfer as well as radiant heat—though rocks dispersed among the heating coils would bring much more radiant heat into the room.

Creating Evenly Distributed Heat

Whatever type of electric heater your sauna uses, you should be able to regulate the temperature of the heater, so the chamber doesn't become too cool or too hot. The size of the heater must be appropriate for the space. If one small unit is supplying heat for a large area, the heater will be forced to operate at higher temperatures. This means that the closer you are to the heater, the hotter you become and the easier it is to get burned (just as you would with a fire).

Within the last decade or so, sauna manufacturers have begun using specially designed infrared heaters that utilize very narrow portions of the far infrared band. As I mentioned in the previous chapter, the wavelengths of FIR have a broad temperature range from −459.67°F (absolute zero) to 470°F (or −273.15°C to 243.3°C), which span from 1000 to 5.6 microns in length. (The hottest wavelengths are the shortest.) The optimal portion of the far infrared radiation spectrum for sauna purposes is just under 9 to a bit over 9 microns, since the normal body temperature of human beings is 98.6°F (37°C), which corresponds to about 9.35 microns. The resonant absorption rate of a water molecule is also about 9.35 microns. Nine microns radiate heat of about 120°F (48.9 °C).

If your sauna's electric heater is in the far infrared range, the potential of being burned is not as great as with an ordinary electric heater—especially if there is more than one heat source in the sauna cabinet or room. This is often the case with FIR saunas. Some manufacturers put several heaters into a sauna, with the heaters occasionally covering an entire wall or even all four walls. This design provides more even heat at even lower temperatures, not only eliminating "cool spots" but lessening the possibility of becoming burned from a concentrated high temperature in any given area. No FIR heaters are built that can accommodate a *löyly* (see below), since temperatures well over 98.6°F (37°C) and even 120°F (48.9 °C) are necessary to make the rocks hot enough to create steam. If you don't mind not having a *löyly*, a sauna containing more than one FIR heater is probably the best choice for evenly distributed heat.

Accommodating a Löyly

Electric heaters that are equipped to accept a *löyly* can be of varied quality. By law, all such heaters are required to use specially insulated metal coils to eliminate the danger of short-circuited wires, which can cause electrical shock or death when water is thrown upon the rocks. However, some heaters are designed to accommodate stones on top of a metal grill rather than among the heating elements themselves. Finnish sauna aficionados say that if the rocks do not make contact with the heating elements, they rarely reach their optimal temperature, thus causing the quality of heat to be harsh. In contrast, the heat imparted by rocks directly touching the heating coils is gentler and smoother and feels much better, because there is more radiant heat. Make sure that the stones can be distributed among the heating elements. This arrangement creates a much better *löyly*, with enough sizzle and vapor to satisfy even the most steadfast Finnish sauna bather.

If you are using a sauna cabinet, the presence or absence of a *löyly* is not relevant because there is no place to put rocks—and anyway, with the head outside of the heating enclosure, you are breathing fresh air, so from a health perspective the presence or absence of moisture is not an issue.

Eliminating Harmful ELF Electromagnetic Fields

Earlier in this chapter I discussed the problem of harmful positive ions generated by some electric saunas. Related to this is the issue of harmful electromagnetic fields. When I interviewed Mikkel Aaland for this book, he strongly expressed his desire for a real fire, even one inside a wood burning stove—not only as an aesthetic preference, but because electrical currents can disrupt the function of the body. It is thought that they do this primarily through the dangerous magnetic fields created when electrons move through electrical wiring.

(Not all electromagnetic fields are dangerous; some are benign or even biologically necessary. For instance, as discussed in Chapter 4, the wavelengths known as far infrared radiation produce life-promoting heat. We would die without FIR.)

The effect of electromagnetic radiation depends on

- *where* on the electromagnetic spectrum the wavelengths lie,
- their *voltage,* or the *force* with which they impact the body, and
- *how* that radiation is being transmitted and administered.

These conditions can literally make the difference between wellness and illness, life and death.

One group of electromagnetic wavelengths known as *extremely low frequency waves* (ELF) is commonly known to be dangerous. The wavelengths of ELF fields range between 0 to 300 hertz (hertz designates cycles per second). ELF is produced by alternating current, not direct current. (The inventor Nikola Tesla used alternating, while his colleague Thomas Edison preferred direct. Most of the world today uses alternating rather than direct current.) B. Blake Levitt, author of the superb book *Electromagnetic Fields: A Consumer's Guide to the Issues and How to Protect Ourselves*, writes:

> Direct current (DC) is the steady flow of electrons in one direction. Alternating current (AC) is an electron flow that changes strength and alters direction within a certain cycle; the AC field collapses and reappears with its poles reversed every time the current changes direction....Direct current creates a steady magnetic field. But with alternating current, each time the direction of the electrons is reversed, or flipped, a powerful magnetic field is created that fluctuates at the same frequency.[12]

When you realize that the body itself generates minute but critical amounts of electrical and magnetic currents as part of its normal functioning, it's easy to see why ELF is so disruptive to the system. Not only is this back-and-forth movement injurious, but the number of cycles per second also has an impact. In North America, electricity is transmitted at 60 hertz. In most of the rest of the world, electricity is transmitted at 50 hertz. But the human body naturally oscillates at 55 hertz! As Levitt points out, "The human body will take on whatever field it is exposed to. Each time you touch a small electric appliance operating at 60 hertz, those same 60-hertz fields will be set up in your body as well."[13] *The reason electromagnetic fields can severely injure living tissue is that they change the rotation and spin of the electrons in the body. This in turn alters the chemical bonds of various molecules in living systems.* Thus neither a 50-hertz nor a 60-hertz rhythm support biological functions. (One might speculate, then, about the possible benefits if electrical current ran at 55 hertz, and was direct instead of alternating.)

Another aspect to the danger of electromagnetic fields relates to the *coherence* of the wave. Some people argue that since the sun is constantly transmitting naturally-occurring radio frequencies, microwaves, and other harmful ELF to the earth, why should we worry?—and that it justifies producing more ELF on the ground. It is true that all this radiation is natural. But radiation from the sun is generally *diffuse*, whereas alternating current is *concentrated. Concentrated radiation is not natural.* For example, you need to purposely focus, augment, and direct electron bombardment to turn on a light bulb. In *Electromagnetic Man: Health & Hazard in the Electrical Environment*, Cyril W. Smith and Simon Best confirm:

> It is just over 100 years since electricity generation started; 60 years since radio transmissions and 40 years since radar and telecommunications entered our environment. [The book was published in 1990.] Like natural fields, man-made fields are limited by the physical properties of the environment. Unlike natural fields, they are highly coherent and can interfere with our bio-signals.[14]

What kind of electrical appliances emit ELF? Anything that plugs into a socket: air conditioners, blenders, coffee makers, computers, copiers, electric blankets, electric clocks, electric heaters of all types, electric ovens and ranges, electric shavers, food processors, hair dryers, irons, laser and inkjet printers, mixers, power drills and saws, refrigerators, stereo equipment, televisions, toasters, vacuum cleaners, VCRs, washing machines and clothes dryers…the list is long. Even phones (corded, cordless and cell) emit ELF.

The harmful effects of ELF radiation are many and varied. In *The Whole Way to Natural Detoxification: The Complete Guide to Clearing Your Body of Toxins*, Jacqueline Krohn and colleagues explain that in the many studies

> exposing cells and animals to ELF fields…electric workers and their children have a higher risk of brain tumors. The incidence of childhood leukemia is higher in children who live near power

lines that carry high voltage. Power-line exposure has also been associated with an increased incidence of suicide. These studies support the hypothesis that ELFs act as a cancer promoter. ELF fields interact with the cell membrane and can affect hormones, calcium exchange, and tissue growth. It is postulated that the ELFs suppress the production of melatonin, a cancer inhibitor, by the pineal gland.[15]

This "postulation" is borne out by other researchers, including Smith and Best, who point out that the pineal gland is particularly sensitive to even minute changes in electromagnetic fields. These authors also cite formal published studies linking the following maladies to ELF electromagnetic fields:

- allergies
- autoimmune disorders, such as lupus erythematosus and multiple sclerosis
- birth defects and genetic abnormalities
- cancers of various types, including brain tumors and leukemia
- emotion and mood changes, including higher percentages of suicides
- eyestrain and headaches
- fatigue and sleep disturbance
- heart attacks
- hormonal abnormalities
- infectious disease increase
- lowered fertility, miscarriages, and pregnancy problems, including stillborn children
- nervous system disorders, including confusion, convulsions, dizziness, hyperactivity, and memory loss
- stress increase and intolerance

Another, important factor that determines harm from electromagnetic fields is the proximity of the person (or animal or conceivably even a plant) to the source of the field. A milligauss is a unit of measurement of the strength of an electromagnetic field. According to tables from the Environmental Protection Agency that are reprinted in Levitt's book, a blender from six inches away emits between 30 and 100 milligauss; an electric can opener six inches away emits between 500 and 1500 milligauss; a hair dryer six inches away emits between one and 700 milligauss; and a ceiling fan 12 inches away emits between three and 50 milligauss.[16] Some sources maintain that even two milligauss is enough to disrupt a person's biological function, and that the maximum safe emission for a person to absorb is only one milligauss.

You can reduce the chance of illness by living away from major power lines and using only those devices that are essential to daily life. For the urban dweller who wants to sweat, however, generally an electrically heated sauna is the only choice. Fortunately, unless you are particularly sensitive to electrical fields, the benefits of sweating will likely outweigh the harmful effects of electromagnetic fields.

Some FIR sauna proponents claim that the use of far infrared naturally minimizes harmful electromagnetic fields, and that it does so almost completely. It is true that compared to conventional heaters, FIR units emit smaller electromagnetic fields. But this is because at lower temperatures, they require less voltage or power—so hence, there is less electricity to create a field. This does not mean that a harmful electromagnetic field is eliminated entirely! However, improvements are constantly being made. One sauna manufacturer, after two years of research, has solved the problem of dangerous electromagnetic fields by constructing his FIR heaters in such a way that emissions are less than one milligauss. (See Appendix B for a listing of sauna manufacturers.) Also, some enlightened appliance manufacturers use sheets of an expensive, composite metal called *mu* that minimizes or virtually eliminates electromagnetic fields (it is not clearly understood how this metal works).

Incidentally, some manufacturers claim that a good quality FIR heater emits so many beneficial negative ions, it offsets the harmful effects of ELF fields. I have not seen any research to either support or refute this statement.

SAUNA BUILDING MATERIALS

There is no simple answer to "What is the best kind of sauna to use?" Everyone has unique tastes and needs. When you're at the gym or your favorite health club, you don't have much choice—the sauna or steam room that's available is the one you use. But if you're thinking of buying your own, this is a matter to consider carefully. Some people like their sauna completely dry. Others crave lots of steam along with the heat, much more steam than the Finns customarily use. And still others prefer a steam bath with the addition of ozone (discussed in Appendix A). Everybody's different, because each person has a different body.

The type of sauna you want, and how often you use it, will determine the materials of which it is made. Not all materials are suitable for all purposes.

Wood Saunas

One of the most popular, common, and traditional materials is wood. Generally, wood is used to build a sauna room rather than a cabinet. Soft woods such as alder, basswood, hemlock, and poplar (also known as aspen) rather than hardwoods are often preferred, because the molecules in hardwoods are more densely packed and thus retain too much heat to comfortably touch after the sauna has been hot for awhile. (However, harder woods such as birch, maple, and oak are sometimes used.) Cedar, a beautiful fragrant wood, is a favorite, since it contains a volatile oil called cedrene (a member of the turpene family), produced by the tree to repel insects and withstand moisture. But the very aromatic oil that makes cedar naturally resistant to rotting contains unsaturated, aliphatic cyclic hydrocarbons that can cause severe allergic and even toxic reactions in sensitive people. After being in such wooden saunas for even brief periods, some bathers—particularly those suffering from multiple chemical or environmental sensitivities—can become very ill with gastrointestinal and respiratory distress, or even neurological disorders including seizures. The turpenes in softer woods like pine, redwood, and spruce can cause similar reactions.

Poplar, which is soft and does not contain turpenes, is a favorite among many sauna manufacturers. However, poplar is exceptionally soft; so it is susceptible to rot, especially with heavy use. Locust, similar to cedar, but without any of the aromatic turpenes that cedar contains, has rot-resistant qualities that make it an ideal wood to use for a sauna. Unfortunately, it is not easily available commercially. Plywood—a synthetic product comprised of thin layers of wood held together with glue—is highly unsuitable and should never be used. Even without being subjected to high heat, plywood emits dangerous fumes. Whatever type of wood is used for the sauna, be aware that many lumber companies use toxic chemicals to preserve the wood that are dangerous to people with chemical sensitivities. A sauna interior should *never* be painted, since the paint will emit fumes when the temperature is high.

To create a truly effective sauna, wood must be kiln-dried to less than 11% moisture. Otherwise, with the constant heating and cooling, the wood will repeatedly expand and contract and eventually crack, thus trapping moisture—and providing an ideal breeding ground for bacteria. (This is why some wooden saunas are equipped with drains or recesses in the floor to collect moisture.)

Although high temperatures are presumed to kill bacteria, a wooden sauna can still become caked with dirt, and reek from the toxins that are sweated out of the skin. Dr. David Root—who has done extensive research on the myriad chemicals found in sweat (primarily of drug users), and whose clinical practice consists of helping such people detoxify (see Chapter 8)—reports that daily use in serious detoxification programs with chemically loaded people will cause even aromatic wood saunas to rot within three years. This, as well as the strong possibility of allergic reactions, is why heavily toxic people with chemical sensitivities or environmental illness should use saunas made of other materials (discussed shortly). Of course, if your system is not too toxic and your heart is set on wood, as long as you are not allergic to turpenes you will probably be very happy with an aromatic wood sauna.

All wood saunas require care. Some people use bleach, detergent, ammonia, or other caustic chemicals to clean the sauna, but I don't recommend that these products be used by *anyone*—not the average person, and certainly not someone who is sensitive to chemicals. Even if you aren't diagnosed with multiple chemical sensitivities or environmental illness, if you are dealing with a chronic or serious illness, or your immune function isn't what it should be, you don't need the added stress of forcing your liver and other organs to eliminate extra poisons. (A source of a very safe and effective cleaner is listed in Appendix B.)

Clean the entire unit—the walls, and especially the benches and floor—at least once a week with plain mild soap (not detergent, which is synthetic and toxic). Alternatively, you can use a mixture of water and white vinegar (one or more cups of vinegar to a 5-gallon bucket of water), or 3% food grade hydrogen peroxide (which kills microbes—and, please note, will also bleach the wood). When you're done cleaning, make sure to turn on the heater, open the door, and let the sauna dry out. This will help preserve the wood. Wood should also be refurbished regularly with food grade oil after it's completely dry. This seals its pores, protecting them from steam and sweat. (In wood, the pores are the openings through which fluids are absorbed or discharged; a wood's grain is the design made by the layers of fibers and the size and arrangement of the pores. Pores may be small and compactly distributed, producing close-grain wood, or they may be large and widely dispersed for open-grain wood.) If you do not react adversely to scents, you can put a few drops of lavender essential oil into either your soap mixture and/or the seasoning oil. Lavender not only smells fragrant, but it has germicidal properties and will help keep your sauna sanitary (especially if some pathogens managed to survive the high heat). You can also use essential oils of tea tree, peppermint, eucalyptus, and neem (a tree from India), which are very powerful germicides.

Make sure that the lumber in your wooden sauna is free of knots. Since knots retain more heat than the wood around them, they can burn you. Also, with the constant expansion and contraction due to heat alternating with cold, the knots will eventually pop out and leave gaping holes. Finally, the boards comprising the sauna walls should be thick enough to minimize shrinkage.

Ceramic, Granite, Marble, and Porcelain Tile Saunas

To avoid the problems from heavy sauna use that you would encounter with wood, other materials such as ceramic, granite, marble, and porcelain tile can be used for the sauna. Obviously, these materials are used to construct rooms. Such saunas generally require very little upkeep, except for a periodic cleaning. The hardiness and imperviousness to rot or deterioration make these substances ideal for serious therapeutic use—although generally, only the better health spas and clinics can afford them.

It is interesting to note that granite has a natural tendency to absorb and emit heat in the far infrared wavelengths. This would make it an exceptionally good (though expensive) material for an enclosed sauna.

Plastic, Fiberglass, and Other Resin Sauna Materials

The only saunas I have seen that are made of plastic are individual cabinets, since their portability requires a material that is more pliable, and lighter in weight, than wood (although a horizontal cabinet made from wood has just been marketed). One problem with many plastics is that they are known to outgas (emit molecules of the plastic into the air), even at room temperature. However, according to the Food and Drug Administration, NASA (the National Aeronautics and Space Administration), and plastics industry standards, a plastic called ABS is relatively stable, and does not outgas after it cools down from having been formed and molded. For this reason, ABS is used to make (among other items) medical diagnostic equipment, medical test kits, refrigerators, and toys. NASA's outgassing test consists of placing the substance inside a vacuum chamber at extremely high heat, and then weighing the material with special precision instruments. If the material is lighter at the end of the test, outgassing has occurred. If there is no weight change, the substance is considered stable.

A September 6, 2002 letter from a General Electric product compliance specialist to a sauna cabinet manufacturer states: "Based on the requirements of your current application, GE Plastics does not anticipate toxic fumes emitting from the [ABS] material under the standard operation conditions."[17] The "standard operation conditions" of ABS is that it is not expected to outgas even if heated to temperatures of up to 140°F (60°C). (Note that the GE product specialist is referring to the temperature of the *plastic*, not the temperature of the air or the sauna heater. It would take an unbearably scorching air temperature to bring the plastic to its upper heat limit.) A conscientious manufacturer will always use a high quality plastic in a sauna. (It should be noted, however, that the heater itself might contain something that outgasses.)

Despite the best manufacturing techniques, or assurances by government and industry that certain medical-grade plastics are safe, some highly reactive people still do not tolerate plastic. Dr. William Rea, author of *Chemical Sensitivity*, observes that chemically sensitive people are often bothered by certain types of plastics, but not all types—and then, not always. Fairly stable hard plastics, he writes, are "relatively odor-free." However, he adds, the plastics should be "self-tested, particularly when warm."[18] Try to test the unit before you buy it. If that is not possible, see if the manufacturer offers a full or even partial money-back guarantee. If you are extremely reactive, saunas made only from more inert materials such as tile, marble, or non-aromatic wood should be used. Be aware that your need for a non-outgassing sauna material must be weighed against the possibility of the wood rotting—particularly if you have a high level of toxins in your system and plan to use the sauna for many hours on a regular basis.

Related to the problem of plastic outgassing is the concern voiced by some researchers about the emission of (harmful) positive ions. I have not seen any scientific data in this area, so am unable to comment. In any case, if the plastic is of a high enough quality, the positive ion discharge into the air might be considerably less. An advantage to plastic is its durability and imperviousness to water; all it requires is a bit of soap (not detergent) to keep it clean.

Fiberglass, which is very strong and similar to plastic (though comprised of different materials), is also used by some sauna cabinet manufacturers. It is especially suitable for steam cabinets that accommodate ozone generators, because (unlike ABS) it is one of only five substances that are impervious to corrosion by ozone. (The only materials that are completely impervious to ozone, and which could be recommended for use in an ozone sauna, are glass, and four synthetic materials. See the "Sauna Style" table at the end of this chapter for a list of the four synthetics.) However, after its creation, fiberglass noticeably outgasses for a few weeks—even up to a year, according to one manufacturer, who holds a patent on a special coating designed to permanently eliminate the outgassing that normally occurs with fiberglass (see the list of sauna manufacturers in Appendix B). Out of consideration for chemically sensitive individuals, the manufacturer should leave the heater on in the unit for at least 24 hours, thus giving it a chance to outgas in the factory at least partially before it is shipped.

If you are planning to use your fiberglass cabinet as an ozone steam sauna, make sure that it is not constructed with glues and adhesives, since ozone will cause the emission of chemical vapors as the bonding agents disintegrate. Incidentally, you *must* use a sauna *cabinet* rather than a room for ozone-sauna therapy, since the level of ozone considered therapeutic irritates the respiratory tract and instead must be absorbed through the skin. (See Appendix A, "A Brief Summary of Ozone.")

Fabric Saunas

Before the recent upsurge of FIR saunas, the only infrared or far infrared devices that most people knew about were either the FIR light bulbs in bathrooms that help keep you warm when you exit the shower, or the FIR lamp in their health care provider's office. When NASA discovered in the mid 1960s that several mineral oxides can produce FIR, these minerals were added to the FIR lamps. Today, there are a number of products that use FIR: hair dryers; blankets, sheets and mattress pads; jackets, mittens, socks, underwear, and other clothing; foot, ankle and leg wraps for sports injuries; car seats and chair cushions; and even FIR creams. The ability of scientists to create cloth with specific FIR properties is pertinent to our present discussion of fabric saunas.

A number of sauna tents have recently begun appearing on the market, reminiscent of the draped cloth canopies of over a century ago. The tents are made of a quilted fabric that is stiff yet collapsible. In all models, the person's head stays outside the tent. None of the dealers with whom I spoke could tell me the exact composition of the fabric, whether or not the tent outgasses or contains glues, how the heater is made, or the durability of the merchandise—probably because most sauna tents are made anonymously in the Orient. It could be determined only that the fabric in most of the imported tents is metallic (some fabric is also advertised as containing ceramic fibers that conduct FIR), and that the heaters are either built in to the fabric or are lamps placed inside the tent. The one United States-based manufacturer (a naturopath) did tell me that her tent consists of a silver metallic mesh outer layer with a carbon-impregnated fiberglass lining and no adhesives or glues. Most sauna tents are designed to accommodate a chair, although the U.S. model is designed for lying down. There is some question as to whether a fabric tent can withstand heavy use by seriously ill people, who need to take lengthy saunas on a continual therapeutic basis—although these tents probably have not been on the market long enough for anyone to discover the answer. The United States manufacturer, who used to work at a clinic that offers ozone therapy to its clientele, says that when ozone was pumped inside their one sauna tent (not hers), the fabric quickly corroded. Also, fluids can leak through the zipper portion of the tent onto the floor.

The sauna tent's price (attractive to consumers on a tight budget), and its portability, will have to be weighed against a need for a sturdier unit.

Ventilation

"One additional facet of sauna construction which is often overlooked, particularly in home installations," writes Virtanen in *The Finnish Sauna*, "is the need for adequate ventilation."

> Avid sauna goers have often encountered poorly designed saunas where oxygen is lacking, where there are foreign substances in the air, for instance dust or mold spores, or where there is a form of pollution produced by exposed electric heater elements, which can charge the air much as the atmosphere becomes charged preceding a thunderstorm [with undesirable positive ions], thereby interfering with proper respiration.[19]

If your sauna room is not ventilated, you'll also inhale carbon dioxide and the volatile chemicals that are expelled from the body. Make sure that your sauna has openings near the top so fresh air can enter the room. A cabinet, by definition, is already ventilated at the head. If you are in a room and have trouble breathing (or the room doesn't contain a vent), open the door to allow the odors and gases to escape.

A vent in a well-constructed sauna room containing a convection heater might reduce the air temperature a little, but the advantages far outweigh the disadvantages. In a FIR, electric light, or other radiant heat sauna, some cooler air should not substantially interfere with the heating effect, since radiant heat goes directly into the body independent of the temperature of the air.

The average consumer has a choice of a wide range of sauna construction materials and styles; but people with full-blown chemical sensitivities must be especially careful in choosing their unit, ensuring that the sauna is free of adhesives, glues, putty, preservatives, varnishes, and dyes—all of which emit fumes when heated. An individual sauna cabinet allows one to breathe fresh air from *outside* the cabinet, instead of the toxic fumes and stale (carbon dioxide-filled) air excreted by a sweaty body. Despite the fact that your head is outside when using a cabinet, it's probably a good idea to make sure that the cabinet is made either of wood, or of ABS and not another type of plastic—especially if you are environmentally ill or sensitive to plastic in general. A sauna cabinet, rather than a room, is also more suitable for someone with any kind of respiratory condition. But if you don't want a cabinet, and plan on spending lots of time in the sauna—say, more than 20 minutes each day—buy or build a room that is well ventilated. This will make a huge difference in how you respond to the therapy.

Size, Shape and Portability

For some people, the socializing aspect of a sauna is very important. How many people do you want your sauna to hold? Do you enjoy the company of just one or two, or many? You also need to consider how much space you have in or around your home. Except for one manufacturer who makes one or two sauna rooms on wheels, the majority of rooms are not portable. The size of a full-body enclosure can range from closet-like structures 3 feet wide by 4 feet long by 6 feet high, to roomy shelters that are 9 feet wide by 12 feet long by 7 feet high. Except for the native sweat lodges which are dome or teepee shaped, most saunas are square or rectangular rooms (although a custom builder can generally fashion any shape you desire).

If you don't have much space in your home, you will probably prefer a cabinet to a full-body enclosure. Cabinets are made to be portable. The upright models are made to fit through a standard doorway. The horizontal cabinets, while requiring more floor space than the upright models, are made to collapse into several pieces.

If you like to socialize with your friends or family, make sure you're comfortable being naked in front of people. A sauna works better without restrictive bathing suits or underwear. If you are the solitary sort who'd prefer to meditate, go inward, doze or rest during your sauna, then you don't need a large room, unless you have the space and the funds for one. If you do decide to purchase a cabinet, do you want to sit or lie down? Individual cabinets can accommodate you horizontally or vertically.

The size and even shape of your sauna can affect the temperature. *The Edgar Cayce Handbook for Health Through Drugless Therapy* states:

> The highest heat in a Turkish bath or sauna is always at the top of the room. People generally sit or lie on the bottom or middle tiers, and when they stand up, as their head reaches the hottest layer of air, they can faint, especially if there is a tendency to a cardiovascular condition that they are not aware of.

Expanding on the above, the authors caution that it is wise to take the "proper precautions" of having someone around "when using extreme heat—whether in tub baths, steam, or sauna. This is one of the reasons [we] prefer the sweat cabinets, where the head is exposed to the air."[20] Of course, "extreme" depends on who is evaluating the temperature; what is comfortable for you might be too hot for me. Chapters 6 and 7 give common sense tips on how to comfortably and safely use any type of sauna.

HEAT SOURCE

You also have to decide what you want to use to supply the heat. Wood burning stoves can be cozy, but impossible in a city apartment. If you're environmentally sensitive, can you handle a gas heater? If you're living a rustic lifestyle in the middle of the country and don't have electricity, you can't buy a unit that plugs into the wall. Finally, more and more people are becoming sensitive to the negative effects of electromagnetic pollution. Even if an appliance isn't turned on, there is electricity running through the wires in the wall. There are many aspects to consider, based on your needs, tastes, environment, and budget.

In my own experience, a FIR-heated sauna confers a completely different sense of sweating than does a dry heat sauna: I feel "cleaner" and more energized with far infrared. However, not everyone feels this way. While doing research for this book, I telephoned a man who happens to live near me and custom builds and installs FIR sauna rooms of all sizes—in homes, attached to homes, or as single, cabin-like outbuildings. In the course of our conversation, I said that it must be wonderful to be able to take a FIR sauna anytime he wanted. (I was hinting that I'd love to be invited for a sweat soon. This was before I obtained my own sauna cabinet.) I was completely unprepared for his response. "Not really," he said in his delightful British accent. "If you want to know the truth, I don't really enjoy FIR saunas." Surprised, I asked him why. "Because the air doesn't get as hot as it gets in a regular sauna," he replied. "I never feel as though I'm *really* sweating. Me, I like a *hot* sauna."

What he meant was that he associated the quintessential sauna experience with heat in the air. Since FIR heats solid objects (and human bodies) rather than air, it was not his optimal choice. He also expressed a preference for some moisture in the sauna—in other words, a *löyly*, which (at least so far) is assembled only for electric heaters that are *not* far infrared. Mikkel Aaland also prefers a *löyly*. Furthermore, Aaland—who spent three years visiting thousands of body heating facilities all over the world to write *Sweat*—likes a sauna comprised of all natural and no synthetic materials.

It is the sauna aficionados (from Finland, I have noticed) who maintain that only saunas using hot rocks are the "real" thing. Hot rocks might have been the only "real" thing at one time. But we are living in the 21ˢᵗ century. Many people do not have access to large rocks roasted in a fire; nor do they have a space in which to place such rocks. I am grateful to the Finns, Native Americans, and other cultures for popularizing sauna therapy to everyone's benefit. However, in an increasingly complex world we sometimes need to make more complex adjustments.

It may be that one's preference in saunas may also depend on body type. According to my own informal survey, people who tend to retain water (and in Chinese medical diagnostic terms are "damp") may prefer a dry sauna, whereas those whose bodies are more dry may express more affinity with moist heat.

The following pages contain photos of many different types of saunas, from small cabinets to roomy cabins; as well as charts that summarize the advantages and disadvantages of the different types of heat sources, the various materials used to construct saunas, and the types of saunas themselves. It is always a good idea to buy either directly from a manufacturer, or from a dealer you trust who will ensure that your sauna will be serviced properly if it breaks.

- Photo essay: pages 136–145.
- Heat Source: pages 146–147.
- Sauna Construction Materials: pages 148-149.
- Sauna, Style 1: pages 150–151.
- Sauna, Style 2: page 152.

Now you know what to look for in sauna design and construction. But before you go out and use or purchase a sauna, please read the next two chapters. They explain who can and who might not benefit from body heating, the best source of heat for your particular health condition, and how to take a sauna. Knowing what precautions to take—for instance, you might need to check with your doctor before starting sauna therapy, or you might require medical supervision during your program—will help ensure that your sauna experience is enjoyable and rewarding.

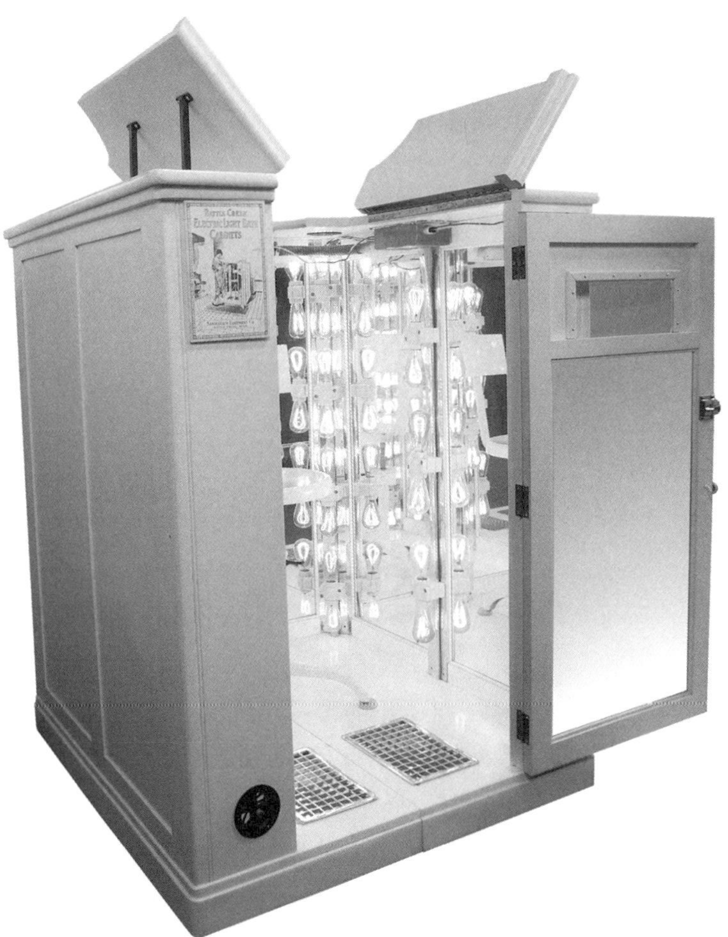

ABOVE: Dr. Kellogg's original electric light bath, where the seated subject was exposed to 32 bulbs. Several of these units are still fully functioning and in use today at the Battle Creek Lifestyle Health Center in Battle Creek, Michigan.

RIGHT: Steam bath cabinets. The early version (top) is a three-piece model made out of metal. The later models (bottom) were made by Bernarr Schaeffer in 1957 for the Battle Creek Equipment Company. Constructed of masonite (comparable to a very dense, hard particle board), wood, and stainless steel, the cabinets had to be painted 10 times, inside and outside, to protect them from degradation by steam. The steam was dispensed from an electrically-fitted aluminum pot, which the consumer had to fill with water before each use. Considered state-of-the-art at the time they were made, the cabinets cost about $500. Among the first dozen cabinets produced, two were sold to the Senate office building. Just before Mr. Schaeffer left Battle Creek in 1961, the company began using fiberglass for the cabinet shells.

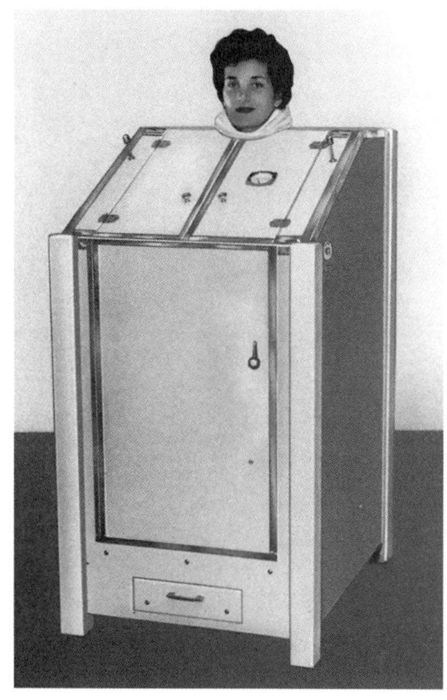
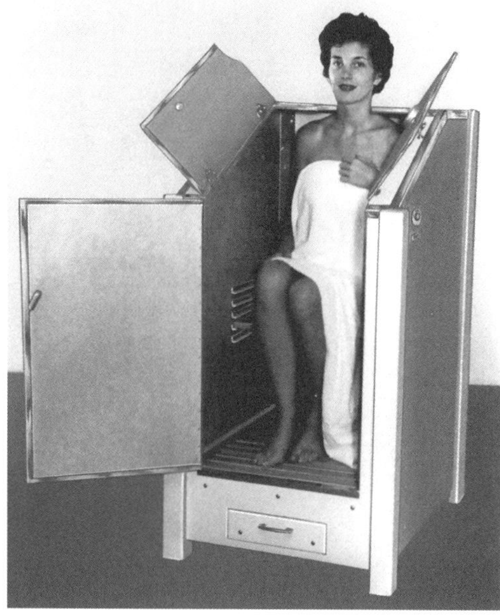
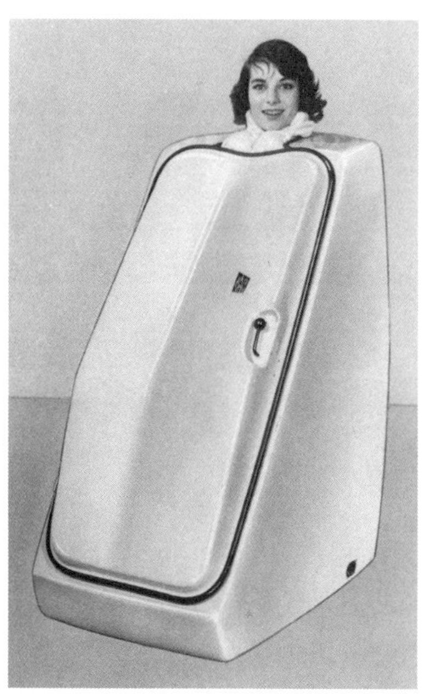
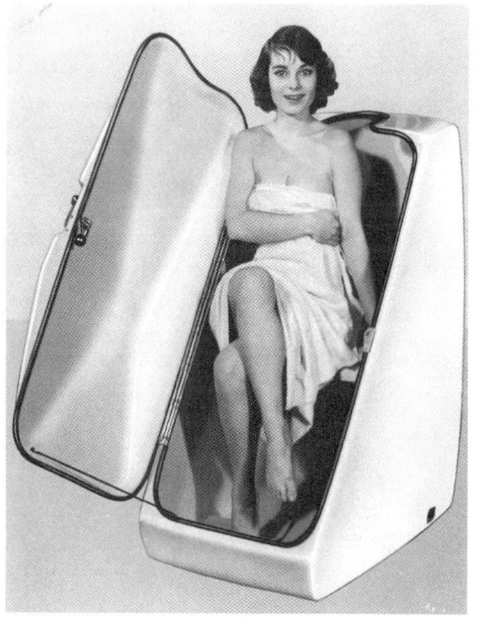

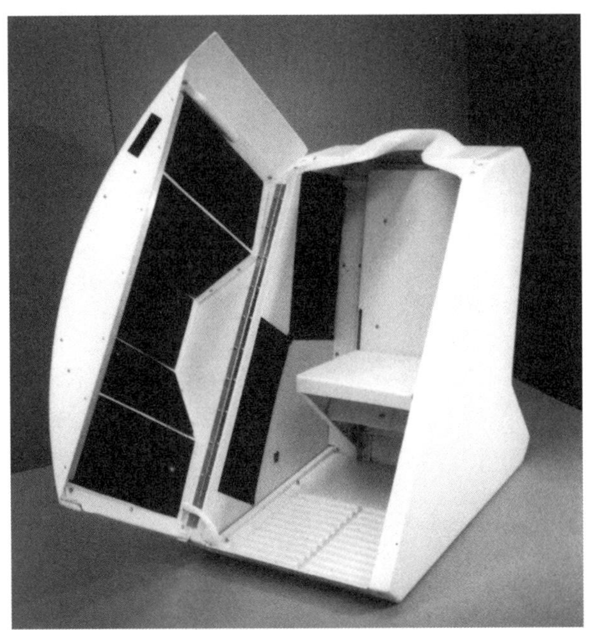

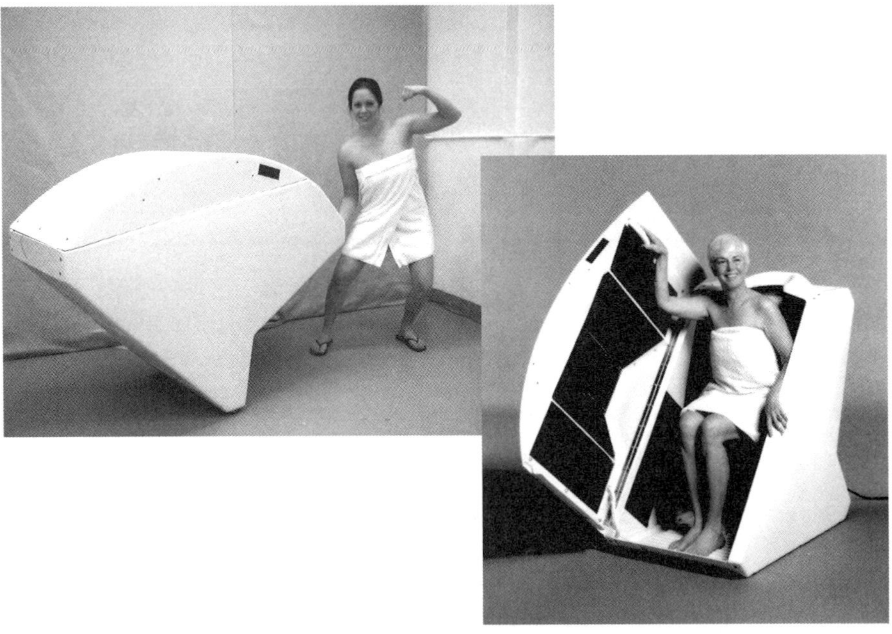

Mr. Schaeffer's newest sauna cabinet, the Saunex. The heat source is not steam, but a series of flat, far infrared heaters. Perfected in 2002, it produces less than 2 milligauss of harmful electromagnetic emissions. Schaeffer, whose sauna-making career was begun in 1948 with the production of a steam cabinet, feels that sauna technology has "greatly improved" since the early days.

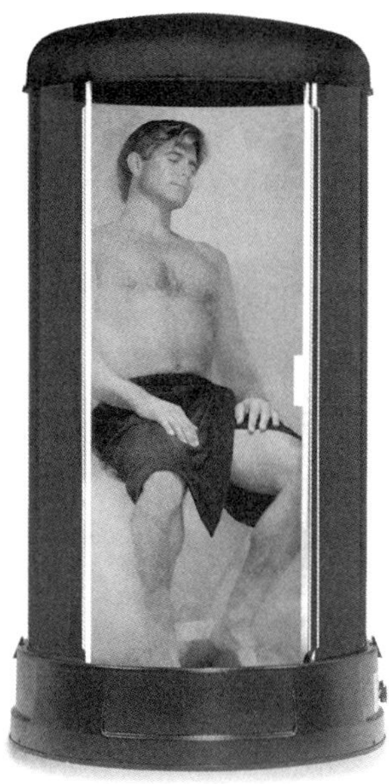
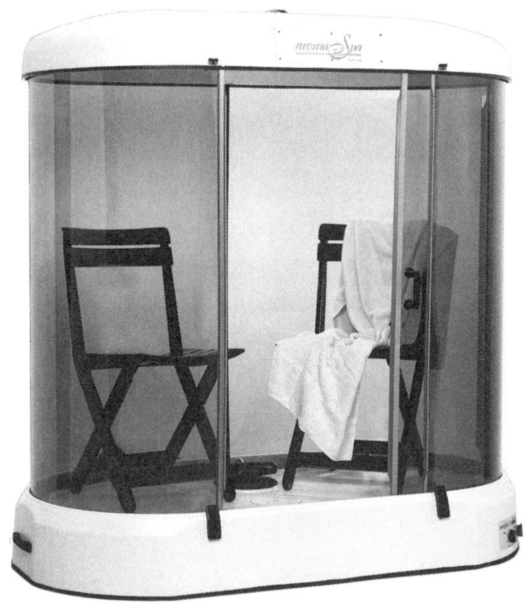

Some modern descendants of the early steam cabinets.

TOP: "Aromatic steam capsules" from AromaSpa. Fully self-contained, they require no plumbing, wiring or special ventilation. The top and base are made of lightweight and durable ABS plastic, and the smoke-tinted walls and doors are made of the same material used in producing airplane windows.

BELOW: The Infra-Therapist. Only 6.7 feet long, 21.5 inches tall, and 31 inches wide, it weighs 100 pounds and is also completely self-contained. It is one of the few horizontal far infrared models on the market. The capsule flips up for easy entry and exit.

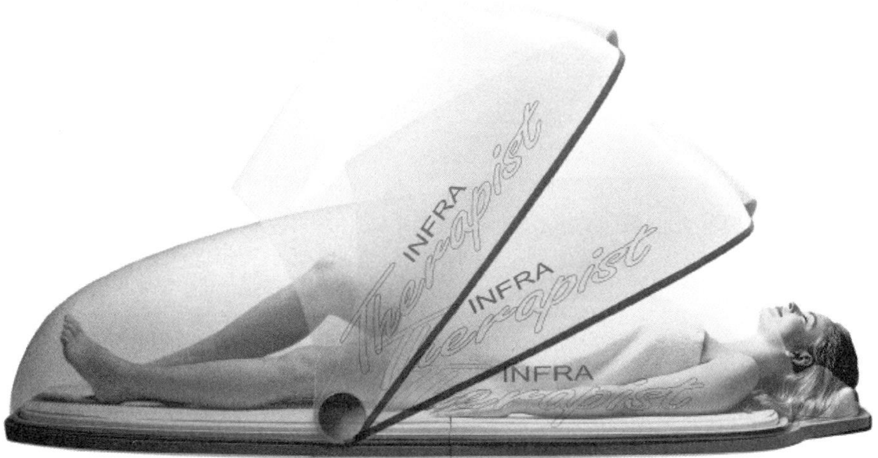

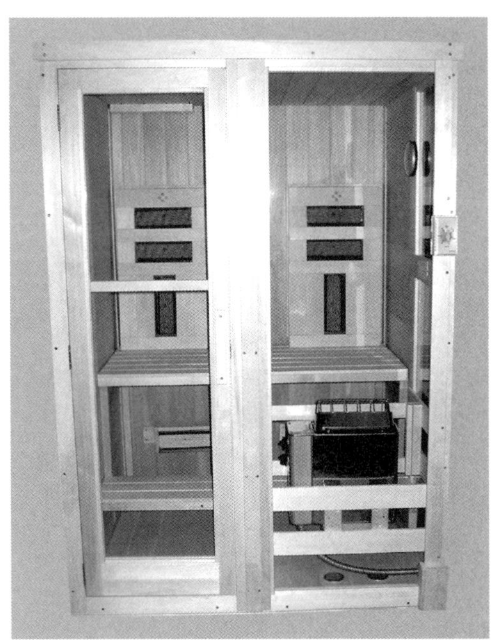

A sauna chamber of white poplar and tempered glass with a ceramic FIR heater, from Heavenly Heat Sauna. Note the heating elements in the back and under the seat of the sauna.

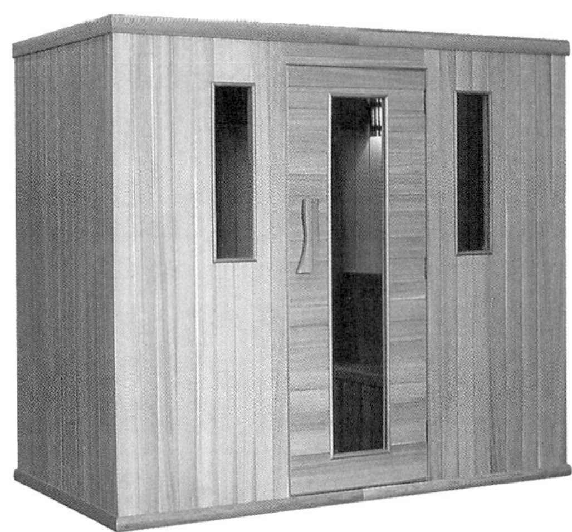

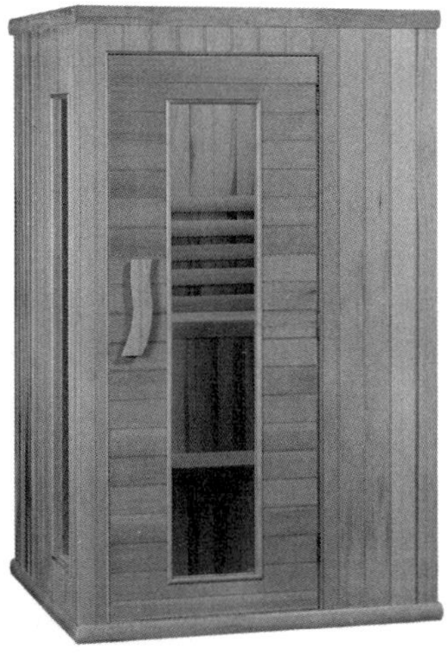

Canadian red cedar infrared sauna chambers that accommodate from one to four people. These can be located inside a house or fit on a porch. Two models from Finn Haven.

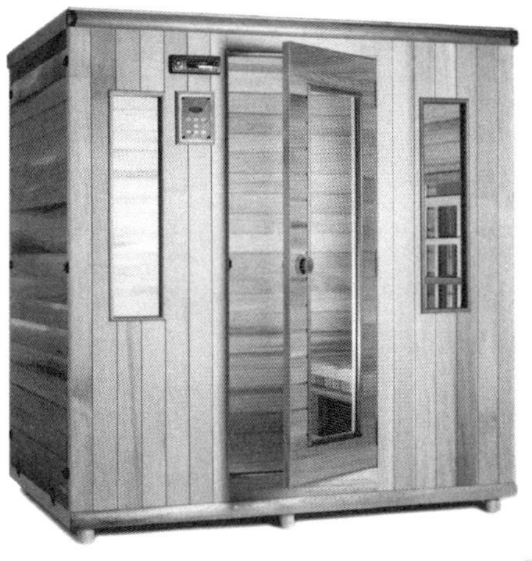

A selection of Health Mate Canadian red cedar infrared saunas. The larger rooms allow the sauna bather to lie down with the feet up if no one else is on the bench.

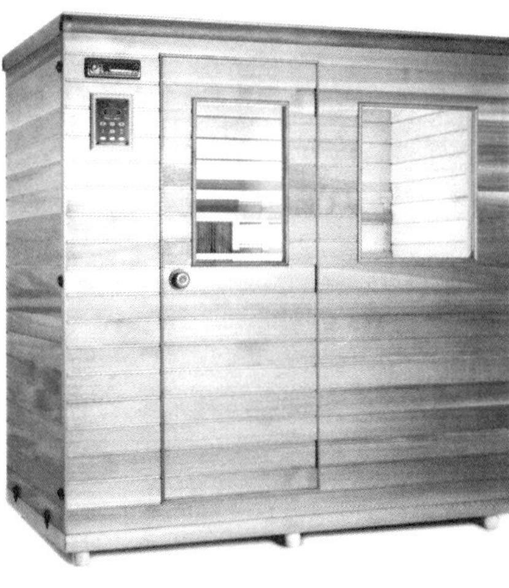

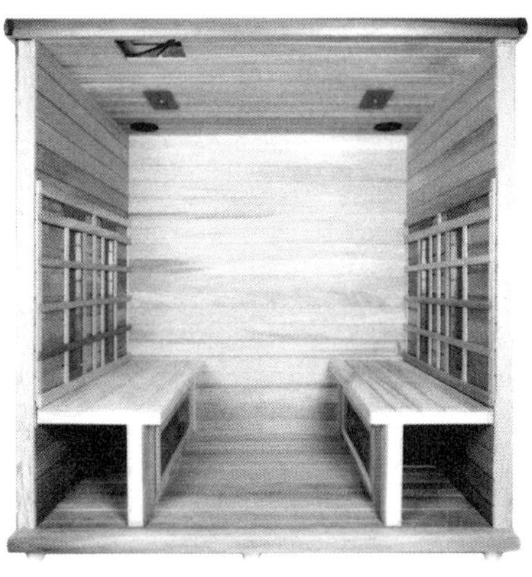

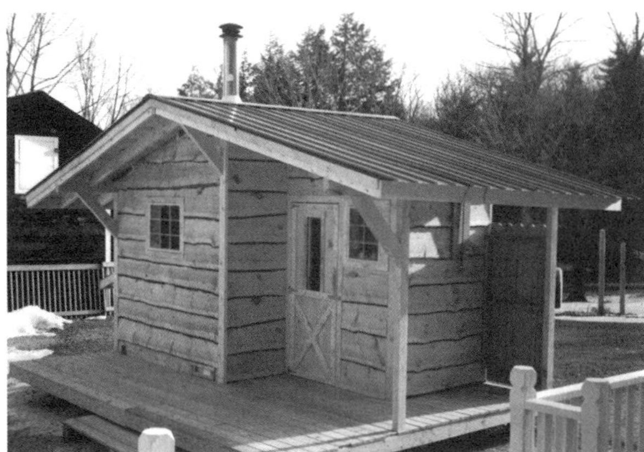

All of the saunas on pages 142-143 were built by Stephen Johnson of Northernlight Sauna. Note the great variety of styles. They are large enough to be small cabins (although smaller chambers are also available).

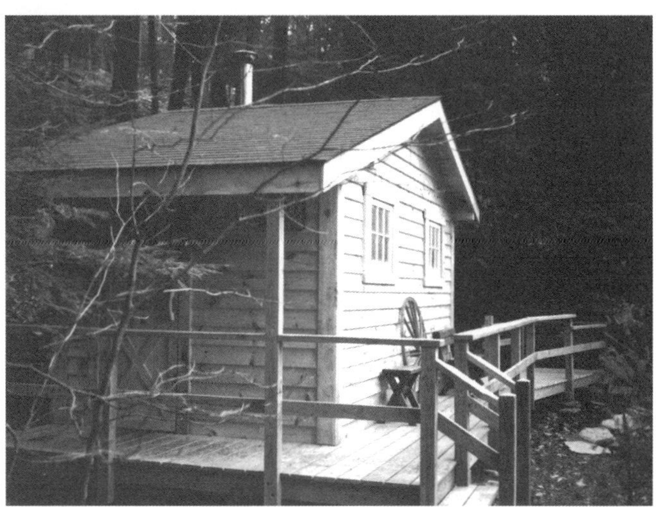

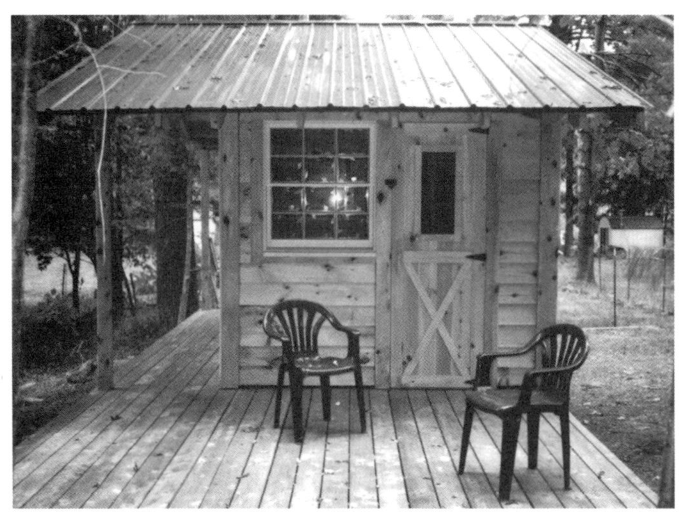

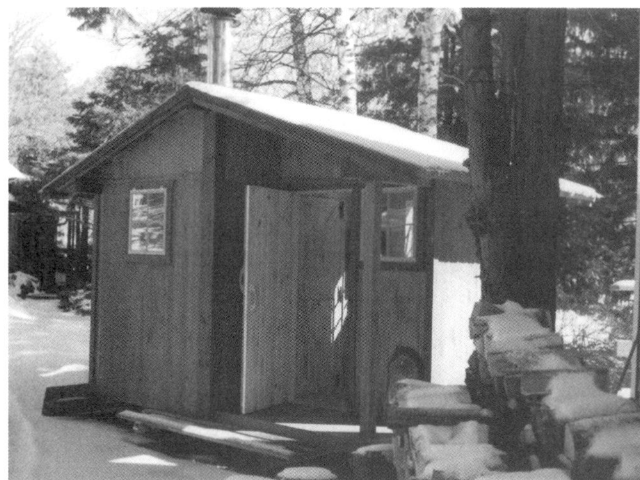

Builder's first personal sauna, located in Rosendale, New York. The roof is metal for fireproofing, and the chimney piping is triple-insulated.

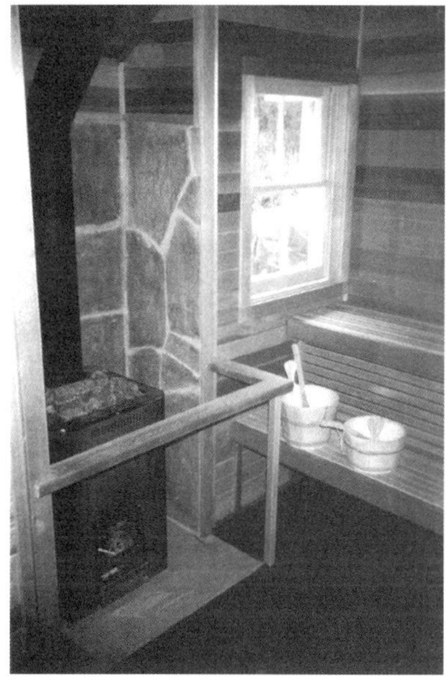

ABOVE: Interior of a typical sauna cabin built by Mr. Johnson. The heater is a Harvia wood stove. One hundred thirty pounds of rocks fill the entire heater. Water can be thrown on the rocks to create a *löyly*, moistening the air.

RIGHT: Close-up of a Harvia wood stove in a cabin just being built, shown before the protective rail has been installed.

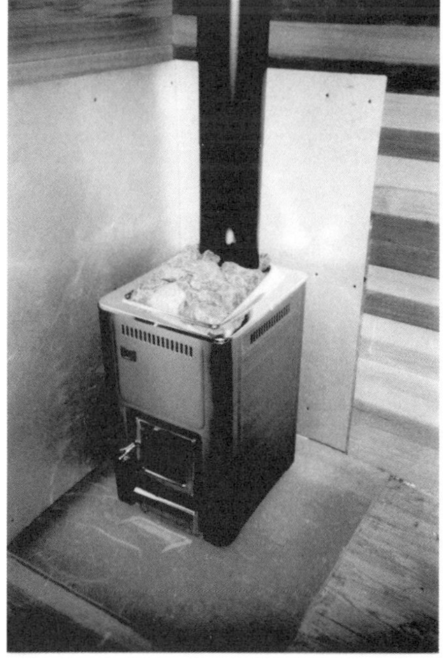

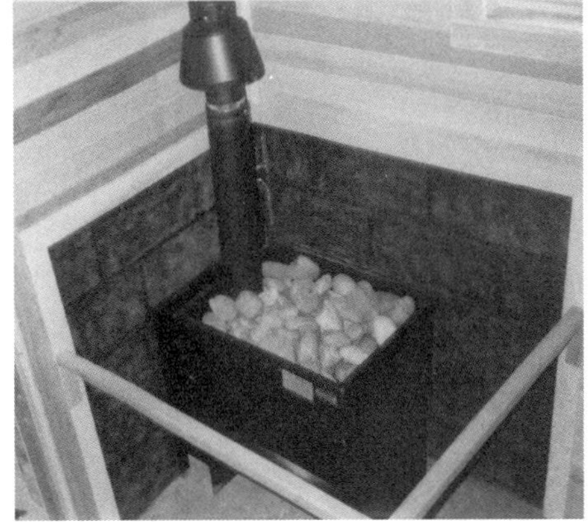

All photos on this page: Interior of Northernlight Sauna cabins.

LEFT: Nippa gas stove. These rocks are polished.

BELOW: Finlandia-Harvia KV electric heater. Sixty pounds of rocks surround the electric elements.

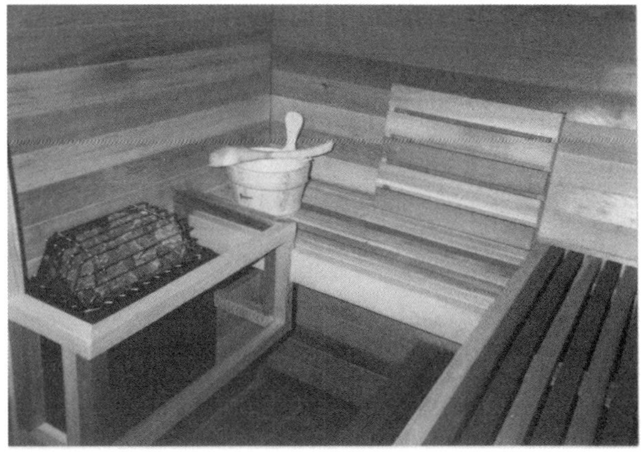

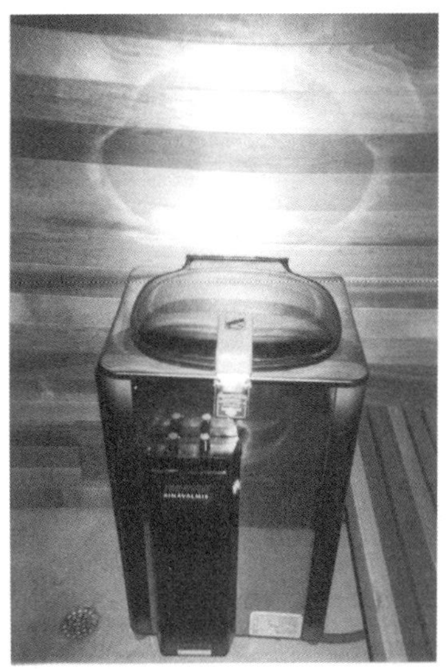

LEFT: Harvia Eveready AV—"the nemesis of electric sauna storage heaters," according to Stephen Johnson. The power in this energy-efficient heater can be left on continually in the low heat mode. More than 200 pounds of well insulated rocks are kept hot, and then the glass lid is opened to warm the sauna.

The Shawangunk I & II

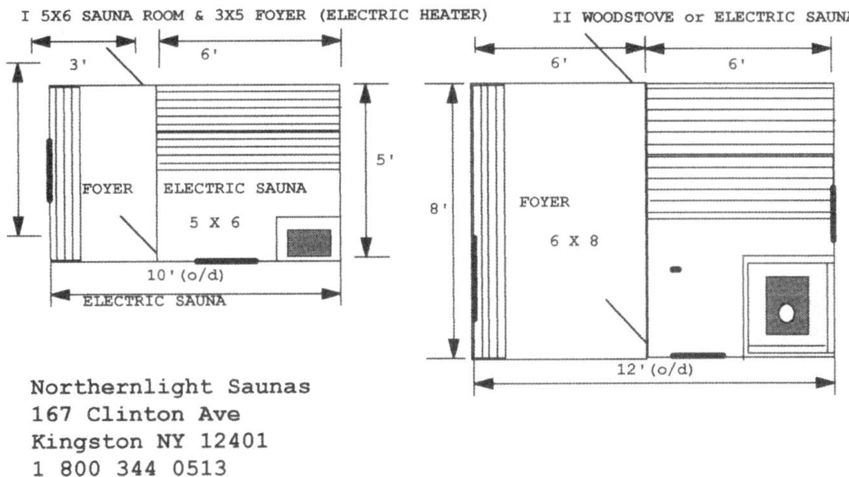

Northernlight Saunas
167 Clinton Ave
Kingston NY 12401
1 800 344 0513

Northernlight Saunas Mohohonk 6x8 room with 5x6 foyer & 3x5 porch plan

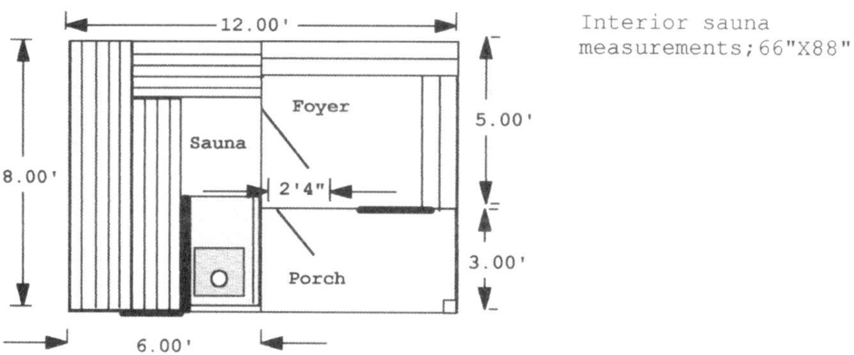

These floor plans for custom-built
saunas are by Mr. Johnson. They show
the work and planning required of any
builder for a custom sauna.

HEAT SOURCE

A detailed evaluation of the different types of electric heaters is not possible. Nevertheless, one can determine somewhat the effect of the heat source based on what type of sauna houses the heater.

	Time spent heating the sauna	Possibility of being burned	Harmful electromagnetic fields	Positive ion emissions (harmful)	Chemical or byproduct emissions	Manageability of heat	Compatibility with steam inside the sauna
Wood Fire, Open or Semi-open *Convection*	One to two hours.	Moderate. Do not touch fire, and avoid flying sparks.	No.	No.	Yes.	Poor to good.	Yes. Bring in water bucket and splash water on skin.
Stove: Fire, Gas, or Wood-Burning Stove *Convection & Radiant*	Thirty minutes to one hour.	Low, as long as you do not touch stove and avoid overfeeding the fire.	No.	No.	Possibly minimal, depending on stove used.	Fair to excellent, depending on stove used.	Yes. Bring in water bucket and splash water on skin.
Hot Rocks (pre-heated, then placed in sauna—used as sole heat source) *Convection & Radiant*	Four to five hours (first the fire must be made, then the rocks must be heated).	Low, as long as you do not touch rocks and avoid throwing too much water onto them (too much steam at very high temperatures can burn the skin).	No.	No.	Possibly, depending on type of rock used; definitely, if herbs are thrown on the rocks.	Fair to good.	Yes. Bring in water bucket and splash water on skin. Water can also be poured onto the stones to moisturize the air.

Electric Heater, Room (non-FIR) *Convection*	Perhaps one hour. Smaller rooms will heat more quickly than large rooms.	Low, as long as you do not touch the heater. Some heaters are specially shielded.	Probably, unless the heater is shielded.	Often yes.	Depends on materials comprising sauna.	Fair to excellent, depending on heater and thermostat sensitivity.	Place pan of water on floor. If heater can accommodate löyly, splash water onto the rocks.
Electric Heater, Room (FIR) *Radiant*	With FIR, air temperature is not important. However, subject will sweat sooner in a small room.	Low, as long as you do not touch the heater. Some heaters are specially shielded.	Probably, unless the heater is shielded.	Possibly yes.	Depends on materials comprising sauna.	Fair to excellent, depending on heater and thermostat sensitivity.	Place pan of water on floor. If heater can accommodate löyly, splash water onto the rocks.
Electric Heater, Cabinet (FIR only) *Radiant*	With FIR, air temperature is not important. Subject will sweat soon.	Low, as long as you do not touch the heater. Some heaters are specially shielded.	Possibly, unless the heater is shielded.*	Possibly yes.	Depends on materials comprising sauna.	Fair to excellent, depending on heater and thermostat sensitivity.	If there is space, place pan of water on floor. Cabinet heaters are not designed to hold rocks for a *löyly*.
Electric Light Bulbs (home built unit) *Radiant*	Ten minutes to one-half hour. But with FIR, air temperature is not important.	Yes, unless screen is used.	No.	No.	Depends on materials comprising sauna.	Fair to excellent.	If there is space, place pan of water on floor.

* At least one manufacturer has eliminated virtually all of the harmful electromagnetic radiation.

SAUNA CONSTRUCTION MATERIALS

Outgassing is commonly known to be a potential problem with plastics, but it can also occur with wood—especially if non-water-based adhesives, glues, putty, and stains are used. All manufacturers should run the sauna at the factory before shipping it to ensure proper function and no (or low) chemical emissions.

	Positive ion emissions (harmful)	Maintenance (should be cleaned at least weekly with heavy sauna use)	Possible harmful chemical emissions and/or outgassing
Wood: Cedar	No.	Mild soap (not toxic detergent); 1 or more cups of white vinegar to 5 gallons of water; or 3% food grade hydrogen peroxide (which might bleach the wood). Run heater after cleaning to dry the wood. Season wood with food grade oil. Freshen wood scent and durability with essential oil of cedar.	The natural oils that give cedar its aroma and make it resistant to rot can cause intense allergic reactions in sensitive people or in those with environmental illness and multiple chemical sensitivity. Most adhesives, glues, putty, preservatives, and stains used in construction are irritants.
Woods, other (soft): Pine, Redwood, Spruce	No.	Mild soap (not toxic detergent); 1 or more cups of white vinegar to 5 gallons of water; or 3% food grade hydrogen peroxide (which might bleach the wood). Run heater after cleaning to dry the wood. Season wood with food grade oil, perhaps containing lavender or other fragrant germicidal essential oil.	The natural aromatic oils in these woods (which make them somewhat resistant to rot) can cause allergic reactions in sensitive people or in those with environmental illness and multiple chemical sensitivity. Most adhesives, glues, putty, preservatives, and stains used in construction are irritants.

Material		Cleaning	Emissions
Woods, other (soft): Alder, Basswood, Hemlock, Poplar (also called Aspen)	No.	Mild soap (not toxic detergent); 1 or more cups of white vinegar to 5 gallons of water; or 3% food grade hydrogen peroxide (which might bleach the wood). Run heater after cleaning to dry the wood, which may rot with frequent use by toxic individuals. Season wood with food grade oil, perhaps containing lavender or other fragrant germicidal essential oil, if you can tolerate scents.	No harmful emissions. Most adhesives, glues, putty, preservatives, and stains used in construction are irritants.
Woods, other (hard): Birch, Cherry, Maple, Oak	No.	Mild soap (not toxic detergent); 1 or more cups of white vinegar to 5 gallons of water; or 3% food grade hydrogen peroxide (note that this will bleach the wood). Run heater after to dry the wood. Season wood with food grade oil, perhaps containing lavender or other fragrant germicidal essential oil, if you can tolerate scents.	No harmful emissions. Most adhesives, glues, putty, preservatives, and stains used in construction are irritants.
Plastic (ABS)	Possibly yes.	Mild soap (not toxic detergent), or 1 or more cups of white vinegar to 5 gallons of water. Do not use hydrogen peroxide, which degrades plastics. Not necessary to dry unit after cleaning.	No outgassing if plastic itself remains below 140°F (60°C). (Air temperature can be much higher.) Most adhesives, glues, putty, preservatives, and stains used in construction are irritants.
Fiberglass	Possibly yes.	Mild soap (not toxic detergent), or 1 or more cups of white vinegar to 5 gallons of water. Not necessary to dry unit after cleaning.	Estimates on when outgassing ends range from three weeks to one year after manufacture. One manufacturer holds a patent on "curing" the fiberglass to eliminate the problem. Most adhesives, glues, putty, preservatives, and stains used in construction are irritants.
Marble, Glass, Granite, Stainless Steel	No.	Mild soap (not toxic detergent); 1 or more cups of white vinegar to 5 gallons of water; or 3% food grade hydrogen peroxide. Not necessary to dry unit after cleaning.	No harmful emissions. Most adhesives, glues, putty, preservatives, and stains used in construction are irritants (but are not likely to be needed for a stone, glass or stainless steel sauna).
Fabric (for commercial tent)	Unknown.	Mild soap (not toxic detergent). Do not use hydrogen peroxide; it might degrade the fabric. Dry after cleaning.	Since fabric is synthetic and chemicals are used in its manufacture, there is usually outgassing. Place in sun to eliminate odors.

Sauna Style: 1

There are only five materials that are resistant to ozone: glass; a polyvinylidene fluoride or PVDF resin (one brand is Kynar™); a fluoroelastomer with excellent resistance to heat, aggressive fuels and chemicals (one brand is Viton); an exceptionally strong polycarbonate plastic (one brand is Lexan™); and polytetrafluoroethylene or PTFE, which is impervious to heat and remains stable (one brand is Teflon™—not to be confused with the coating for pans that prevents food from sticking).

	The space required by the unit	Body position	Privacy	Can person breathe fresh, cooler air	Compatibility with ozone therapy
Room (for any number of people)	Large space indoors or outdoors.	Person sits. May lean or even lie down if room is large enough.	No, not if others are also using the sauna.	No.	Incompatible (regardless of material comprising the sauna), because the therapeutic amounts required for detoxification should not be breathed.
Individual hard-shell cabinet (the head sticks out), upright	Small space (good for indoors).	Person sits with head outside cabinet.	Yes.	Yes.	Compatible (as long as cabinet is lined with ozone-impervious material), since the head is outside the cabinet. Seal hole with a towel. Ozone will, however, cause chemical emissions from any adhesives or glues used in construction.
Individual hard-shell cabinet (the head sticks out), horizontal	Relatively small space (good for indoors), but requires sufficient floor room.	Person lies down with head outside cabinet.	Yes.	Yes.	Compatible (as long as cabinet is lined with ozone-impervious material), since the head is outside the cabinet. Seal hole with a towel. Ozone will, however, cause chemical emissions from any adhesives or glues used in construction.

Tent (the head sticks out), upright	Small space (good for indoors).	Person sits in chair with head outside tent.	Yes.	Yes.	Since the head is outside the tent, the person does not breathe ozone (as long as hole is sealed with a towel). However, ozone will degrade fabric in time, as well as cause chemical emissions from any adhesives and glues used in construction.
Tent (the head sticks out), horizontal	Relatively small space (good for indoors), but requires sufficient floor room.	Person lies down with head outside tent.	Yes.	Yes.	Since the head is outside the tent, the person does not breathe ozone (as long as hole is sealed with a towel). However, ozone will degrade fabric in time, as well as cause chemical emissions from any adhesives and glues used in construction.

SAUNA STYLE: 2

	Suitability for heavy use (every day, six or more hours)	Maintenance	Average cost
Room: for two or more people, clinical use	Saunas meant for continual therapeutic use are best made of tile, porcelain, steel, granite, and/or marble—materials that are durable, not allergenic, and require minimal upkeep. Wood rots easily from excessive wastes and moisture. Even aromatic woods, whose natural oils make them fairly resistant to rotting, do eventually rot with heavy use—and anyway, as their oils are allergenic to sensitive people, these woods are not recommended for clinical use.	Clean regularly with mild soap (not toxic detergent). Spray with 3% food grade hydrogen peroxide to disinfect (this does bleach wood). If sauna is made of wood, turn on heat after cleaning to dry the wood and keep dry when not in use.	$3000 to $10,000 and up, depending on size, sophistication of design, and materials.
Room: for two or more people, home use only	Limited, non-therapeutic use offers more (and cheaper) options in materials than clinical use (see above). If the users are not too toxic, wood can be a viable choice. If one can tolerate aromatic wood, this is an even better choice than odorless wood, as its natural oils help prevent rotting. With consistent, proper care and for limited home use, any wooden sauna should last for a reasonable time.	Clean regularly with mild soap (not toxic detergent). Spray with 3% food grade hydrogen peroxide to disinfect (this does bleach wood). If sauna is made of wood, turn on heat after cleaning to dry the wood and keep dry when not in use.	$2500 to $4000 and up, depending on size, sophistication of design, and materials.
Individual: Hard-shell cabinet (the head sticks out), upright or horizontal	ABS, fiberglass, or similar plastic-like materials are strong and durable and unable to rot; so they are suitable for continual therapeutic use providing the user is not sensitive to that particular plastic.	Clean with mild soap (not toxic detergent). Do not use hydrogen peroxide on ABS, as this will eventually degrade it. Fiberglass cabinets intended for use with ozone will automatically be sterilized, so simply wipe with damp cloth and soap or essential oils.	Both types: $2500 to $3000.
Individual: Tent (the head sticks out), upright or horizontal	A fabric sauna is meant to be used for short periods in the home, rather than for long therapeutic periods in a clinical setting.	Regularly clean with mild soap (not toxic detergent), and expose tent to air. Be careful not to rip fabric. Do not use hydrogen peroxide or ozone; this will destroy the fabric and cause glues and adhesives to outgas.	Upright: $550 to $750. Horizontal: $700 to $900.

NOTES

1. Mikkel Aaland, *Sweat* (Santa Barbara: Capra Press, 1978), 14.

2. John O. Virtanen, *The Finnish Sauna: Peace of Mind, Body and Soul* (Withee, Wisc.: O-W Enterprise, 1998), 183.

3. John Harvey Kellogg, *Light Therapeutics: A Practical Manual of Phototherapy for the Student and the Practitioner, Revised Edition* (Battle Creek: The Good Health Publishing Co., 1910), 104-105.

4. Ibid., 107.

5. Ibid., 110-111.

6. Ibid., 66.

7. Ibid.

8. Ibid., 65–67.

9. Ibid., 67.

10. Ibid., 67-68.

11. Ibid., 68.

12. B. Blake Levitt, *Electromagnetic Fields: A Consumer's Guide to the Issues and How to Protect Ourselves* (San Diego: Harcourt Brace & Company, 1995), 47–48.

13. Ibid., 54.

14. Cyril W. Smith and Simon Best, *Electromagnetic Man: Health & Hazard in the Electrical Environment* (London: J.M. Dent and Sons, Ltd., 1990), 45.

15. Jacqueline Krohn, et al. *The Whole Way to Natural Detoxification: The Complete Guide to Clearing Your Body of Toxins* (Point Roberts, Wash.: Hartley & Marks Publishers, Inc., 1996), 85.

16. Levitt, op. cit., 254-258.

17. Pius Thriveni, personal letter as General Electric Product Compliance Specialist, September 6, 2002.

18. William J. Rea, *Chemical Sensitivity, Vol. 4: Tools of Diagnosis and Methods of Treatment* (Boca Raton: Lewis Publishers, 1997), 2330.

19. Virtanen, op. cit., 176.

20. Harold J. Reilly and Ruth Hagy Brod. *The Edgar Cayce Handbook for Health Through Drugless Therapy* (New York: Berkeley Publishing Group, 1986), 308.

CHAPTER 6

Who May Use the Sauna
and Who Should Not

*To say yes, you have to sweat and roll up your sleeves
and plunge both hands into life up to the elbows.*

JEAN ANOUILH, FRENCH PLAYWRIGHT (1910–1987)

One of the first questions people ask about sauna therapy is, "What medical conditions are compatible with sauna use, and which are not?" As with many things in life, the answer is, "It depends." The question really should be, "*Who* can use the sauna?", because a medical condition can manifest very differently in two individuals. As a general guideline, you need to consider the particular circumstances of the *user*, rather than restrict or forbid sauna use according to the *condition*. Most people may freely use the sauna (following standard commonsense sauna protocol, of course); others may use the sauna if they take certain additional precautions; and only a very small percentage should avoid saunas altogether. And the circumstances of the last group are not fixed. One's state of health can change enough so that body heating is no longer harmful, but beneficial. Much to my surprise, all of the physicians whom I interviewed about their sauna detoxification programs discussed in detail in Chapter 8, told me that, almost without exception, anyone can use the sauna—even those with delicate health conditions—*as long as they are receiving proper medical supervision.*

The emphasis in this book is on do-it-yourself sauna therapy for those who desire relaxation and restoration of energy and body function through the elimination of systemic toxins. The following list is meant only as a guide to see if you might need to take precautions. *If you have a serious or chronic illness, always see your doctor—or some qualified health care provider who is knowledgeable about body heating—before using the sauna.*

Adrenal stress

"Adrenal stress" is a general term for overwork and exhaustion of the adrenal glands. This is implicated in a large number of conditions, including chronic fatigue and depression. Heat stimulates the adrenals to increase their secretion of several different hormones, including cortisol. With adrenals that are too depleted, intense stimulation will only drain them more, and ultimately make them nonfunctional. However, if the adrenals are merely tired but still have some level of function, sauna bathing might help, particularly if toxins are preventing the glands from functioning properly. This is why it is necessary to consult with a qualified health professional who can determine adrenal stress levels. With people too ill to use the sauna, after the adrenals are nourished and even just slightly rejuvenated, sauna therapy can help.

Artificial joints

Discomfort can indicate either harm or healing, so consult with your doctor to make sure that body heating is not causing damage.

Brain tumors

According to Dr. T. R. Shantha at Integrated Medical Specialists in Stockbridge, Georgia, sauna therapy is generally not advised for people with "very large" brain tumors—as well as a history of recent surgery in that area—because the heat can make a brain tumor swell, thus causing cerebral edema. However, someone with a "very small" brain tumor can benefit from mild sauna therapy *if a cabinet only is used, if the body temperature does not exceed 100°F (37.8°C), and if the treatment is medically supervised.* For such a person, low-level body heating can improve circulation, carry immune bio-chemicals and other therapeutic agents close to the tumor, enhance lymphocyte activity near the site, and remove metabolic toxins surrounding the site.

Cardiovascular problems

In America, sauna manufacturers—fearing lawsuits from warranted or unwarranted liability—explicitly advise people with cardiovascular problems not to use the sauna. However, research indicates that sauna therapy can be helpful in certain situations. A two-week Japanese study was recently conducted by M. Imamura and colleagues with 25 men who had at least one risk factor for heart disease. After 60°C (140°F) sauna therapy for 15 minutes per day, followed by 30-minute bed rest covered with a blanket, the subjects had the thickness of their artery lining measured by ultrasound. The test showed a 40 percent reduction of the inner lining of blood vessels—leaving more room for the blood to flow, which in turn lowers blood pressure. Vascular endothelial function was discernibly improved, the researchers report, "suggesting a therapeutic role for sauna treatment in patients with risk factors for atherosclerosis."[1] Far infrared saunas, which are very popular in Japan, were used.

The article "Benefits and Risks of Sauna Bathing," appearing in *The American Journal of Medicine*, is based on a large database of 130 studies of Finnish saunas. The authors state that "long-term sauna bathing may help lower blood pressure in patients with hypertension and improve the left ventricular ejection fraction in patients with chronic congestive heart failure," although they add that additional research is needed to conclusively confirm this. They mention that sauna bathing is contraindicated in cases of "unstable angina pectoris, recent myocardial infarction, and severe aortic stenosis," but add that sauna therapy is safe "for most people with coronary heart disease with stable angina pectoris or old myocardial infarction."[2] (Note their observation that "Very few acute myocardial infarctions and sudden deaths occur in saunas, but alcohol consumption during sauna bathing increases the risk of hypotension, arrhythmia, and sudden death, and should be avoided."[3])

Dr. William Rea, founder of the Environmental Health Center in Dallas, Texas, also discusses myocardial infarction in *Chemical Sensitivity*. "As long as water is used to maintain circulating [blood] volume and replenish electrolytes, myocardial infarction as a result of heat depuration [cleansing or purifying] is unlikely. Reports from Finland, which has one of the highest myocardial infarction rates in the world, show that sauna use rarely precedes infarcts."[4] Rea does not specify what type of sauna is used.

Finally, a 1995 study in *Circulation* on sauna therapy for people with congestive heart failure concludes that "thermal vasodilation can be applied with little risk if appropriately performed and may provide a new nonpharmacological therapy for CHF [congestive heart failure]." Significantly, in this experiment (as with the first), the sauna is equipped with a FIR heater.

> A major reason why warm-water or sauna bathing has been considered inappropriate for patients with CHF is the concern that cardiac work increases. Therefore, in the present study, the effects of thermally induced sympathetic hypertonia and various bath-related activities were minimized; the warm-water bath temperature was set at a comfortable 41° C [105.8° F], and a bathtub with automatic motion was used. None of our patients complained of excessive heat stimulation. In the sauna experiment, a far infrared-ray sauna was used at a room temperature of 60° C [140° F] to prevent thermal stimulation due to high-temperature air inhalation. This temperature is lower than that of a conventional sauna. As a result…sauna bathing [was] safely accomplished without arrhythmias, dyspnea, or angina occurring.…[5]

Of course, the person with congestive heart failure should be examined carefully before sauna treatment. Dr. Shantha, who has experience using the sauna for people with this condition, emphasizes, as do other doctors, that there are degrees of severity. "If it is a mild condition, and it is being treated effectively so the person does not have symptoms such as atrial fibrillation [tremors in some of the chambers in the heart], edema [water retention] of the legs, or resting angina [pain and blockage around the heart], the sauna can be beneficial. Full-blown congestive heart failure, however, where the coronary arteries are heavily compromised, can put a strain on the heart and result in severe damage and even death."[6] Cardiovascular problems are complex and generally serious. *If you have heart problems, consult with a physician who is experienced in sauna use and is capable of assessing your particular situation.*

Children and infants

Most American sauna manufacturers, fearing lawsuits due to justified or unjustified liability, advise against infants and children using the sauna. Yet in countries like Finland where people grow up using saunas, babies two years old (and occasionally younger) are regularly introduced to the custom for short periods of time. In the *Annals of Clinical Research*, Ilkka Vuori states categorically that "Sauna is not a risk to…infants."[7] And a 2002 study by Rissmann and colleagues found that infants between three and 14 months of age, after being placed in a swimming pool for 15 minutes, adapted very well to a three-minute sauna bath with no ill effects from heat stress.

Nevertheless, it's important to remember that children are not simply smaller adults. Their systems are not fully developed, so it is wise to take some precautions. The previously mentioned article "Benefits and Risks of Sauna Bathing" cites a study of the effects of sauna bathing in 81 healthy children two to 15 years of age, in a 10-minute sauna bath at 70°C (158°F).

> Most respiratory, hormonal, and cardiovascular changes were similar to those of adults [although]…The ability to maintain stroke volume…was impaired, especially in younger children (aged 2 to 4 years), who had the greatest increase in heart rate. Cardiac output was increased in older but not in younger children. Systolic and diastolic blood pressures did not change during sauna bathing but dropped immediately afterward, and 2 children fainted.[8]

It appears that children under 12 (as well as infants, of course) are the most vulnerable to critical systemic changes during body heating. Children eight years old or younger might feel dizzy or nauseated, especially if exposed for too long a time at too high a temperature. Plus, if they already have dermatitis or middle ear infections, the sauna might exacerbate these conditions. In "The Sauna and Children," appearing in the *Annals of Clinical Research*, the authors report that the "thermoregulatory range" of the infant is "fairly narrow," and the "ability to regulate body temperature by sweating matures only at puberty....Exposure to the raised [sauna] temperatures...can cause thermoregulatory imbalances in children." The reason for this may partly relate to the fact that children have less skin surface per pound of weight than do adults.

Yet despite the need to take special care of children in the sauna, body heating appears to be so beneficial that it is worth assessing a child's level of heat tolerance. The authors of "Benefits and Risks of Sauna Bathing" add:

> Interestingly, most children in our study seemed to tolerate heat stress in a sauna fairly well. This accords with the clinical experience of Finnish children's hospitals, where the commonest problems related to sauna bathing are accidental burns....Our data show that Finnish children, who are accustomed to sauna bathing, tolerate the Finnish sauna bathing well, *if the bathing time is appropriate to the individual child's ability to cope with the raised temperature.*[9] [emphasis added]

The above data points to the need for the child's caregivers to use commonsense when bringing children into the sauna. *Do not allow young children to use the sauna without adult supervision.* Even in Finland, children under seven years old are rarely allowed to enter the sauna alone; and healthy infants are brought in for no more than five minutes. Used judiciously, body heating can be beneficial to young people.

Claustrophobia

You might find an enclosed sauna room acceptable only if it is exceptionally large, and/or has a glass door so you can see out. If a room doesn't appeal to you, consider a cabinet so your head can remain outside.

Cochlear implants

Hearing-impaired individuals who receive surgical implants for the inner ear may find that the portion closer to the exterior does not tolerate humidity very well. Avoid steam rooms and high-moisture saunas. For your comfort and peace of mind, consider using a sauna cabinet instead of a room. In any case, you must wait until the area has healed before using any type of sauna.

Dental fillings

Holistic dentists disagree as to whether silver-mercury amalgam fillings should first be removed before sauna therapy is undertaken. While it is commonly recognized that the mercury in fillings is highly toxic, it is also true that improper removal of such fillings can actually cause more damage than if they had been left alone. (If the gums and nose are not shielded during the filling removal, mercury vapor is inhaled or leaks into the gum tissue.) For some people, the metal fillings do not seem to emit enough mercury vapor into the mouth to make them immediately dangerous (although longer-term effects would be harder to perceive). A number of mercury-toxic sauna bathers report being extra sensitive to heat, in which case a FIR sauna would probably be preferable to a higher-temperature, non-FIR sauna. A few people have reported losing their fillings in FIR rooms, leading to speculation that the deep penetration of far infrared radiation might have loosened the adhesions that bond fillings to teeth. However, such reports are rare. If any of this concerns you, use a sauna cabinet rather than a full-body enclosure.

Drugs, prescription

Dr. David Root, the director of a California clinic that specializes in sauna therapy to help clients detoxify from both prescription and "recreational" ("street") drugs (see Chapter 8), says that sauna bathing can augment the absorption rate of prescription drugs. This is especially true of drugs administered through transdermal skin patches, because the increase in circulation from body heating brings substances into the cells extraordinarily fast. Drugs such as insulin can affect you in unexpected and drastic ways if they are utilized by your body at an abnormally fast rate. On the other hand, Root cautions, it is also possible for medication to be sweated out of the body quickly, thus creating a deficit. Someone for whom medication doses are critical—such as people with epilepsy, diabetes, or depression—should be carefully monitored by a doctor. (It is never a good idea, Root adds, to suddenly stop taking prescription medications if a person is dependent on them.) Finally, people taking steroids (such as those with lupus) should not use the sauna at all, because steroids commonly prevent the blood vessels from dilating. *Consult a knowledgeable health care practitioner, and also your pharmacist, before using a sauna.*

Epilepsy

It can be very dangerous to be inside a sauna when you have a seizure. Consult with a qualified medical professional.

Eye problems, specifically acute inflammation

The delicate mucous membranes of the eyes can become irritated by excesses of heat, dryness, or moisture. Therefore, precise regulation of the air in your sauna is important. Use a sauna *cabinet*, which does not expose the eyes to the sauna air, and consult your doctor.

Fever

This depends on how high the fever is, and whether you are receiving medical supervision. If your fever is already high, being in the sauna may make you overheat to dangerous limits. (See the information on heatstroke in the next chapter.) If your fever is low enough, sauna therapy can be helpful. Use a sauna cabinet, rather than an enclosed room, to keep the temperature of your brain as low as possible.

Heart conditions

See "Cardiovascular Problems."

Hemophilia or a tendency to hemorrhage

Heat from a sauna can cause the superficial blood vessels to dilate, which could induce bleeding. Check with your doctor.

Hyperthyroidism

An overactive thyroid gland causes an increase in metabolism, which makes the heart beat faster. Body heating also speeds the heart rate, so don't overdo your sauna time and make sure you are under a doctor's care. Some holistic practitioners recommend low heat, short periods of time (about 15 or 20 minutes, maximum), and sauna use of not more than twice a week.

Implants

See "Cochlear implants," "Metal pins or rods," and "Silicone implants."

Inflammatory conditions

Not everyone with an inflammatory condition feels better with sauna therapy. According to H. Isomäki, about 25% of women with fibromyalgia find heat detrimental. Most men with fibromyalgia find it helpful. Those who react badly to sauna therapy generally feel better at first, and have an inflammatory reaction the next day. However, an inflammatory response can be avoided by cooling off thoroughly with cold water directly after sauna use. An initial inflammatory reaction might also indicate the beginning of a healing response rather than a negative backlash, so check with a qualified health care provider who is familiar with sauna therapy and your particular situation.

Injuries (sprains, pulled muscles, etc.) that are very recent

In most cases, the injury should not be exposed to heat for the first forty-eight hours—or at least until the swelling subsides. However, some people initially feel much better with heat than with cold, so you will have to experiment to see what is best for you.

Lupus erythematosus

This autoimmune disorder causes heat sensitivity in the skin. However, all of the doctors I interviewed for this book stated that sauna therapy can be helpful for people with lupus (as long as they are not taking steroids). Obtain medical supervision from someone familiar with sauna therapy.

Menstruation

Heating of the low back area during a woman's menstrual period may temporarily increase the flow. However, the relief from menstrual cramps can be immediate, so most woman don't mind a little extra discharge.

Metal pins or rods

Consult with your doctor to make sure that body heating will not cause discomfort or harm. Discontinue use if you experience pain near your implants.

Multiple sclerosis

Many people with MS don't sweat easily, if at all. Due to the degeneration of myelin (the fatty covering on the nerve cells), the neurological messages of the autonomic (involuntary) nervous system are incomplete or entirely absent—including messages that the body needs to perspire. If a non-sweating person is in the sauna for a long enough period, a buildup of interstitial fluid is created when the blood plasma seeps between the cells without being excreted by the sweat glands. Then the body temperature rises to a dangerous extent, since without perspiration there is no outlet for the heat. The conventional medical opinion is that people with MS should never take saunas. However, physicians who regularly use saunas in their practice have told me that even people with MS who tend not to perspire can be helped enough so that their bodies *learn* to sweat. (This suggests that other aspects of neurological functioning might be restored as well—if not with saunas, then through other means.) Make sure that the unit is not too hot, your body temperature is allowed to rise gradually, you leave when you feel warm, and, of course, *you are under strict medical supervision* from a doctor skilled in this area. You can even use a FIR sauna and keep your clothes on. However, if you find that your symptoms worsen from sweating/body heating, discontinue using the sauna.

Nosebleeds

See "Respiratory Disorders."

Older people

Vuori bluntly states that sauna bathing is not a risk "to old people."[10] However, people tend to have more health concerns as they grow older. Therefore, use common sense, pay attention to how you feel, and if necessary, have someone in the room with you. See a doctor if you feel worse after body heating.

Overheating

If you are already excessively overheated, cool off before entering the sauna. If you tend to become overheated too quickly, make sure that the sauna temperature is not too hot—you will still benefit.

Pacemakers

Check with your doctor and the manufacturer of your pacemaker.

Pregnancy

This pertains to pregnant women who are generally healthy and are not heavily loaded with toxic metals, organic chemicals, pathogens, and other poisons. In America some sauna manufacturers, fearing lawsuits about warranted or unwarranted liability, categorically advise pregnant women against using the sauna. But this may needlessly deter pregnant women from a healthy, pleasurable experience. The scientific studies I found agree that, with a few exceptions, a pregnant woman can derive great benefits from the sauna without harming the fetus.

In an *Annals of Clinical Research* article, the authors write: "Up to 90% of pregnant women in Finland regularly visit the sauna until the expected time of delivery," adding that "formerly it was not unusual to give birth in the sauna."[11] Vuori, in the same journal, writes that the "vast experience [of Finns] has proven, in our minds, that sauna is not a risk to a pregnant mother or to her unborn child."[12] The more recent "Benefits and Risks of Sauna Bathing," based on a database of 130 studies of Finnish saunas, states that sauna bathing is safe "during the uncomplicated pregnancies of healthy women." Hypertensive women are advised not to use the sauna since uterine vascular resistance increases during pregnancy, making them and their unborn children high-risk for various health problems.[13] The authors advise pregnant Finnish women to use the sauna for about six to 12 minutes per session—although later in the article, the authors concede that sessions can be longer.

This data suggests that sauna use is reasonably safe during pregnancy—and also that worry plays a large factor in one's comfort level. Europeans, with a more extensive history and experience of body heating than

Americans, are much more relaxed and knowledgeable about sauna use. *Note that the above data applies to Finnish saunas that use hot rocks and contain moderate amounts of moisture in the air.* Some researchers hypothesize that since FIR penetrates and heats the body more deeply than hot air, it might not be advisable during pregnancy; but at this time we simply do not know for sure. Conceivably, a FIR sauna could be highly beneficial to the fetus—after all, the FIR wavelengths in the 9 micron range are needed to hatch eggs.

Again, the above data citing sauna safety applies to women who are reasonably healthy. If the mother's system is toxic, sauna therapy can harm the fetus because all the wastes circulating in her bloodstream will cross the placenta. Dr. David Root, who helps people detoxify from drugs, emphasizes that in his program, under no circumstances is sauna detoxification therapy administered to a pregnant woman.

By the way, there have been no studies showing that body heating impedes fertility in women. Nor have I seen studies showing that sauna therapy improves fertility in women. Sauna use does not appear to hinder fertility in men—although heating the testicles will temporarily lower the sperm count. (Keeping the testicles cool for a few days corrects the problem.) Sauna therapy may prove helpful if one is infertile due to bodily toxins, chronic infection, or impaired hormonal function.

Prescription drugs

See "Drugs, prescription."

Respiratory disorders

The mucous membrane lining of the lungs becomes irritated by excessive heat, excessive dryness, *and* excessive moisture, so precise regulation of the air in your sauna is important. The "Benefits and Risks of Sauna Bathing" article indicates that sauna therapy is not harmful to—and may even benefit—people with asthma and chronic bronchitis; although serious chronic illnesses like pneumonia and conditions such as nosebleeds might be exacerbated by sauna use. However, this applies to *full-body enclosures* as opposed to sauna *cabinets*, which allow you to breathe regular room temperature air. There is some evidence that FIR in an enclosed room may be acceptable if the temperature is not too high. You may want to consult a doctor before entering a sauna.

Silicone implants

This pertains to people who have undergone breast enlargements, or have prosthesis implants for the ear, jaw, nose, etc. Despite reassurances of safety from the manufacturers of these implant plastics, there is extensive documentation that over time, implants leak toxic waste into the body. Some sauna manufacturers warn that not only does silicone absorb FIR and thus produce (unspecified) negative reactions in the body, but exposing the body to heat—from either a hot air *or* a steam sauna—can cause the silicone to leak and/or change its shape.

From the above data, it would seem that under no circumstances should a person with silicone implants use a sauna. However, doctors William Rea and Deborah Baird provide another perspective. In an article in the *Journal of Nutritional & Environmental Medicine*, they discuss a study of people with TMJ alloplastic implants, who "exhibit similar multi-system complexes to breast implant patients" (even though their "symptoms and signs seem to be universally more diverse than in either the breast implant or chemically sensitive patient without implants"). They suffer from "a dysfunction of their immune system as well as dysfunction of the autonomic nervous and central nervous systems," with symptoms that include "severe pain, short-term memory, fatigue, fibromyalgia…GI [gastrointestinal] disturbances, GU [genital-urinary] dysfunction, recurrent sinusitis, increased cardiovascular dysfunction, tinnitus, and seizures." Rea and Baird are very clear that "the jaw implant materials are not the 'inert' material that they are touted to be, with the body reacting accordingly with inflammatory responses causing the aforementioned symptom complex." They conclude that "The patient will always have a permanent handicap: a persistent toxic chemical irritant (synthetic jaw implant) that cannot be eliminated," since in this case it is not feasible to have the implant removed.

Nevertheless, in view of the array of debilitating symptoms, it makes sense to embark on a detoxification protocol whenever possible. The authors emphasize that "Heat, exercise and massage…are more rapid ways of releasing many primary and secondary offending incitants that have already been stored in fat. Treatment should only be under the direct supervision of a physician since initial complications can be severe."[14] If you have implants, be aware that the permanent presence of a noxious material in your body will make you more reactive to other irritants than usual—so vigilant attention to a lifelong detoxification program is indicated, under the careful eye of a knowledgeable physician.

Stroke

Dr. Shantha advises waiting three to six months for the condition to stabilize; otherwise, heating the body may cause the brain to bleed again. Begin with mild heat and short session times, and gradually increase the temperature and duration of sauna sessions. Be sure to see your doctor regularly for checkups, if not supervision.

The charts on the following pages list many symptoms and ailments for which people might seek sauna therapy. Circles and dots in the charts indicate which changes caused by sauna therapy are crucial in helping the condition heal, which are useful in helping the condition heal, and which might or might not help the condition heal. In those cases where sauna bathing might harm the person, could actively prevent the condition from healing, or requires precautionary measures, the charts contain explanatory text. *Please note that these charts are general guidelines. Nothing applies to everyone always.* It is up to each person to use common sense and decide for him or herself how to best use a sauna. If you don't have enough information, find the appropriate person to advise you. Since this book is oriented toward those who are not being supervised by a doctor, I chose to err on the side of caution and list all possible contraindications.

Some details about disease may surprise you. For instance, the disabling or killing of microbes is listed as one of the changes induced by sauna therapy. Many laypeople and even doctors express surprise at the number (and type) of symptom pictures that involve microbes. But in the last few decades, medical researchers have discovered that microbes play a major role in many disease pictures that one might not ordinarily associate with pathogens. For instance, the *Gonococcus* bacterium has been implicated in some forms of arthritis. One researcher found *Chlamydia pneumoniae* in the spinal fluid of 90% of the people he tested with multiple sclerosis. And it is now understood that a major cause of stomach ulcers is the microbe *Heliobacter pylori*. For detailed information on how microbes relate to the onset of illness, see *The Handbook of Rife Frequency Healing*.

It is impossible to list all known symptom pictures (diseases) in these charts. If you don't see a specific symptom picture listed, look for something similar or see the very last chart, which contains an assortment of conditions that do not fit neatly into the other categories. There are actually very few health problems that cannot be helped (or would become worse) with sauna therapy. Considering the variety and number of health conditions that exist, the circumstances under which the sauna should not be used are very few.

Now that you have a good foundation in sauna therapy, in the next chapter I will tell you exactly how to put yourself in the hot seat.

	Medical Condition	Increases cardio-vascular activity, enhancing circulation	Increases norepinephrine, beta-endorphin and possibly thyroxin production, raising metabolism and increasing waste removal and nutrient absorption	Increases white blood cell production, helping the body eliminate toxins, foreign proteins and microbes	Increases production of enzymes (needed by white blood cells)	Relaxes muscles, reducing pain	Kills or disables microbes
Blood and Cardio-vascular Disorders Saunas increase the amount of hemoglobin in red blood cells, augment its ability to carry oxygen, and cause it to release oxygen faster.	**Angina Pectoris, unstable**	Ask your doctor! If your condition is stable, Far infrared at very low to moderate temperatures for a brief time may be helpful and relieve pain due to the dilation of the blood vessels. But you should be under medical supervision, at least initially.					
	Aortic Stenosis, severe	Not advised! Far infrared at very low temperatures briefly may be helpful, but ask your doctor first.					
	Arterio/athero Sclerosis	●●	●	●●	●●	●●	●
	Cardiac Arrhythmia	Not advised! Far infrared at very low temperature for a brief time may be helpful, but check with your doctor first. Do not dive right into cold water after perspiring; cool off slowly to avoid risk of cardiac arrhythmia.					
	Cardiac Edema	Ask your doctor.					
	Cerebral Thrombosis	If condition is unstable, do not use sauna. If condition is stable, consult with your doctor after receiving a thorough medical examination.					
	Blood Pressure, high	Doctors disagree about harm, since heat can raise uncontrolled high blood pressure to the extent that stroke results. Consult with a doctor knowledgeable about your condition and sauna therapy.					
	Blood Pressure, low	●●	●	●●	●●	●●	●

Notes	Condition						
If capillaries break due to dilation, leave the sauna and next time try a lower temperature. Radiant heat (FIR) is more effective than thermic heat in dilating blood vessels, and might be safer. Drinking alcohol can cause death! Cooling too suddenly can increase cardiac arrhythmia risk.	**Circulation Impairment**	●●	●●	●●	●●	●●	●●
	Congestive Heart Failure *Only under medical supervision*	●●	●●	●●	●●	●●	●
	Frostbite	●●	●●	●●	●●	●●	●●
	Hemophilia	People with hemophilia should not use the sauna; the dilation of blood vessels may cause them to bleed.					
	Leukemia	●●	●●	●●	●●	●●	●●
	Myocardial Infarction: acute/ recent	Not advised! Check with your doctor first. If you do decide to use the sauna, make sure you are supervised and do not cool off too quickly.					
	Myocardial Infarction: old (stable)	●●	●●	●●	●●	●●	●
	Varicose Veins	●●	●	●	●	●●	●

Key

●● Function is crucial in helping condition heal

● Function is useful in helping condition heal

○ Function might or might not help condition heal

Gastro-intestinal Tract

Many digestive problems involve pathogenic microbes. That is why this category responds well to sauna therapy.

Medical Condition	Increases cardio-vascular activity, enhancing circulation	Increases norepinephrine, beta-endorphin and possibly thyroxin production, raising metabolism and increasing waste removal and nutrient absorption	Increases white blood cell production, helping the body eliminate toxins, foreign proteins and microbes	Increases production of enzymes (needed by white blood cells)	Relaxes muscles, reducing pain	Kills or disables microbes
Appendicitis	This condition requires immediate surgery. However, using the sauna afterward will help the body heal much faster. And regular use of sauna may prevent the problem before it starts.					
Botulism / Food Poisoning	●●	●●	●●	●●	●●	●●
Candida and other Fungal Infections	●●	●●	●●	●●	●●	●●
Colitis, Crohn's Disease, Irritable Bowel	●●	●●	●●	●●	●●	●●
Constipation	●●	●●	●●	●●	●●	●●
Diarrhea, Dysentery	●●	●●	●●	●●	●●	●●

	Condition						
Too much heat at digestive area can destroy enzymes and divert needed blood away from the area, thus slowing digestion—so do not eat for 2 hours before entering the sauna, or else eat very lightly.	Heartburn / Flatulence / Gas	●●	●●	●●	●●	●●	●●
	Hemorrhoids	●●	●	●●	●●	●●	●
	Indigestion	●●	●●	●●	●●	●●	●●
	Leaky Gut	●●	●●	●●	●●	●●	●●
	Nausea, Vomiting	●●	●●	●●	●●	●●	●●
	Parasites, Protozoa and Worms	●●	●●	●●	●●	●●	●●
	Stomach Disorders	●●	●●	●●	●●	●●	●●
	Ulcer	●●	●●	●●	●●	●●	●●

Key

●●   Function is crucial in helping condition heal

●   Function is useful in helping condition heal

○   Function might or might not help condition heal

	Medical Condition	Increases cardio-vascular activity, enhancing circulation	Increases norepinephrine, beta-endorphin and possibly thyroxin production, raising metabolism and increasing waste removal and nutrient absorption	Increases white blood cell production, helping the body eliminate toxins, foreign proteins and microbes	Increases production of enzymes (needed by white blood cells)	Relaxes muscles, reducing pain	Kills or disables microbes
Reproductive System and Urinary Tract Problems These areas are so close together, that what affects one may affect the other. Infections in these regions can spread rather easily.	**Bladder / Urethra Infection, Cystitis**	●●	●●	●●	●●	●●	●●
	Breast Conditions	●●	●●	●●	●●	●●	●●
	Childbirth *Use low temperature*	●●	●●	●●	●●	●●	●●
	Cysts in Ovaries/ Fallopian Tubes	●●	●●	●●	●●	●●	●●
	Endome-triosis	●●	●●	●●	●●	●●	●●
	Kidney Infection/ Inflammation	●●	●●	●●	●●	●●	●●

Some physicians believe that menstruation may function to eliminate waste from the entire body, not just from the uterus. Thus menopausal women may especially benefit from sauna use.	Menopause	●●	●●	●●	●●	●●	•
	Menstruation Problems	●●	●●	●●	●●	●●	●●
	Pregnancy	Cultures with no history of regular sauna use advise against use during pregnancy. However, pregnant Finnish women routinely use it in moderation safely. Consult your doctor.					
	Prostate Conditions	●●	●●	●●	●●	●●	●●
	Sexually Transmitted Diseases, all	●●	●●	●●	●●	●●	●●
	Testicle Conditions	●●	●●	●●	●●	●●	●●
	Vaginitis / Ovary Problems	●●	●●	●●	●●	●●	●●

Key

●● Function is crucial in helping condition heal

● Function is useful in helping condition heal

○ Function might or might not help condition heal

Injuries: Joint, Fascia, Ligament, Muscle, Tendon, Skeletal, and Tissue Damage

For the first 48 hours after injury, most people feel better applying cold than heat.

Medical Condition	Increases cardiovascular activity, enhancing circulation	Increases norepinephrine, beta-endorphin and possibly thyroxin production, raising metabolism and increasing waste removal and nutrient absorption	Increases white blood cell production, helping the body eliminate toxins, foreign proteins and microbes	Increases production of enzymes (needed by white blood cells)	Relaxes muscles, reducing pain	Kills or disables microbes
Arthritis, all	●●	●●	●●	●●	●●	●●
Back pain, all	●●	●●	●●	●●	●●	●
Bursitis	●●	●●	●●	●●	●●	○
Carpal Tunnel	●●	●●	●●	●●	●●	○
Fascitis, Hardening	●●	●●	●●	●●	●●	●●
Fibromyalgia	●●	●●	●●	●●	●●	●●
Frozen Shoulder	●●	●●	●●	●●	●●	●
Inflammation (all types)	●●	●●	●●	●●	●●	●
Joints	●●	●●	●●	●●	●●	○
Ligament pull	●●	●●	●●	●●	●●	○

People with fibromyalgia sometimes feel pain after saunas, but this can be a healing response. If it's not, cold packs can alleviate the inflammation.

Inflammation is not infection, but excessive stagnation may cause infection.

Condition						
Lumbago	●●	●●	●●	●●	●●	●
Muscle ache, pull or spasm	●●	●●	●●	●●	●●	●
Neck pain	●●	●●	●●	●●	●●	●
Repetitive Stress Injury	●●	●●	●●	●●	●●	○
Rheumatism	●●	●●	●●	●●	●●	○
Skeletal pain	●●	●●	●●	●●	●●	○
Sprains, Strains, Stiffness	●●	●●	●●	●●	●●	○
Tendinitis	●●	●●	●●	●●	●●	○
Whiplash *See a doctor / chiropractor*	●●	●●	●●	●●	●●	○

Key

●● Function is crucial in helping condition heal

● Function is useful in helping condition heal

○ Function might or might not help condition heal

Nervous System / Brain Disorders

Medical Condition	Increases cardio-vascular activity, enhancing circulation	Increases norepinephrine, beta-endorphin and possibly thyroxin production, raising metabolism and increasing waste removal and nutrient absorption	Increases white blood cell production, helping the body eliminate toxins, foreign proteins and microbes	Increases production of enzymes (needed by white blood cells)	Relaxes muscles, reducing pain	Kills or disables microbes
Anxiety and Stress	••	••	••	••	••	••
Autism	••	••	••	••	••	••
Bell's Palsy	••	••	••	••	••	••
Brain Tumor	For very small brain tumors only, use a sauna cabinet (not enclosed chamber), if the body temperature does not exceed 100°F (37.8°C), and if supervised by a doctor.					
Cerebral Palsy	••	••	••	••	••	••
Depression	••	••	••	••	••	••
Dizziness	People subject to dizzy spells should use sauna only if supervised by qualified health care practitioner.					
Encephalitis	••	••	••	••	••	••
Epilepsy	Most modern heath care practitioners say that people with epilepsy should not use the sauna. But Dr. Kellogg successfully treated this condition with cold applied after the sauna, and strict diet.					
Fainting	People who faint should use the sauna only when supervised by a qualified health care practitioner.					

Alternating with cold packs may help. Even though high heat is not advised for multiple sclerosis, in many cases the presence of chronic viral and bacterial infections indicate a moderate, supervised use of the FIR sauna.

Autistic children often respond well, as they are usually filled with toxic chemicals. People with Parkinson's and similar diseases may also respond well.	**Mental / Behavioral Problems**	●●	●●	●●	●●	●●	●●
	Multiple Sclerosis	Since some people with Multiple Sclerosis have a hard time sweating, many health care practitioners advise against sauna therapy. However, medically supervised FIR sauna therapy at low levels might be helpful.					
	Neuralgia, Neuritis	●●	●●	●	●●	●●	○
	Paralysis	●●	●●	●	●●	●●	○
	Parkinson's disease	●●	●●	●●	●●	●●	○
	Raynaud's	●●	●●	●●	●●	●●	○
	Sciatica (nerve pain caused by misplaced bone)	●●	●●	●	●●	●●	○

Key

●●   Function is crucial in helping condition heal

●   Function is useful in helping condition heal

○   Function might or might not help condition heal

	Medical Condition	Increases cardio-vascular activity, enhancing circulation	Increases norepinephrine, beta-endorphin and possibly thyroxin production, raising metabolism and increasing waste removal and nutrient absorption	Increases white blood cell production, helping the body eliminate toxins, foreign proteins and microbes	Increases production of enzymes (needed by white blood cells)	Relaxes muscles, reducing pain	Kills or disables microbes
Respiratory Conditions The delicate mucous membranes lining the respiratory tract become inflamed if the air is too hot, dry or moist. If using a sauna room, make sure the heat source is clean and not smoky.	Allergies	●●	●●	●●	●●	●●	●●
	Asthma	●●	●●	●●	●●	●●	●●
	Bronchitis	●●	●●	●●	●●	●●	●●
	Cold	●●	●●	●●	●●	●●	●●
	Cough	●●	●●	●●	●●	●●	●●
	Emphysema	●●	●●	●●	●●	●●	●●
	Hay Fever	●●	●●	●●	●●	●●	●●
	Infections, all types	●●	●●	●●	●●	●●	●●
	Laryngitis	●●	●●	●●	●●	●●	●●
	Nasal Congestion	●●	●●	●●	●●	●●	●●

For severe problems, use a cabinet so you can breathe unheated air. Also try an aromatherapy diffuser with essential oils such as eucalyptus, lavender, lemon, peppermint, and tea tree.	**Nosebleeds** *Use a cabinet*	••	••	••	••	••
	Pneumonia	••	••	••	••	••
	Runny nose	••	••	••	••	••
	Sinus Infection	••	••	••	••	••
	Sneezing	••	••	••	••	••
	Sore throat	••	••	••	••	••
	Swollen Glands	••	••	••	••	••
	Tonsillitis	••	••	••	••	••
	Tuberculosis	••	••	••	••	••

Key

••   Function is crucial in helping condition heal

•   Function is useful in helping condition heal

○   Function might or might not help condition heal

	Medical Condition	Increases cardio-vascular activity, enhancing circulation	Increases norepinephrine, beta-endorphin and possibly thyroxin production, raising metabolism and increasing waste removal and nutrient absorption	Increases white blood cell production, helping the body eliminate toxins, foreign proteins and microbes	Increases production of enzymes (needed by white blood cells)	Relaxes muscles, reducing pain	Kills or disables microbes
Skin Conditions Since the skin is a major organ of elimination, there might be a systemic condition that needs attention as well as what is expressed locally by the skin.	**Abscesses, Boils and Lesions**	●●	●●	●●	●●	●●	●
	Acne and Pimples	●●	●●	●●	●●	●●	●●
	Atopic Dermatitis and Eczema *Some people itch, but proper washing will eliminate the problem*	●●	●●	●●	●●	●●	●●
	Bacterial Infections	●●	●●	●●	●●	●●	●●
	Bruises	●●	●●	●●	●●	●●	○
	Burns	●●	●●	●●	●●	●●	●
	Cholinergic Urticaria	Sauna use may cause intense itching of the skin. FIR sauna at very low temperatures might be helpful. Consult with your doctor.					

Studies showing that sauna use can aggravate certain skin conditions and cause itching also find that the itching is harmless. If you use soap, make sure it is free of detergents and additives, and that it does not leave a film. Moisturizers should be similarly pure.	**Cuts and Abrasions**	●●	●●	●●	●●	●●	●
	Dermatitis	●●	●●	●●	●●	●●	●●
	Fungal Infections	●●	●●	●●	●●	●●	●●
	Hives	●●	●●	●●	●●	●●	●
	Insect Bites	●●	●●	●●	●●	●●	●●
	Lupus Erythematosus	Health professionals differ as to whether heat is good for people with lupus. Supervised FIR sauna therapy at very low levels can bring results, but make sure you are supervised by a health care provider. Dr. Kellogg regularly used ultraviolet radiation, finding it safe and effective. If you are taking steroids, the sauna cannot be used because the drugs prevent the blood vessel from dilating.					
	Moles	●●	●●	●●	●●	●●	●●
	Nail Infections	●●	●●	●●	●●	●●	●●
	Psoriasis	●●	●●	●●	●●	●●	●
	Rashes	●●	●●	●●	●●	●●	●
	Warts	●●	●●	●●	●●	●●	●●

Key

●● Function is crucial in helping condition heal

● Function is useful in helping condition heal

○ Function might or might not help condition heal

	Medical Condition	Increases cardio-vascular activity, enhancing circulation	Increases norepinephrine, beta-endorphin and possibly thyroxin production, raising metabolism and increasing waste removal and nutrient absorption	Increases white blood cell production, helping the body eliminate toxins, foreign proteins and microbes	Increases production of enzymes (needed by white blood cells)	Relaxes muscles, reducing pain	Kills or disables microbes
Other Conditions Most of these conditions require the care of a licensed health care provider.	**AIDS**	●●	●●	●●	●●	●●	●●
	Alcoholism	●●	●●	●●	●●	●●	●●
	Anorexia Nervosa *A bit of food in the stomach will help prevent fainting*	●●	●●	●●	●●	●●	●
	Cancers, all types *Make the sauna as hot as possible*	●●	●●	●●	●●	●●	●●
	Chemical Exposure: cigarettes, drugs, glue, metals, poor diet, paint, solvents etc.	●●	●●	●●	●●	●●	○

Chemical sensitivity conditions are often caused or exacerbated by toxic chemicals, so sufferers respond very well to sauna therapy as part of an overall wellness program. Microbes often proliferate where there are toxic chemicals.	**Dental Problems** *See a dentist*	●●	●●	●●	●●	●●	●●
	Diabetes *Don't overheat*	●●	●●	●●	●●	●●	●●
	Drug Addiction	●●	●●	●●	●●	●●	●●
	Environmental Illness (EI)	●●	●●	●●	●●	●●	●●
	Eye problems, including inflammation	With all sauna bathing, it is important to keep the head (and the eyes) cool. A sauna room is not appropriate, but a cabinet might be useful for some people and conditions. Check with your doctor.					
	Fatigue, Low Energy	●●	●●	●●	●●	●●	●●
	Gangrene *Warm gradually; use ice or cold water after. See a doctor!*	●●	●●	●●	●●	●●	●●

Key

●● Function is crucial in helping condition heal

● Function is useful in helping condition heal

○ Function might or might not help condition heal

Other Conditions (continued)

Chemical and heavy metal toxicity can cause or contribute to any illness, including allergies, depression, chronic fatigue, fibromyalgia, gastrointestinal ailments, infections, insomnia, migraines, neurological disorders, and weight problems.

Medical Condition	Increases cardiovascular activity, enhancing circulation	Increases norepinephrine, beta-endorphin and possibly thyroxin production, raising metabolism and increasing waste removal and nutrient absorption	Increases white blood cell production, helping the body eliminate toxins, foreign proteins and microbes	Increases production of enzymes (needed by white blood cells)	Relaxes muscles, reducing pain	Kills or disables microbes
Gingivitis (gum infection)	●●	●●	●●	●●	●●	●●
Gout	●●	●●	●●	●●	●●	●●
Headache, Migraine *After, apply cold to head*	●●	●●	●●	●●	●●	●●
Heavy Metal Toxicity	●●	●●	●●	●●	●●	●●
Hepatitis / other Liver Ailments	●●	●●	●●	●●	●●	●●
Hormone Dysfunction	●●	●●	●●	●●	●●	●●
Hypoglycemia *Don't overheat; leave if faint or dizzy*	●●	●●	●●	●●	●●	●●

Massage might help since it helps move the poisons out of the dense lymph and into the venous bloodstream to be excreted.	**Infections, all types**	●●	●●	●●	●●	●●	●●
	Insomnia	●	●	●	●●	●●	●
	Lyme Disease	●●	●●	●●	●●	●●	●●
	Lymph Problems	●●	●●	●●	●●	●●	●●
	Multiple Chemical Sensitivity	●●	●●	●●	●●	●●	●●
	Obesity	●●	●●	●●	●●	●●	●●
	Stroke *Only if stabilized; wait 3 to 6 months*	●●	●●	●●	●●	●●	●●
	Thyroid, Overactive	Similar to procedure for underactive thyroid. However, use lower heat and less time (10 or 15 rather than 30 minutes), as heat speeds up the metabolism and an overactive thyroid is already too speedy.					
	Thyroid, Underactive/ Hashimoto's Thyroiditis	●●	●●	●●	●●	●●	●●

Key

●● Function is crucial in helping condition heal

● Function is useful in helping condition heal

○ Function might or might not help condition heal

NOTES

1. Masakazu Imamura et al, "Repeated Thermal Therapy Improves Impaired Vascular Endothelial Function in Patients with Coronary Risk Factors," *Journal of the American College of Cardiology* 38 (October 2001), 1083.

2. Minna L. Hannuksela and Samer Ellahham, "Benefits and Risks of Sauna Bathing," *The American Journal of Medicine* 110 (February 2001), 118.

3. Ibid.

4. William J. Rea, *Chemical Sensitivity, Volume 4: Tools of Diagnosis and Methods of Treatment* (Boca Raton: Lewis Publishers, 1997), 2439 and 2441.

5. C. Tei et al, "Acute Hemodynamic Improvement by Thermal Vasodilation in Congestive Heart Failure," *Circulation* 91 (10): 2582-90.

6. T.R. Shantha, personal communication, March 3, 2003

7. Ilkka Vuori, "Healthy and Unhealthy Sauna Bathing," *Annals of Clinical Research* 20: 217.

8. Hannuksela, op cit., 126.

9. E. Jokinen, E.L. Gregory, and I. Välimäki, "The Sauna and Children," *Annals of Clinical Research* 20: 283-286.

10. Vuori, op. cit.

11. K. Vähä-Eskeli and R. Erkkola, "The Sauna and Pregnancy," *Annals of Clinical Research* 20: 279.

12. Vuori, op. cit.

13. Hannuksela, op. cit.

14. Deborah N. Baird and William J. Rea, "The Temporomandibular Joint Implant Controversy: Its Clinical Implications," *Journal of Nutritional & Environmental Medicine* 9: 209-222. Reprint, page 15.

CHAPTER 7

How to Take a Sauna

A sweat suit is never worn in the sauna.

L. RON HUBBARD
CLEAR BODY, CLEAR MIND, 1990

Despite the obvious benefits of hot and warm soaks—such as muscle relaxation, pain relief, and increase in circulation—"there is something about an ordinary container of hot water," Licht writes in *Therapeutic Heat and Cold*, "which is too commonplace to be considered therapeutic by patients when they encounter it in a hospital or physician's office. When the hot water is placed in a vessel of special shape or material, it is accepted as therapy more readily by physician and patient alike."[1] The packaging may seem important—but fundamentally, it is the heat that heals.

We can apply the above psychology to sauna therapy. Body heating is actually very simple. People have done it for centuries because it feels good and gets results. Our ancestors did not need the external validation of scientists conducting studies on the effectiveness of sweating. Their own experience (which today we call empirical evidence) proved that building fires or putting hot stones in enclosures was beneficial. Yet in modern times, even those not requiring medical supervision often want or need a doctor to tell them what to do. "If my doctor tells me that it's okay," or "if it's medically necessary," the person says, "I'll take saunas"—forgetting that custom and cultural familiarity are as much a part of medicine as is science.

Depending on information from outside sources is not necessarily a negative thing, particularly when it's about something unfamiliar. But people who place their health in the hands of others because "that's the way it's done"—or because they don't trust their own experience, senses, or ability to learn—are less likely to heal, or heal completely, than those who educate themselves and make their own decisions. That's because participation in one's own health care stimulates the body's immune response. To me, one of the main advantages of sauna therapy is that you don't need special training to benefit from it. By following some basic guidelines and common sense, you can help rejuvenate your system—and even heal long-standing complaints—by giving yourself the opportunity to sweat. The body has a wonderful capacity to heal itself, if we only give it the chance.

With that in mind, here are guidelines to a successful sweat program. *They are only guidelines.* Each reader must decide for himself or herself if s/he has health problems that require medical supervision.

While You Are Considering Sauna Therapy

1. ***Before you ever approach a sauna, please review Chapter 6 for a full list of medical conditions and other circumstances that you need to know about before undergoing sauna therapy.***

   Many people who visit their local health clubs never bother to think about whether or not they are "candidates" for sauna therapy. If this includes you, please read Chapter 6 carefully, and if necessary, see your health practitioner before proceeding to use the sauna! Although the sauna is safe for most people under most circumstances, there are certain conditions under which people should not use the sauna at all, or may use the sauna only within certain parameters. *If you have a chronic or serious illness, consult a doctor who is knowledgeable about sauna therapy to make sure that you can safely use this modality.* Remember that all disease conditions are exacerbated (if not caused) by toxic chemicals in the environment, so even a tiny concentration like 1 ppm or 2 ppm can have negative consequences. Volatile chemicals (whether natural or synthetic, lipid- or fat-soluble) easily diffuse through the olfactory (nose) cell membranes and eventually migrate to the brain, bloodstream, or both.

2. *If you are taking prescription medication, check with both your pharmacist and your doctor to make sure that you can use the sauna.*

As noted in Chapter 6, heat can react in unexpected ways with prescription medications. Increased efficiency in circulation can cause medication to enter the bloodstream and bodily tissues more rapidly—in which case, the dosage may have to be decreased. On the other hand, sweating can cause the medication to be excreted more quickly from the system, in which case the amount may have to be increased, or the timing of your doses may need adjustment. *If prescription medication is in your bloodstream and you want to do sauna therapy, seek supervision from a physician!*

3. *After you have clearly established that sauna therapy is appropriate for you, examine the sauna you intend to use to see if it is suitable for you.*

How is the sauna built, and with what materials? Are there any materials to which you might negatively react? Is the seating comfortable? Is there adequate ventilation? What is the heat source, and is it compatible with your needs? Does the sauna accommodate water vapor? If so, how much? Have aromatic oils been used in it? If so, are they pleasing or irritating to your system? And what cleaner is used to disinfect the sauna? Chapter 5, "Construction of the Sauna," explains everything you need to know about these issues. Whether or not the sauna is right for you can make the difference between an enjoyable, healing experience and an unpleasant one.

Now, with all the preliminaries answered to your fullest satisfaction, you are ready to begin your sauna experience.

JUST BEFORE THE SAUNA SESSION

1. *Do not eat a large meal for at least one to two hours prior to using the sauna. But make sure that there is some food in your stomach.*

The process of digestion normally redirects some blood from the rest of the body to the stomach and abdomen. A sufficient intestinal blood flow encourages the gut in its peristaltic action (the wavelike, rhythmical motions that squeeze and move the food down the digestive tract). An adequate blood flow also helps the stomach secrete sufficient hydrochloric acid (which is needed to digest protein). But when heat is applied directly to the abdomen, and even generally to the rest of the body as well, much-needed blood is diverted away from the digestive organs to the capillaries at the surface of the skin. Once this occurs, your food will tend to simply lie in the stomach and ferment. The conflicting agendas of digesting and perspiring help explain why many people do not feel hungry on very hot days. They also help explain why people who eat large meals before entering the sauna don't sweat as easily as those with emptier bellies. The body prioritizes its needs; so when food must be digested, it doesn't easily give up its blood supply to the surface of the skin.

On the other hand, it is common for one to feel faint (and even nauseated) if one uses the sauna without having any food at all in the stomach, because blood sugar levels can dip too low. If you feel hungry just before entering the sauna, eat a small amount of something that is easily digestible (generally a carbohydrate, such as fruit, raw vegetables, sprouts, nuts, or sprouted bread). Some health care professionals believe that faintness in a sauna can be caused by electrolyte imbalance; so make sure your mineral intake is sufficient. (See Chapter 3 for a more detailed discussion of electrolytes, as well as Dr. Lawrence Wilson's book *Nutritional Balancing and Hair Mineral Analysis*.)

2. *Do not drink alcohol.*

Just as it is unwise to drive a car or operate heavy machinery when under the influence of alcohol, you should not drink before using the sauna. Alcohol is a systemic depressant. Even a low level in the blood-stream can markedly decrease judgement, balance, and neuromuscular coordination, dulling your responses so much that you may not be coherent enough to leave the sauna if you start to overheat.

Alcohol also increases the concentration of stress hormones in the blood and urine. Since sauna use by itself causes the body to increase its production of certain hormones, the higher hormone levels from the two sources combined can produce undesirable and unknown effects. The changes induced by alcohol in the balance of hormones, neurotransmitters, and other bodily substances alters the function of the entire cardiovascular system. This can cause elevated or low blood pressure, rapid heartbeat, and/or irregular heartbeat. Whereas sauna bathing is therapeutic partly *because* of its intensified effect on the cardiovascular system, when combined with alcohol consumption, the work load on the heart is so dramatically increased that rapid heart rate or even heart failure may occur. Finally, alcohol is a diuretic. The last thing you want to do before entering a sauna is deplete your body's water stores!

Hospital emergency room staffs know the painful consequences of someone drinking too much alcohol quickly and then falling asleep. The alcohol shuts down breathing and heart functions, and the person dies within a few hours. It's easy to doze off in a hot sauna. You don't need the added stress or danger of alcohol ingestion.

In "Benefits and Risks of Sauna Bathing" in *The American Journal of Medicine*, a database review of 130 studies of Finnish saunas shows that within a one year time span, the vast majority of sudden deaths connected to sauna bathing (which comprised only 1.7% of sudden deaths overall from all sources) were due to complications directly or indirectly connected to *alcohol consumption*. In another article, "The Sauna and Alcohol" in *Annals of Clinical Research*, the authors write that "The most unfortunate accidents related to sauna are those when an intoxicated bather passes out in the sauna or drowns while swimming after sauna bathing."[2] If you have been drinking, wait at least 24 hours, until the effects of the alcohol have worn off—and *then* use the sauna to detoxify. You'll need it.

3. Do not take other "recreational" drugs.

Tranquilizers, stimulants, and hallucinogens alter the body's metabolism and may not interact well with the heat of the sauna. Also, your responses to both your inner and outer environments can be dangerously altered so that you are unable to respond appropriately. If you are taking prescription medications, consult your pharmacist and your doctor to make sure you can use the sauna. See page 191 earlier in this chapter.

4. Do drink plenty of water beforehand.

Don't wait until you're dehydrated before replenishing your bodily fluids. Begin *before* entering the sauna. "In a study of subjects' abilities to perform mental exercises after heat-stress induced dehydration," research scientist Susan M. Kleiner writes, "a fluid loss of only 2 percent of body weight caused reductions in arithmetic ability, short-term memory, and the ability to visually track an object by 20 percent compared to their well-hydrated state."[3] She recommends drinking two cups of fluid two hours before exercise, four to six ounces every 15 to 20 minutes during exercise, and 16 to 20 ounces (2 to 2½ cups) of fluid, for every pound of body weight lost during exercise, when you have completed your exercise program.

Alcoholic, caffeinated, and carbonated beverages don't count as part of your fluid intake since they can act as diuretics and actually cause water loss. (The body must use part of its water stores to flush out the chemical wastes from the system.) Naturally *or* synthetically sweetened juice doesn't count either, since it too is a diuretic (extra water goes into the bloodstream to dilute the excessively high levels of glucose and flush it out through the urinary tract). In addition, a high chemical or sugar content directs the blood flow to the stomach at the expense of lessening the blood volume to the muscles elsewhere, which can result in cramping. Note that under normal circumstances, the body handles a fluid intake at the rate of four ounces every half hour, since more than that floods the kidneys too much. So you might want to ration your water intake accordingly, increasing the amount as you begin to sweat.

Keeping yourself hydrated stimulates the production of various hormones and helps speed metabolism in the right way. "Efficient sweating will prevent the core temperature from rising more than a degree or two, and this is essential," University of Toronto physiology professor William A. MacKay notes. "If your core temperature rises as high as 104° F [40° C], the extra energy needed to fuel the high metabolic rate will come out of your muscles and not your fat cells."[4]

5. ***If you are extremely overheated from prior exercise, heavy physical labor, being in the sun, or for any other reason, rest for about 15 minutes and allow your body to cool to an appropriate level before entering the sauna.***

Heatstroke is the absolute extreme of body heating and should be avoided. Too much heat from any source will give you heatstroke. See pages 197–198 for a list of heatstroke symptoms and first aid measures.

That said, it should be noted that one particular detoxification program (discussed in the next chapter) actually requires that the person exercise immediately before using the sauna. In this protocol, the person is under the care of a physician.

6. ***Remove all jewelry: watches, necklaces, rings, earrings, body piercing metal.***

If metal gets hot enough, it can burn your skin. Also, tissues swell when the body is heated, so you may find that your rings will hurt or even become stuck on your finger.

7. ***Shower or bathe.***

Your sweating experience will not be optimal if your skin is already covered with a film of toxins. Showering also helps keep the sauna clean (which is even more important if more than one person uses it). A thin layer of water on your skin (but not too much) can help accelerate the sweating process, so don't dry off completely after you shower.

8. ***Give the sauna enough time to get hot.***

If you are burning wood for a fire, the sauna can take up to 45 minutes to get hot. If you use stones heated in a wood fire (such as for a Native American sweat lodge), you may require three to five hours to heat the lodge, starting from when you first light the fire to when you place the stones inside the chamber. If the heat source for your sauna is a conventional electric heater, depending on the size of the room, the time required for pre-heating can range from 20 to 45 minutes.

If the heat source is a FIR heater, the need to warm the air is not important—unlike with a hot air sauna—since far infrared radiation raises the temperature of the body without heating the air. (Most of the heat in the air of a FIR-heated room is caused by the *reflection* of FIR from the walls back into the room.) However, some people like to wait anyway—10 minutes when using a FIR cabinet and about 30 minutes for a FIR room—because they do not feel that they are in a "real" sauna unless the air is heated above 95° or 100°F (35° to 37.8°C). Most people sweat more with a FIR heater than with a conventional hot air heater. However, if you like extravagantly hot air temperatures, you may prefer a conventional electric heater, wood, or rocks as your heat source.

Keep in mind that people who are very ill might not be able to tolerate high heat, particularly when they start their sauna protocol. If this applies to you, be comfortable and start slowly. Also, many people do not require very high heat in order to begin sweating. For such individuals, a FIR sauna at low temperatures may be ideal. The goal is not to see how long you can endure a high temperature; the goal is to sweat. So be sensitive to the environment that is optimum for your particular sweating experience.

Whether you prefer low or high heat, the shock of sudden, very high heat (relative to what your system can tolderate) has the *opposite* effect of what's desired: it shuts down the body's sweating mechanism. The blood vessels suddenly constrict, the skin tightens, and stiff muscles and joints can become irritated. *Make sure that the sauna is not too hot for you before you enter.*

During the Sauna Session

1. Leave the sauna if you feel uncomfortable.

"Uncomfortable" is subjective, based on your tolerance and wellness quotient. A little discomfort in the sauna is to be expected, especially if you are very toxic. However, be aware of signals of needing to leave. You might be suffering from either dehydration or moderately severe heat exhaustion if you have the following symptoms: breathing problems, dizziness or lightheadedness, energy loss or weakness, fatigue, headache, loss of appetite, muscle cramps, nausea, nosebleeds, thirst, or dark urine with a strong odor.

If you are suffering from heat exhaustion, drink fluids. Immerse yourself immediately in cool, *shallow* water, or place a cold wet cloth against your face or wrapped around your head and neck. (Recent studies question the wisdom of immersing yourself in extremely cold water, as this may cause the capillaries to rapidly constrict, thereby inhibiting the cooling process.) Lie down, or sit with your head bent to your knees, to bring the flow of blood to your brain. When your breathing normalizes and your body starts to cool, drink fruit juice or eat a piece of fruit to quickly increase your blood sugar level. Maintaining a stable blood sugar level is crucial for the brain, which cannot extract glucose from the body's tissues and depends on adequate amounts of glucose circulating in the blood to function properly.

Heat exhaustion is the result of mild to moderate overheating. However, if your body temperature is too high and your skin feels dry, this is a sign that your brain is so overheated that its internal thermostat has ceased operating. Dry skin means that your skin circulation has shut down and the sweating process is no longer functioning. At this point, you are no longer suffering from simple heat exhaustion, but much more dangerous heatstroke. Besides the previously noted fatigue, faintness and headache, symptoms of the more extreme heatstroke include dim vision, excessive dizziness (also called vertigo), mental confusion and disorientation, difficulty swallowing, and hot and flushed skin (although some doctors say that this can alternate with the cold, clammy "goosebumps" skin typically associated with heat exhaustion rather than heatstroke). In addition, the pulse rate can increase to as much as 160 beats per minute. Prolonged cases of heatstroke can induce unconsciousness and convulsions. Eventually, brain damage and death can occur rapidly if the process is not reversed.

"The treatment of heatstroke," Guyton and Hall write, "is to reduce the body temperature as rapidly as possible," through the removal of all clothing, the application of cool water on all surfaces of the body, and blowing air across the body with a fan. "Experiments have shown that this treatment can reduce the temperature either as rapidly or almost as rapidly as any other procedure, though some physicians prefer total immersion of the body in water containing a mush of crushed ice."[5] *Heatstroke is a true medical emergency, requiring medical attention. If you think that you or someone else might be suffering from heatstroke, call an ambulance immediately.*

I am telling you about heatstroke not to scare you, but to help you have a safe and enjoyable sauna experience. Stop when you have had enough—sauna bathing isn't an experiment to see how much heat you can tolerate. As Hillila reminds us, "Sauna-taking should never be an endurance contest or test of manliness [sic]. The aim is not to simulate the pains of purgatory or the pangs of hell but rather to produce a feeling of well-being."[6] People who are older, infirm, are taking drugs of any kind, or have delicate health conditions, need to be especially careful to prevent overheating.

Incidentally, you are not likely to experience heatstroke in a far infrared sauna, since unlike other types of units it does not heat the air.

2. *Keep plenty of drinking water with you at all times, and be near a shower, pool, or bucket of cool water for rinsing.*

This is common sense, but sometimes people forget. It's important to have enough water to drink and splash on yourself at all times, to counteract the effects of dehydration and overheating. Use these practical guidelines based on Kleiner's recommendations and adapted for sauna use: drink four ounces of water every half hour, for two hours before your sauna session, and another four ounces just before you step into the sauna. Drink another two ounces in 15 minutes. Once you have begun to sweat, depending on how much you are perspiring, drink four to eight ounces every 15 to 20 minutes during your sauna session. (The pH of your water should be at least 7.0, preferably higher. See the following chapter for more information.)

3. **Bring in plenty of towels—to wipe off sweat, and also to sit on.**

It is always a courtesy to others to sit on a towel; other people don't want your sweaty toxins. Mopping up your sweat from the surrounding area with a towel helps make the sauna experience more pleasant for others—and yourself, when you next use the sauna. There is also a psychological benefit to keeping the bench dry and hygienic for the next session.

4. **If possible, sauna bathe nude—or else wear a minimum of lightweight, loose-fitting clothing.**

Some public saunas and sweat lodges require that participants wear clothing. You might obtain acceptable results if loose, light clothing is worn, but the ideal situation is no clothing. This may seem difficult if you are not used to being nude, and feel shy about undressing in front of other people. However, there is a very good reason to be naked. Covering the body can prevent sweat from either evaporating or evaporating quickly. Also, if you sweat profusely, clothing can become clammy and uncomfortable, and detract from what would otherwise be a pleasurable experience. Rather than miss a positive sauna experience—or suffer any heath repercussions—it might be better to confront cultural inhibitions about nudity.

On the other hand, some people are easily chilled, or feel too ill to undress. For these folks, far infrared is a good heat source because it is easily transmitted through clothing, and can provide benefits even if clothes are worn.

5. **Make sure to leave the sauna periodically to shower, sponge bathe, splash water on yourself, or jump into a pool or cool bath.**

If you get too sweaty, leave the sauna and shower to remove the perspiration and toxins from your skin. Even though you are wiping off your sweat with a towel, cold water is an important part of sauna bathing for three reasons. First, the body reaches a limit in the amount of heat it accepts before the beneficial effects of the sauna become liabilities. (That is why Dr. Kellogg kept an electric fan in his electric light baths, and periodically gave his clients sponge baths.) Second, you need to eliminate the toxins that have been secreted through your skin. You don't want your pores to become blocked, and you don't want the waste material to be reabsorbed into the skin. Third, as I discussed in Chapter 2, the thyroid is stimulated to produce thyroxin (its metabolism-quickening hormone) by cold in contrast to heat; so the application of cold after body heating may be beneficial for those wanting more efficient thyroid function. *Incidentally, do not dive head first directly from the sauna into cold water!* The shock to the system can severely impair motor and perceptual function, and even be lethal.

6. *Be careful not to burn yourself.*

You can get burned in a sauna if you are too close to the heat source. (There are some exceptions. One manufacturer of a FIR sauna cabinet, for instance, has made burn-proof heater covers that can be touched without harming the skin; see Appendix B.) According to A. Papp of the Burn Unit at Kuopio University Hospital in Finland, a seven-year analysis of 598 burn patients treated at that hospital's burn unit showed that one in four people acquired the burns when in a sauna. Fifty-four percent of those burn cases required operations. Significantly, 40% of the burn cases had been drinking alcohol. This is one more reason not to drink when taking a sauna.

There is also a remote possibility of getting burned by the sauna seat, especially if it is made from high-density hardwood. The molecules of such woods tend to be packed tightly together, making them trap heat. Make sure that your heat source is compatible with the sauna's building materials.

7. *You may want to have someone checking on you periodically, especially if you are ill, frail, or recovering from an illness.*

If someone else cannot be with you, either inside the sauna or in the room, make sure that they are within hearing distance in case you experience any negative reactions and need help.

8. If your sauna allows you to lie down, get up slowly to avoid dizziness and/or fainting. Even from a sitting position, exit the sauna slowly.

Systemic heating has brought much more blood than usual to the body's surface. This, with the slower-than-usual return of the blood to the heart, means less blood supply to the head. Furthermore, explains naturopath Marian Porter:

> When toxic waste is being released from the cells, it enters the bloodstream in the form of excess mucous and proteins. This is normal and necessary…[but] can cause a temporary thickening of both the lymph and blood.…This condition can influence circulation to such an extent that standing up too fast might cause a delay in oxygen reaching the brain.…If you are experiencing dizziness, stand up very slowly, keeping your head down as you rise. This symptom subsides after frequent cleansing.[7]

9. Don't overdo the amount of time you are in the sauna, especially if you are chronically ill, physically exhausted, or a beginner to this kind of therapy. Also, start with lower temperatures.

How long you should stay in the sauna depends on your constitution, your current physical condition, and even the heat source. People use a sauna for periods as brief as 10 minutes and as long as several hours (which includes short breaks for resting and showering). Virtually every sauna authority agrees that if you are not used to sweating, begin with a session of shorter duration. Medical doctor Lawrence A. Plumlee writes in *Sauna Detoxification Therapy*:

> We do not know why some patients get worse for long periods after sauna. It is thought to be due to toxic damage from remobilized chemicals. Perhaps enzyme systems are poisoned instead of improved by increased toxins in the blood. Hans Selye and others observed that the same stressor which heightened physical performance could lead to illnesses if the stresses were prolonged or excessive. Users of the sauna would

do well to remember this. *Wise patients do not rely solely on their doctors, but also monitor their own symptoms to challenge their bodies without incurring excessive stress. Experience is often the best teacher.*[8] [emphasis added]

Many people, though not all, feel markedly better after their sauna sessions. You might feel worse from the re-circulating toxins and need to remain in the sauna to pass this discomfort point. And you will probably need more than one session to feel relief. See the next chapter for more information on specific approaches to detoxifying with a sauna.

Incidentally, if you find that you are not sweating easily, it may be that *the sauna is too hot.* As I explained in Chapter 2, the body shuts down its sweating mechanism if exposed to too much heat for too long a period. Try lowering the temperature and see what happens. You may find that you achieve the best sweat with FIR heat, which penetrates the body well even at low temperatures.

10. *If you want a sauna session that's longer than 20 or 30 minutes, give yourself ample time for breaks.*

During these intermission periods, rest. Also wipe yourself with a cool wet cloth, or bathe or shower in cool or cold water, to prevent overheating and to wash away the toxins from your skin so they don't get reabsorbed.

Directly After the Sauna Session

1. *Replenish the water lost through perspiration.*

Some people sweat two quarts or more in the sauna. Have water handy at all times. The water should be properly filtered so that it is free of contaminants including microbes, detergents, chlorine, fluoride, and insoluble minerals. Dr. Kleiner recommends drinking 16 ounces of water for every pound lost during exercise; so this would translate to one ounce of fluid for every ounce of body weight you lose during a sauna. If you do not weigh yourself, estimate how much water you lost—or simply drink until you are no longer thirsty.

2. *Replenish the minerals and vitamins lost through perspiration.*

Minerals are vital nutrients because they convey electrical charge in the body and are the constituents of thousands of enzymes. Without minerals, the body cannot function properly. There is some debate as to whether or not people undergo extensive mineral loss after they have been sweating on a regular basis. Kleiner states that after the first few times of perspiring, the mineral loss is kept to a minimum and one loses mostly water. Other sources, such as Dr. Wilson and some companies that manufacture electrolyte formulas, disagree. Everyone is unique, so monitor your responses carefully. In my own experience, I have found that many minerals are indeed lost through sweating—and that this loss continues even with continued prolonged sweats.

People lose more minerals than just sodium. The body can compensate for sodium loss after a while and retain it in the tissues, but potassium will still need to be replaced. According to some sources, three times as much potassium is needed as sodium (leg cramping and vocal hoarseness are signs that potassium levels are too low). Most people need replacements not only of potassium, but also calcium, chloride, and magnesium. Those with environmental illness, and related conditions like fibromyalgia, may excrete more magnesium than normal.

Although it is commonly acknowledged that people lose minerals through perspiration, not enough attention is given to the loss of both fat- and water-soluble vitamins. Dr. David Root (whose sauna therapy protocol is discussed in the next chapter) observes that copious amounts of *all* nutrients are excreted, along with the toxins, when one is on an intensive detoxification program. Make sure you supplement your diet regularly with mineral *and* vitamin supplements. It is strongly recommended that you consult a qualified health care practitioner to help you determine your nutritional needs.

3. *Rest, either lying down or sitting, for five to 15 minutes.*

Sweating has put your system through a rigorous workout, so you need time to normalize.

4. *If you are ill, do not cool off too quickly.*

For most people, this is not a problem, but some people with coronary conditions such as acute myocardial infarction may need to be more careful. *If you have a heart condition, seek medical supervision before undergoing sauna therapy.*

5. *Take a bath or shower with warm or cool water, and brush your skin.*

You have just put your system through a rigorous workout to get rid of toxins. You don't want to leave these wastes on your skin to get re-absorbed. Use warm water but not hot—hot water will open the pores too much and cause the toxins and dirt to seep right back into the skin. A layer of grime sticking to your skin will also keep the heat inside your body and make you tired. There is some controversy about whether or not soap should be used. Conventional commercial soaps leave a film on the skin and clog the pores. However, there are a few cleaners on the market made from natural ingredients that do not leave a film. Make sure the soap label does *not* say "anti-bacterial," because by law any soap with that designation must contain a registered pesticide—which, by definition, is poisonous. (A source for a pure, bio-compatible cleanser that does not contain noxious chemicals, does not clog the pores, and can also be used to clean any sauna, is in Appendix B.) After rinsing, brush your skin and scalp with a loofah or natural bristle skin brush. This will help maintain the health of your skin by improving the circulation.

6. *Replenish the oils that were eliminated through the skin.*

Some people like to receive massage right after their sauna. It's relaxing, helps move the lymph and flush out even more toxins, and helps replace the beneficial oils in the skin that were lost through sweating. Three of my favorite skin oils are coconut, lanolin, and jojoba. *Coconut* is well absorbed into the skin. It has strong anti-viral, anti-bacterial, and anti-fungal properties, and even affords protection against the sun. *Lanolin,* which is secreted by the oil glands of sheep (and gathered without causing any pain or harm to the animal), very closely resembles human sebum (the secretion produced by the skin to protect itself). Some people are allergic to lanolin, so test one small patch of skin to make sure you can tolerate it before covering your entire body. *Jojoba* is not really an oil, but is pressed from the seed of the Jojoba shrub found in the desert. It, too, closely resembles human sebum, has a nice texture, and is well liked by those who do not want to use animal products. Other beneficial oils are apricot kernel, almond, and sesame. It's worth buying organic oils, because after all, whatever is absorbed through the skin goes right into the bloodstream as though you had eaten it.

Some health practitioners suggest that eating oil is a better way of replenishing the body's stores. A balance of cold-pressed flax, olive and coconut oils, and mercury-free fish oils, is a good choice.

7. *Eat some nourishing, easily assimilated food.*

Many people find that they are very hungry on leaving the sauna, since an effective body heating session can speed the metabolism. Wait 15 or 20 minutes for the blood to return to your stomach so you can digest your food, and then eat. Rapidly absorbed food such as fruit will provide the system with immediate energy by raising the blood sugar level. But not everyone can handle even more carbohydrates after a sauna. Pay attention to what you need; it might be some concentrated animal protein.

8. *Clean the sauna and leave the door open to dry out.*

You entered the sauna to get rid of waste from your body. Those toxins are not good for the sauna, either. Use a pure mild soap, not toxic synthetic detergent. If you can tolerate scents and are not chemically sensitive, you might want to spray the room or cabinet with essential oils such as eucalyptus, lavender, lemon, or peppermint. These oils are antiseptic and germicidal as well as fragrant.

Sauna bathing can provide you with much-needed relaxation. It is a vital part of any detoxification program. And it can be an enjoyable social experience, helping to restore and rejuvenate you at a less tangible (but equally important) spiritual level. Whatever type of sauna you use, following the above guidelines will help ensure the benefits, pleasures, and cleansing properties of body heating for years to come.

Notes

1. Sidney Licht, "History of Therapeutic Heat," in *Therapeutic Heat and Cold, Second Edition: Volume Two of the Physical Medicine Library*, ed. Sidney Licht with Herman L. Kamenetz, (New Haven: Elizabeth Licht, Publisher, 1972), 205.

2. R. Ylikahri, E. Heikkonen, and A. Suokas, "The Sauna and Alcohol," *Annals of Clinical Research* 20: 287.

3. Susan M. Kleiner, "Can '8-a-day' Keep Cancer Away? The Latest News On Water, Health And Performance," http://www.nutrifit.org/8aday.html#signs (accessed September 26, 2001).

4. William MacKay, personal communication, October 2001.

5. Arthur C. Guyton and John E. Hall, *Textbook of Medical Physiology*, Tenth Ed. (Philadelphia: W.B. Saunders Company, 2000), 977.

6. Bernhard Hillila, *The Sauna Is…* (Iowa City: Penfield Press, 1988), 22.

7. Marian Porter, "Dr. Porter's Health Notes" (newsletter of The Oxygen Spa, Silver Spring, Md., November 17, 2001).

8. Lawrence A. Plumlee, "Introduction," in *Sauna Detoxification Therapy: A Guide for the Chemically Sensitive,* ed. Marilyn McVicker (Jefferson, N.C.: McFarland & Company, Inc., Publishers, 1997), 10.

Detoxification Programs for Getting Well and Staying Well

*Miracles sometimes happen, but more often they're made of faith
and will and hope and imagination, to say nothing of sweat.*

BING CROSBY AS HARVEY IN THE MOVIE *HIGH TIME* (1960),
WRITTEN BY FRANK AND TOM WALDMAN

In holistic or complementary health facilities, whenever the word *toxin* is used, *detoxification* follows. What does it mean to detoxify? Is it the same as an illness? If not, what is the difference between detoxifying and disease? And what comprises a successful detox program? Can everyone benefit from one?

As discussed in Chapter 3, toxins can be classified into two general groups: *endogenous* (biological waste materials, either created within the body or from microbes), and *exogenous* (created outside of the body, such as chemicals and heavy metals). When the system becomes overloaded from these waste products, the body's ability to function is impaired—sometimes so seriously that illness develops.

Since the liver is a major detoxification organ of the body, this chapter will first describe how it works and what it needs to do its job. Then some effective detoxification programs that include regular use of a sauna will be explored. At the end are guidelines for staying well once you have recovered your health.

DETOXIFICATION EXPLAINED

The Liver, a Major Detoxification Organ

The liver is one of the most powerful structures in the body—so powerful, in fact, that it is the only body part that can easily regenerate itself if it's badly damaged. And it has a correspondingly mighty job, that of neutralizing toxins. Most researchers classify the liver's cleansing processes into two parts: Phase I and Phase II detoxification (sometimes with an intermediary step in between). In Phase II especially, the liver produces enzymes that break down harmful chemicals into more benign and manageable substances that the body can either eliminate or reuse. The process by which harmful materials are rendered harmless is fairly complex, but a simplified description will give you some idea of what occurs.

In the Phase I stage, certain enzymes change toxins through *oxidization* (combining them with oxygen), *reduction* (breaking them down into simpler components), or *hydrolysis* (creating acids and bases through chemical alteration). The substances that result from the processing of the original chemicals are called *metabolites*. If the metabolites from Phase I detoxification are still injurious to the body—and they often are—they undergo Phase II detoxification. In Phase II, other enzymes further convert the toxins into a water-soluble form. The water-soluble waste then exits the liver into the bloodstream, where it is ultimately filtered by the kidneys and excreted through the urinary tract. Sometimes the water-soluble waste in the bloodstream is absorbed into the large intestine through the intestine wall, where it then leaves with the feces.

If toxins remain fat-soluble and cannot be made water-soluble, the route of elimination is different. Inside the liver, the fat-soluble material attaches to *bile*, a substance that the liver produces (bile has receptors for fat). The bile then travels, as it normally does, via a short passage into the gall bladder, and next into the duodenum portion of the small intestine. From there, the fat-soluble toxins are pushed down through the intestinal tract into the large intestine, to be eventually excreted with the feces.

"Phase II must be functioning in balance with Phase I to transform the intermediate metabolites to non-toxic, excretable end-products, thus successfully completing the detoxification process," points out Mark Percival in "Nutritional Support for Detoxification." "Proper functioning of both of these phases is critically important, because the intermediate metabolites produced during Phase I may actually be more harmful than the original toxins."[1] One example of this is a component of cigarette smoke that is inert before Phase I processing, but which actually becomes carcinogenic after being partially dismantled by Phase I enzymes. That is why if Phase I occurs without being accompanied by a complete Phase II process, people can actually feel worse than before the transformation cycle began.

Phase I detox can cause considerable oxidative stress. This means the production of free radicals, which are extremely unstable substances due to the way their electrons are arranged. The electrons in the outer shell of any atom are responsible for chemical reactions. They produce new compounds by binding to the electrons of other atoms. The article "Understanding Free Radicals and Antioxidants" describes how the behavior of electrons can produce free radicals:

> The innermost shell [of the atom] is full when it has two electrons. When the first shell is full, electrons begin to fill the second shell. When the second shell has eight electrons, it is full, and so on. [The number of electrons increases the further out they are in the atom's outer shells.] *The most important structural feature of an atom for determining its chemical behavior is the number of electrons in its outer shell.* A substance that has a full outer shell tends not to enter in chemical reactions... [and is called inert]. Because atoms seek to reach a state of maximum stability, an atom will try to fill its outer shell by gaining or losing electrons to either fill or empty its outer shell... [or by] sharing its electrons... with other atoms in order to complete its outer shell. Normally, bonds don't split in a way that leaves a molecule with an odd, unpaired electron [an electron that is not balanced by the same number of protons in the nucleus

of the atom]. But when weak bonds split, free radicals are formed. Free radicals are very unstable and react quickly with other compounds, trying to capture the needed electron to gain stability. Generally, free radicals attack the nearest stable molecule, "stealing" its electron. When the "attacked" molecule loses its electron, it becomes a free radical itself, beginning a chain reaction. Once the process is started, it can cascade, finally resulting in the disruption of a living cell.[2]

In *The Complete Book of Enzyme Therapy*, Anthony Cichoke describes the myriad problems that can be caused by free radicals:

> Free radicals lead to faulty metabolism of proteins, including DNA and enzymes, by oxidizing cells so that they practically rust....Free radicals can inactivate enzymes in the cell membrane. This damages the membrane, interfering with the cell's ability to take in nutrients and expel wastes. They can cause lipid peroxidation in cell membranes, in which the protective lipid layer of the cell is oxidized, which damages it. This causes body fat compounds to become rancid and release even more free radicals.[3]

The free radical damage created as the body detoxifies illustrates the complexity and precision of liver function. If, during any phase, the liver cannot produce enough enzymes and other biochemicals to efficiently break down the toxins, whatever has not been neutralized—be it the original toxin or a metabolite of that toxin—goes right back into the bloodstream and lodges in the fat tissue. Therefore, it is vitally important to support the liver so that it can complete its entire detox cycle. (Incidentally, free radicals can also be produced and augmented during exercise and sauna therapy.)

Liver support means obtaining plenty of the right nutrients, including those with antioxidant properties. "Antioxidants," writes Cichoke, "protect the body from free-radical damage by helping the body repair cellular damage caused by free radicals or by intercepting the free radicals before they can do any harm."[4] Below is a list of nutrients, some of which have antioxidant properties. All of them help protect the liver, and provide materials for the creation of enzymes and other bio-chemicals, during Phase I of the detoxification cycle.

Note that I do not suggest amounts for these nutrients. *Natural Detoxification* by Jacqueline Krohn and Frances Taylor, *Detoxify or Die* by Sherry A. Rogers, and *The Chemistry of Success* by Susan Lark and James A. Richards (all listed in the Bibliography) give dosage recommendations for various nutrients. I am not reporting suggested doses because the authors suggest different amounts. And everyone is unique and has different needs, depending on their constitution, environment, state of health, and toxin level (among other factors). A lot more is involved in nutrition counseling than one might think. For instance, one person may assimilate calcium lactate well, while another person may better absorb the mineral in its calcium carbonate form. It is wise to thoroughly educate yourself. But it's also a good idea to consult a knowledgeable health care practitioner about the amounts and types of supplements that will work best for you—especially if you have a chronic or serious illness. Now here are the nutrients:

- B-complex vitamins (all)
- catalase
- copper
- flavonoids
- folic acid
- iron
- magnesium
- vitamin C
- vitamin E
- selenium
- superoxide dismutase, or SOD (some sprouted grains such as barley contain high amounts of SOD)
- zinc

During an intermediate phase, in addition to the above, the liver can be supported with:

- vitamin A
- coenzyme Q_{10}

And for Phase II, people add:

- amino acids: methionine, glutathione, cysteine, and N-acetyl cysteine (NAC)
- glutamine
- glutathione

◆ sulfur (and foods high in sulfur, such as the cruciferous vegetables broccoli, cauliflower and cabbage, and beans, eggs, garlic and onions)

Other nutrients that support the liver include essential fatty acids (EFAs), and herbs such as dandelion and milk thistle (also called silymarin).

A critical point about liver support (and detoxification programs in general) must be mentioned. In order to do its job, the liver requires a particular ratio between dietary proteins and carbohydrates. Even if the carbohydrates are complex—for instance, made from whole grains instead of refined white flour—they are still starch, and capable of unbalancing the system. Fresh juice (a popular item during a cleanse) is another food that can easily unbalance the protein-carbohydrate relationship if it is high in sugars. Fruit juices have an obviously high sugar content and are therefore unacceptable (unless heavily diluted in water); but the sugar content of some vegetable juices such as carrot is equally high. Green grass drinks, popular due to their beneficially high chlorophyll content, are excellent for all phases of liver detoxification *provided they are low in sugar*. This means that wheatgrass, a cloyingly sweet grass drink, may not be the best choice during a detox program or fast. Sugars—whether naturally occurring or not—in a high enough concentration will tax the body. They will even prevent the detox process from taking place entirely.

"Protein deficiency states can often result in decreased liver detoxification of many drugs and other chemicals," Percival emphasizes. "Fasting, which involves protein restriction, can result in lowered detoxification ability and actually increase the potential for more active secondary toxins to be produced from the liver."[5] Without adequate proteins, carbohydrates interfere with the production of anti-inflammatory, immune-enhancing substances. And without these immune-enhancing chemicals, the body's increased production of inflammatory hormones causes pain and other undesirable symptoms. Too many carbohydrates also prevent certain liver enzymes from working properly.

Of course, people are different. A diet that works well for one person can have the opposite effect on another. However, a toxified individual needs to restrict carbohydrate intake. Be careful what you eat if you want to provide your liver with the optimal support. You cannot sweat out many toxins if the liver cannot break them down first.

Illness as a Detoxification Response

The study of perspiration can be viewed as a window into a much larger picture: the efficiency with which the body eliminates its waste materials. The efficiency of the waste removal system is generally a very reliable indicator of one's state of health. I explain detoxification in *The Handbook of Rife Frequency Healing*:

> [I]llness is the body's attempt to clear out toxic debris. For instance [in addition to raising the rate of metabolism and enzyme activity], fever is a strategy the body devises to literally "cook" to death microbes that cannot survive in high heat. Coughing is a natural reflex of the respiratory tract to expel germs that have become embedded in the mucous membrane lining of the lungs. The production of excess mucous itself is the body's way of trapping microbes and other debris that might otherwise seep into the bloodstream. A sore throat indicates that the lymph nodes in the neck are swollen from the extra white blood cells they have created to fight an infection somewhere in the body. Vomiting and diarrhea can be wonderful defenses of the body against poisons (whether from spoiled food or dangerous chemicals) that have gotten into the stomach and threaten the life of the organism. An eruption of hives, boils or a rash means that there is too much waste for the body to handle internally (such as through the urinary tract), and it must be removed through the skin. A sneeze is the body's way of trying to expel foreign particles (such as dust or pollen) that have migrated up through the nose, and so on. Thus, when people try to alleviate or altogether abolish "symptoms"—which are merely the body's ways of trying to eliminate what doesn't belong in it—too often they stop a process that (as long as the symptoms are not life-threatening) should have been allowed to finish. *When you prevent the body from doing its job—that is, when fevers, coughing, sore throat, vomiting, diarrhea, rashes, sneezing, etc. are unduly suppressed—many of the toxic waste materials remain.* If the waste materials happen to be living microbes, they may exist at what is called a "sub-clinical" level—too low to be detected

by standard allopathic tests, but nonetheless present in enough quantity to make a sensitive person feel unwell.[6]

When you use a detox technique such as sauna therapy to help you eliminate stored waste, you might feel ill, because your system is going through an elimination cycle all over again. In this sense, a detoxification response resembles an illness. This is why some people undergoing sauna therapy experience uncomfortable or painful symptoms such as the ones above, as well as diarrhea and/or constipation, disorientation, dizziness, exhaustion, headache, irritability, lethargy, runny nose, and muscle weakness. Old, noxious material is being pulled out of the fat cells and other tissue, and it's floating around in the bloodstream before being eliminated from the body.

Healing Crisis (Detox Response) Versus a Disease Crisis

If a detox response and a disease state feel similar, many people legitimately ask, what is the difference between the two? In *Nutritional Balancing and Hair Mineral Analysis*, Dr. Lawrence Wilson points out that with a healing crisis (detox response), old symptoms are often retraced, or felt all over again, indicating "an incompletely healed event....Healing reactions often produce unusual symptoms, such as a cold or sore throat but without fatigue."[7] In his experience, if a person following a particular dietary, supplement, and lifestyle change program feels better and more energized, and then suddenly does not feel well, this probably indicates a healing response. Naturopath Marian Porter observes that with a disease crisis, one's elimination processes are sluggish and incomplete; whereas with a healing crisis, elimination processes are greatly improved.

A *healing crisis* can be defined, then, as a state in which the body rids itself of accumulated waste and then revitalizes itself. A *disease crisis* can be defined as a state in which the body attempts to rid itself of accumulated waste, but because of extreme weakness, inefficiency, and/or too many poisons, is no longer able to revitalize itself. *The line between a detox and a disease response is crossed when the body can no longer eliminate poisons, and as a result begins to degenerate instead of regenerate.* Sometimes radical intervention is required, wherein the body is given substitutes for its own ability to function (drugs, surgery) until it can function on its own. *If, despite sauna therapy and the other protocols that you are doing, you continue to feel bad with no relief from your symptoms—or you feel worse and even more depleted—you may be experiencing a disease crisis and should see a qualified health care professional immediately.*

Interestingly, many of the herbs and spices that people use to cleanse—when used in large enough amounts—induce or increase perspiration. These include cayenne pepper, cinnamon, ginger, and peppermint. The essential oils of these plants, provided you are not allergic or chemically sensitive to them, can produce excellent results. Be sure to obtain good quality nutritional supplements, since nutritional deficiencies play a huge role in whether or not the body can absorb and assimilate food, and eliminate wastes.

DETOXIFICATION PROGRAMS

The L. Ron Hubbard Sweat Purification Program

Some of the most important research on eliminating systemic toxins was conducted by the late L. Ron Hubbard in conjunction with scientists from the United States Environmental Protection Agency (EPA). Unfortunately, Hubbard has received almost no recognition for his remarkable work with niacin in conjunction with the earliest publicized sauna therapy. For decades, this program helped thousands of people eliminate poisonous chemicals from their bodies. Niacin (also called nicotinic acid or Vitamin B-3) is known as the "flushing" vitamin because it causes the skin to redden or become flushed due to capillary enlargement and increased blood flow. It also makes the skin feel itchy and prickly. If people take high enough doses of B-3, they sometimes also feel nauseated, dizzy, disoriented, and even mentally unstable and volatile. For these reasons, niacinamide—a close relative chemically to niacin that does not cause skin flush or other symptoms—has become a popular substitute. However, it turns out that this "flushing" property unique to niacin is not only crucial to the detoxification process, but indicates that a detoxification process is actually occurring.

Hubbard's research on niacin, begun in 1950, explains how this detox process works. In *Clear Body, Clear Mind: The Effective Purification Program*, he wrote:

> Odd manifestations occurred when this vitamin [niacin] was administered to individuals. Its most startling effect was that it would turn on, in a red flush, a sunburn on the person's body in an exact pattern of a bathing suit! These were very neat patterns. The bathing suit outline was unmistakable.
>
> What kind of "educated vitamin" was this that caused bodies to turn on a flush exactly like a previous sunburn, showing the exact pattern of a bathing suit outline?[8]

Could it be, Hubbard wondered, that niacin in itself does not cause a flush, but instead *causes the body to start discharging old waste materials that had been stored in the fatty tissue?* What if these people were simply recovering from a prior case of sun poisoning, acquired from too much sunbathing while in a swim suit? The subjects in this research program took carefully controlled dosages of niacin. At a 200 mg. (milligram) dose, the "sunburnlike" flushes eventually disappeared, at which point the dose was increased to 500 mg. At a 500 mg. dose, the flushes recurred, but with less intensity, at which point the dose was increased to 1000 mg. (which equals one gram). At a 1000 mg. dose, there was a small reaction for several days, at which point the dose was increased, and so on. Finally, at a 2000 mg. dose, Hubbard reported, there were no more niacin flush "side" effects. "The person would feel fine, his 'sunburn' would be gone, and he would experience no more flush from the niacin."[9]

Both British and American pharmacopoeia agencies, Hubbard also pointed out, "advertised" that the niacin flush—presumably an intrinsic characteristic of the vitamin—is inherently negative to the body, and thus the vitamin is "toxic" in large amounts. "But if niacin was toxic," the author asked, "how was it that the more you 'overdosed' [on] it the sooner you no longer experienced the sunburnlike flushes from it?"[10] Those in orthodox medicine circles hypothesized that this was an example of the body's adjusting to unfavorable conditions by repressing the symptoms, and thus appearing asymptomatic. But this hypothesis was completely unsatisfactory, in view of the bathing suit outline on the test subjects!

Nevertheless, Hubbard's revealing evidence was mostly ignored by mainstream doctors and scientists. They didn't consider Hubbard qualified to do research, regardless of how carefully he designed his experiments or how coherent and rational his observations were.

Six years later, Hubbard had the opportunity to gather even more compelling data when working with subjects who had been exposed to fallout from atomic bomb tests, atomic accidents, and materials that had been part of an old atomic bomb explosion. "In 1956," he wrote, "niacin was reacting differently on people than it had in 1950, and the effects were more severe."

> People on the research program in 1950 had experienced only past sunburn flushes. In 1956, people on the research program, while experiencing a flush, were also experiencing nausea, skin irritations, hives, colitis and other uncomfortable manifestations, on the same vitamin and in the same dosages as had been used in 1950.[11]

One highly significant detail is that some of the same people participated in both Hubbard's earlier and later research. What had changed? Only the newly developed health problems the subjects brought with them to the second research project! The first group of research subjects, who needed to recover from sun poisoning, developed symptoms uniquely related to sun exposure. The second group manifested symptoms specific to atomic radiation poisoning (as well as more symptoms in general) because they had been exposed to nuclear waste. Hubbard's explanation 50 years ago was convincing then, and seems equally convincing today—that niacin is an effective and powerful catalyst that induces the body's detoxification response without itself becoming transformed in the change. Niacin's use in sauna therapy is also a wonderful choice because its dilation of surface blood vessels allows heat to escape.

Then in 1977, Hubbard noticed many young people who had smoked marijuana, taken LSD (lysergic acid diethylamide), and/or been addicted to narcotics, and now wanted to quit. So he devised his Sweat Purification Program to help them eliminate their drug cravings. His program, administered under the supervision of medical doctors, consisted of controlled, escalating doses of niacin, along with other vitamin and mineral supplements whose amounts were based on need *but were also proportional to the amount of niacin taken*, as the extra niacin could unbalance the system. (The B-vitamins must always be in the correct ratio to each other; otherwise, deficiency diseases can result.) Hubbard also insisted on exercise in the form of running to stimulate the circulation; sauna therapy; sufficient water to replace the fluids lost through sweating; plenty of fresh vegetables, both raw and very lightly cooked; and adequate restful sleep, eight hours a night average. Most people took two to three weeks to complete the Sweat Program, although some required a longer period of time. For those who were very ill, frail or in poor physical condition, to prevent overexertion Hubbard advised a gradual increase in the amount of time they exercised, and a gradual increase of their sauna time as well. The sauna therapy and exercise were coordinated in one five-hour period daily, consisting of 4 to 4½ hours of sauna therapy for every 20 to 30 minutes of running. The ratio was important, Hubbard wrote. "The bulk of the period is best spent in the sauna after the circulation has been worked up by running. In other words, the five-hour period is *not* 50 percent exercising and 50 percent sauna. The program gives best results with a much lower percentage of time exercising and a much higher percentage in the sauna."[12] Interestingly, Hubbard reported that a dry rather than a wet sauna "proved to be the most successful in inducing profuse sweating in most people"—although he freely acknowledged that since people's responses to sauna therapy are very individual, "there is no regulation on the program that outlaws the use of a wet sauna…the whole idea is to use the system which permits the person to sweat the most."[13] People left the sauna periodically to cool off for five or 10 minutes.

Here is Hubbard's report on what happened to the drug addicts who took niacin:

> Taken in sufficient quantities, niacin appears to break up and unleash LSD, marijuana and other drugs and poisons from the tissues and cells. It can rapidly release LSD crystals into the system and send a person who has taken LSD on a "trip." (One fellow who had done the earlier Sweat Program for a period of months, and who believed he had no more LSD in his system, took 100 milligrams of niacin and promptly turned on a restimulation of a full-blown LSD experience.)[14]

The ability of fatty tissue to store, for an unlimited time period, either the original intact poison or its incompletely processed metabolites, explains the re-occurrence of symptoms that drug users experience. Since fat cells tend to get replaced rather slowly in the system compared to other components (such as muscle or red blood cells), toxins can remain dormant for years or even decades. Once the fat cells do get broken down, they quickly release the stored drugs and/or their metabolites back into the bloodstream. The materials are now free to travel to all of the body's cells—including the brain—where (depending on their chemical makeup and degree of breakdown) they can *re-stimulate the same receptor sites as if the person had just taken the drug.* This is why even people who stopped taking drugs years ago might experience flashbacks now of past drug trips. This is also why drug levels in blood and urine—levels that may have been minimal or even non-existent—suddenly increase during a detox program before lessening and finally vanishing. Finally, this explains why people on a drug detox program often feel a sudden, fresh craving for the drug: the chemicals have been liberated from fat cells and are circulating throughout the bloodstream, free to latch on to any convenient receptor site. As the toxins are completely eliminated from the body, the residual drugs in the blood and urine, and the person's cravings and flashbacks, disappear at last.

Hubbard was very aware of how a detoxification program for drug and other substances worked, so he was not troubled by sudden increases of symptoms. In fact, he welcomed them, since this meant that his subjects were finally clearing harmful substances from their bodies. It was often necessary to remind people not to be concerned about symptoms as long as they were following the protocol; the body was in a healing crisis rather than a disease crisis. Niacin, Hubbard emphasized, "apparently does not do anything by itself. It is simply interacting with niacin deficiencies which already exist in the cellular structure. It doesn't turn on [cause] allergies; it appears to run out [eliminate] allergies." However, taking niacin is not without its risks. The symptoms that result from taking niacin can be quite horrifying. Hubbard described seeing a "full-blown" case of skin cancer appear in someone who took high enough dosages. Apparently the condition was latent in the body, and was thus able to be "turned on." "If that should happen," Hubbard advised, "the handling [of the condition], by observable fact, has been to continue the niacin until the skin cancer has run out [run its course] completely."[15]

Allowing the body to completely eliminate its poisons is important for the success of any detox program. It is tempting to want to stop the process—if indeed it can be stopped—particularly if you are experiencing many and varied symptoms that are uncomfortable and even scary. However, if you are truly undergoing a detoxification response, *keep going* until the symptoms subside. You might be able to slow down the rate of elimination—after all, the goal is to cleanse, not suffer. Or, you might be able to speed up the response. But if you try to stop it permanently, without addressing the waste products that are still in your body, you will eventually suffer from their presence. Fortunately, sweating is an easy and efficient way to detoxify with a minimum of stress. In fact, sauna therapy is desirable *because* the act of perspiring relieves the detox burden from so many systems in the body.

Another potential problem with a detox program, which Hubbard articulated quite clearly, is that imbalances of the body could be misinterpreted as effects of the sauna therapy itself—a common mistake made by laypersons and health care practitioners alike. This is why you might want to learn as much as possible about sauna therapy (as with any health protocol you are using). The better informed you are, the better prepared you are for any kind of reaction.

Be aware, too, that during a detox program the body can become unbalanced due to the lack of proper support—be it dietary, emotional, or other. This is usually how the person got sick in the first place. Hubbard addressed the nutritional aspect. "What could slow down the Purification Program, and make it appear incomplete would be a nutritional failure—a failure to flank the niacin on either side by sufficient amounts of the other needed vitamins and minerals in proportion, and a failure to provide food intake which included vegetables (with their vitamin and mineral content) and oil."[16] (Oils will be discussed in the following paragraph.) Again—and this cannot be emphasized enough—it is imperative to take other vitamins along with the niacin, especially all of the B-complex, since flooding the system with some B vitamins while omitting others can produce severe conditions due to deficiencies. In the journal *Medical Hypotheses*, D. W. Schnare and colleagues write that "the reported side effects of niacin may actually be the creation of other vitamin and mineral imbalances…*as negative side effects were not noted when correct proportions were administered.*"[17] [emphasis added]

David Root, David Katzin, and David Schnare explain why consuming oil is an important part of Hubbard's program. Ordinarily, "as the fat-soluble toxic chemicals are released into the bloodstream [from various tissues in the body], many of them are carried to the gut where they are released intraluminally" (in other words, they pass from the bloodstream back through the intestinal wall into the small intestine). "There, they are reabsorbed into the lipophilic [fat-loving] bile acids and recirculated back through the liver." (A cluster of veins runs directly from the small intestine to the liver; their purpose is to deliver the contaminated contents of the intestine to the liver for cleaning before the stuff is then discharged back into the bloodstream.) However, in many people, the liver is already toxified and overextended with its cleanup jobs. "The polyunsaturated oil," the authors explain, "tends to retard this recirculation effect and allow[s] the toxic substances to be [directly] excreted through the colon."[18] The extra large amount of oil consumed at one time (between two and eight tablespoons)—too much for the body to digest and use as food—instead binds to the toxins that are lipid-soluble and leaves straight through the colon. The liver, bypassed entirely in this process, is thus prevented from becoming even more toxified. Since there are still plenty of toxins circulating through the bloodstream, this precaution is a sensible one.

A blend of ordinary heat-processed vegetable oils were fed to Hubbard's detox subjects. Heating oils at high temperatures—the manner in which most vegetable oils are produced—creates free radicals and other harmful substances. Today, given our knowledge of the dangers of heat-processed fats, more healthful oils such as *cold*-processed coconut and olive are often substituted, just in case any of the oils happen to be absorbed by the body. (Krohn and Taylor point out in *Natural Detoxification* [2nd ed.] that the body "exchanges" flaxseed, evening primrose, and black currant seed oils "for contaminated fat, which is eliminated through bile excretion and feces."[19] The first edition of the book advises that people known as slow oxidizers, who lose weight slowly, do better with evening primrose oil. For an excellent source of information about fats, see Mary Enig's *Know Your Fats: The Complete Primer for Understanding the Nutrition of Fats*.)

Hubbard, and the later practitioners who administered his program, are said to have worked with 100,000 drug addicts. The results are impressive. A number of reports on Hubbard's detoxification program, authored by medical specialists with impressive credentials, have been published since the mid 1980s. In Chapter 3, I discussed successful clinical trials conducted with police officers who, through their handling of confiscated drugs such as PCP, developed symptoms of drug abuse because the substances had gotten into their bodies through inhalation. These sweating programs used the Hubbard method. Other studies have been done with people who were detoxified from chlorinated pesticides and herbicides, PCBs, and radiation (due to exposure during a nuclear reactor accident in Chernobyl in 1986). Vietnam veterans exposed to Agent Orange (a nasty chemical used to defoliate the vegetation in the Vietnamese jungles to make the enemy more visible) were also detoxification research subjects.

As was also mentioned in Chapter 3, a study of Hubbard's protocol was conducted on Michigan residents who had been heavily exposed in the early 1970s to the fire-retardant chemical PBB (polybrominated biphenyl). Dr. Max Ben gives an account of this study in *National Safety News*.

> The fire-retardant was accidentally substituted in place of a nutritional supplement for farm animals. The contamination of meat, milk, and a variety of other foods resulted in the ingestion of the chemical by virtually the entire population of Michigan... [In this study] participants were first extensively tested to determine the levels of PBB, PCBs, and other toxic substances in their bodies....The toxic levels were established by quantitative analysis of adipose tissue (fat) samples, using solvent extraction and gas chromatography/mass spectrometry....Following the completion of the prescribed *Hubbard Regimen*, the participants were again tested. Dr. David Schnare, a policy analyst for the U.S. Environmental Protection Agency, who took part in the Michigan study, stated that the Hubbard program brought about an immediate average reduction in approximately 20 per cent of all 16 chemicals studied.

Even more significant, however, were the results of a four-month follow-up examination that revealed an average reduction of more than 40 per cent for all chemicals. Dr. David Katzin, medical director at a Los Angeles clinic, which delivers the Hubbard program, stated that the follow up analysis "might possibly indicate that the *Hubbard Regimen* rehabilitates a natural mechanism for the elimination of toxins from the body."[20]

One of the most recent—and equally relevant—reports on the Hubbard program comes from Dr. David Root. Root, a retired colonel from the United States Air Force, is a physician with a background in occupational medicine and Public Health. On November 20, 1998, Dr. Root presented a "Statement Before the Presidential Special Oversight Board for Department of Defense Investigations of Gulf War Chemical and Biological Incidents."

> Since 1982, I have been using a detoxification program to treat patients who have been exposed to fat-soluble chemicals, either at work or from environmental sources. This program, developed by L. Ron Hubbard in 1978, has over the last 15 years been evaluated and used by a growing number of professionals throughout the world who have examined its use in relieving the aftereffects of chemical exposure and found it to be very effective. To my knowledge, there is no other peer-reviewed method for reducing the body burden of fat-soluble toxic chemicals. Papers documenting the efficacy of the Hubbard program have been published by such organizations as the World Health Organization, the Royal Swedish Academy of Science, the Society for Occupational and Environmental Health and others....The Hubbard detoxification program has [even] long been upheld as compensable under state and national workman's compensation laws.[21]

Despite resistance from the mainstream medical establishment, a growing number of enlightened doctors, naturopaths, orthomolecular physicians, and other health care providers are offering detoxification programs that include not only niacin, but other substances that have proven track records in helping many people feel better. One popular method, called *chelation therapy*, consists of the oral or intravenous administration of vitamins, minerals, herbs and other substances that bind to toxic metals in the body so that they can be "escorted" out through the urine or sweat. Intravenous chelation can be expensive; a complete round costs anywhere from $2000 to $2500 (although surgery or continuous doctor visits can be a lot more pricey—and much less effective).

Oral chelation agents, which cost far less, include food grade diatomaceous earth in capsules; DMSA (dimercaptosuccinic acid, which is sold both as a supplement and as a drug); specially processed chlorella in tincture form; and the herb cilantro. So far, the chlorella (with its cell walls broken down for easy absorption) and cilantro are showing the most promise in easily and successfully removing mercury from the brain. (Make sure the cilantro is grown in nontoxic soil; otherwise, it absorbs the heavy metals from the dirt, and people eating it then ingest heavy metals along with the plant.)

Of all the substances that can be used for detoxification, niacin may be an underutilized choice. There are several advantages to using this vitamin: even the synthetic form works well, it is inexpensive, you always have a barometer of what's going on in your system, and you can adjust the dose accordingly. A motivated and informed layperson might conceivably put himself or herself on an abbreviated version of Hubbard's demanding regimen. However, if you have a serious or chronically unmanageable health condition, you should seek supervision from a qualified health care practitioner. Appendix B lists doctors who offer sauna therapy. Of those, a few work with the Hubbard program.

Several doctors who use sauna therapy in their practice consented to be interviewed for this book. Below are some highlights of their detoxifying protocols.

The HealthMed and Narconon Detox Programs

Hubbard's Sweat Purification Program is used exclusively at Dr. David Root's HealthMed clinics on the east and west coasts of the United States (California and New York state), and at Narconon, which has drug detoxification centers in the United States and abroad.

Dr. Root—who has co-authored some of the groundbreaking studies (mentioned throughout this book) of the chemicals in people's sweat and body tissues—uses the Hubbard program at his health centers because, he says, it is the most effective detoxification method he has ever found. The procedure is simple but elegant:

- Each day the program begins with the participant taking a single dose of 100 mg. of niacin. The amount gradually increases, so that by the end of the two or three week period, the client can tolerate considerably more. The final niacin intake might be one gram. In some instances, up to five grams can be ingested without much discomfort.

- The client is weighed. During the sauna therapy time, as much water is drunk as desired. At the end of the day, the client is weighed again. If his or her weight varies by more than one-quarter pound, the client drinks more water to make up for the difference. Possible weight loss from a decrease in fat is not part of the equation here. It is assumed that virtually all decrease in weight is due to water loss.

- The client aerobically exercises for a period ranging from 20 to 30 minutes, according to ability and comfort level, to increase the heart rate. The ratio of exercise to sauna is 20 to 30 minutes of exercise for every 4 to 4½ hours of sauna time.

- The client then enters a sauna for about 20 minutes; although this time period can vary between as low as 15 minutes and as high as (but not to exceed) 30 minutes. After working up a copious sweat, the client exits the sauna for about five or 10 minutes to shower, and again enters the sauna. This cycle is repeated five to seven times over the course of a five-hour daily program.

- Everyone takes mineral salts (including sodium and potassium), and vitamin supplements (including vitamins A, B-complex, C, and D). Dosages vary according to the level of niacin the client is taking. The higher the level of niacin taken, the more one must replace other B-vitamins, as excesses of one B-vitamin alongside lower levels of other B-vitamins will unbalance the system and cause nutritional deficiency symptoms. (Incidentally—and this is an important point—Krohn, Taylor, and Prosser write that not only do drugs and toxins by themselves create nutritional deficiencies, but since "drug and chemical residues persist in the body for a long time, they can continue to deplete these vitamins while stored."[22])

- Two to eight tablespoons of blended vegetable oils are ingested once daily—either at the end of the sauna treatment, or up to within a few hours after the sauna is taken. A typical oil blend might be cold-pressed soy, walnut, peanut, and safflower, with lecithin added.

● Besides the above, an essential aspect of this protocol is adequate sleep.

Dr. Root uses an all-tile sauna room, about 8 feet x 14 feet, well ventilated at the top, with two tiers of benches and a dry convection heater reaching temperatures between 140°F (60°C) and 180°F (82.2°C). As noted in Chapter 5, Root's experience with wooden saunas—even the hardier, aromatic woods—is that they rot after a few years due to the amount of waste excreted through the sweat and the necessary daily cleaning with water. Tile is one of the few materials that does not succumb to rot or mold. It is also easy to clean. Over the long periods of time that the client is in the sauna, Dr. Root reports, the amounts of toxins leaving through the skin will sometimes be so high that the towels will turn black. An adult male generally sweats out four or five quarts per day on the program, and an adult woman sweats out about three or four quarts. When required by court order, urine drug screens are performed on drug abuse clients on a weekly basis during treatment, and at court-ordered intervals after treatment. Sometimes, drugs are detected after the program has begun. Since the clients are no longer taking drugs, it is clear that any drugs in the urine had been stored in the fat and remained undetected until coaxed from the tissues.

A surprising array of illnesses respond positively to sauna therapy—conditions that one might not initially associate with external toxins at all. "Of the three people with multiple sclerosis whom we've treated," Root recalls, "two had been exposed to chemicals. These two experienced a significant reduction of their symptoms after going through the detox program, indicating to me that some cases of MS may be initiated by chemical exposure."[23]

Do people often get severe detoxification responses while they are purging their system of poisons? Some possible reactions, Dr. Root notes, initially can seem alarming—loss of memory and balance, impaired cognitive ability, irritability, even stuttering—but, *as long as the client remains in the sauna to continue the sweat,* these symptoms leave after about a half hour. Sometimes the reactions can be very strong, but they leave rapidly. This suggests both the far-reaching effects of chemicals and the efficacy of sweating as a cleansing protocol. (Not all people on cleansing programs pass through their detox symptom phase so quickly, though. The speed with which HealthMed clients cycle through their detox crisis may be due to the intensity of the Hubbard program, the long periods of time that they remain in the sauna, and the nutritional support that they receive.) The few cases Dr. Root will not treat are pregnant women (because of the increased hazard to the fetus); people who are currently taking psychotropic drugs (since they require specialized supervised care); and people who are on prescription drugs with narrow therapeutic ranges, such as anti-epileptic medicine (critical to one's health) or steroids for lupus (steroids block the niacin-related dilation of blood vessels).

Narconon's drug detoxification centers (which, unlike HealthMed, are affiliated with the Scientology organization) also follow the Hubbard protocol. These centers do not admit people who have taken certain prescription drugs. Instead, prescription drug users are sent to facilities that are more medically oriented because some of these drugs can be very dangerous and cause serious medical problems when exiting the body. For instance, sudden withdrawal or a radical change in the dosage of some psychotropic medications can cause personality shifts and seizures. Drug addictions are treated as physiological rather than psychological cravings. In lieu of psychotherapy, the participants are given lessons in "life skills"—which is why the clients are never referred to as "patients" (which in the allopathic medical model denotes diseased people)—but rather, "students." They are literally being re-educated to live without drugs.

No matter where the Hubbard program is administered, the success rate is documented as high. Dr. Root observes that a significant 72% to 75% of the participants remain drug-free, as evidenced by follow-up reports over a period of five years.

The Environmental Health Center Detox Program

Dr. William Rea's protocol is well known in holistic circles. Once a conventional doctor (his training was in cardiovascular diseases and general surgery), Rea became ill with multiple chemical sensitivity. After finding no relief from allopathic medicine, he underwent a holistic detoxification program. It was so successful that he changed his professional focus to natural medicine, establishing the world-renowned Environmental Health Center in Dallas, Texas. For 25 years, Rea has helped over 40,000 people with environmental illness and multiple chemical sensitivity, lupus, neurotoxicity, cardiac problems, and cancer, among other conditions. About 10 years ago, Rea and his colleagues began using saunas, both Swedish (hot air) and far infrared. Made of wood, glass and ceramic, the saunas emit temperatures varying from 120°F to over 160°F (48.9°C to over 71.1°C). Different people have an affinity for different types of saunas, Rea notes. The success of one type of sauna over another depends on the unique characteristics of the person, *not* the illness.

Although sauna manufacturers customarily give a list of conditions that contraindicate sauna use (probably to avoid possible liability), Rea has discovered that, with adequate medical supervision, almost everyone can and does benefit from sauna therapy. Multiple sclerosis (discussed in Chapter 6) is a good example. Most doctors unfamiliar with sauna therapy categorically claim that body heating is dangerous for people with MS because typically, the sweating mechanism is damaged. However, if the temperature inside the sauna is increased gradually, people with MS can *learn* to sweat and thus have a successful therapeutic sauna experience. Their symptoms will actually go into remission as the environmental toxin load is lessened and the immune function is strengthened. People with a history of seizures can also use the sauna, as long as they are closely supervised. Likewise, for Rea, cardiac problems are not necessarily a deterrent. The only people who absolutely should not use the sauna, he says, are those who have suffered damage to their brain's thermostatic control. Incidentally, Rea believes that people should not use the sauna, alone and unsupervised, without first being tested and monitored in a physician's office. However, his caution may be explained by the fact that he tends to see clients who have not been helped by other modalities and come to him only after they are seriously ill.

I find it significant that Rea uses niacin in his detoxification programs. "Twenty-five to thirty percent of chemically sensitive individuals are deficient in [vitamin] B$_3$," he observes. A niacin deficiency can cause a host of symptoms such as canker sores and dermatitis, indigestion and nausea, depression and memory impairment, headaches and insomnia, limb pain and inflammation—and a "failure to detoxify xenobiotics [substances foreign to the body] effectively"! For those who cannot absorb niacin by mouth, Dr. Rea provides preservative-free niacin injections daily, which he says severely chemically sensitive people require "to function optimally." Fortunately, "Niacin supplementation has a wide margin of safety." Even oral administration of six grams of niacin per day "has not produced any toxic manifestations."[24] Considering that the average American diet is highly deficient in niacin—and considering the increased levels of toxic chemicals in our food, water, air, personal care items, and household cleaners—the range and number of symptoms associated with a Vitamin B_3 deficiency is not surprising.

The Battle Creek Lifestyle Health Center Detox Program

The Battle Creek Lifestyle Health Center, a faithful descendent of Dr. Kellogg's first clinic, emphasizes the principles of clean air, pure water, and healthful food. Various forms of hydrotherapy and other detoxification methods are used. The staff also helps clients to improve their lifestyle so they can avoid recurrence of illness in the future. Among the customized supplements that are given is bovine colostrum, the thin watery fluid secreted by a nursing mammal for about 48 hours before the actual milk flows. Colostrum is popular because it contains transfer factor, the ingredient that stimulates the production of more efficient, and more of, "killer" white blood cells that devour biological toxins. Since transfer factor is present in all colostrum—whether the nursing mammal is a cow, goat, sheep, or human—this highly effective support of the body's immune response crosses the species barrier. (Some people are allergic or otherwise reactive to the milk proteins in colostrum. Concentrated transfer factor alone is available as a supplement, listed in Appendix B.)

Many of Battle Creek's clientele are afflicted with heavy metal toxicity—especially from mercury, due to the preponderance of silver-mercury amalgam used to fill dental cavities. Others have asthma, autoimmune conditions such as lupus, coronary diseases, diabetes, obesity, and psoriasis.

The two staff doctors—Bruce Hyde and Jeff Gates—both feel that a variety of saunas can make a detoxification program successful. As each person is unique, there are individual responses to different methods of inducing sweat. Some clients find a method and stay with it. Others switch from one method to another until they find what most supports them, given their particular condition at the time. The center regularly uses several of Dr. Kellogg's original electric light baths, which are in excellent, operational condition. Steam cabinets are also used, some of which are equipped with ozone (particularly helpful for infections and wounds). In the doctors' experience, FIR rooms should be avoided not only by people with implants, but also those with dental fillings—as there have been some reports that the deeply penetrating FIR can loosen adhesive that bonds a filling to a tooth. (A far infrared cabinet does not pose this problem, as the head remains exposed to fresh air.) At Battle Creek, it usually takes between five and seven sauna sessions to achieve an optimal immune response in the body.

The center's long history of hydrotherapy has continued into the present. The staff alternates hot and cold treatments. Sometimes the heat is dispensed as a hot water foot bath. Other times, with the client lying on a massage table, hot fomentation packs (to stimulate blood flow) are placed along the spine or across the abdomen and topped with towels, and the entire body is then covered with a sheet. The alternation of heat and cold (five minutes of each, in continuous cycles) creates a pumping action, Hyde remarks, which dramatically improves circulation and immune response. Heat draws white blood cells to wherever it is applied, and cold stimulates the white blood cells to recirculate.

Another deceptively simple procedure is an activated charcoal and ground flax seed poultice. The charcoal draws toxins out through the skin that sauna sessions might not elicit if the client does not sweat for long enough periods of time. Equal parts of charcoal and flax seeds are mixed with enough water to make a slurry, or runny paste. (Flax seeds are used because they absorb and hold water.) The mixture is then wrapped in cloth, with the permeable side touching the skin, and the client lies down with the poultice, often overnight. "It's a little messy," Dr. Hyde volunteers, "but there's a remarkably high record of compliance. These poultices are extremely effective." A major focus of all these natural treatments is to stimulate blood flow. "Perfect health requires perfect circulation," is an unofficial motto at Battle Creek Lifestyle Health Center.

SpiritMed: Additional Protocols

Dr. Walter Crinnion, a naturopath with a background in environmental medicine, has extensive experience in treating his clients with sauna therapy. Today, Crinnion teaches other health care professionals how to recognize and deal with toxic overload, and how to use the sauna as part of a general wellness program. He emphasizes that people who are seriously chemically overloaded should *not* begin sauna sessions right away, because it causes the toxins stored in the tissues to be dumped into the bloodstream with no reliable outlet. "If you haven't worked with the client's exit routes, the person gets worse," he warns. "With chemically sensitive individuals, you must make sure that their stool is flowing properly and they're having more than one bowel movement a day."[25] Consequently, two other protocols that Dr. Crinnion sees as essential before allowing sick people to enter the sauna are colon irrigation (colonics) and hydrotherapy.

Colon irrigation removes impacted fecal material from the walls of the colon and helps restore the motility of the large intestine. As described in *The Handbook of Rife Frequency Healing*:

> The person lies down on a table and a trained professional, using special equipment, gently places a tube up past the anal muscle into the rectum. This allows the water to flow into the descending colon, across the transverse colon (horizontal at the belly button), and around through the ascending colon as much as comfort will allow. When the abdominal area gets too full, the water leaves through the tube, out through another attachment into the building's plumbing system. Colonics allow water to pass high into the colon….To help expedite the passing of waste, the colon therapist should massage the belly and the outside of the thighs (which contain reflex points for the colon and thus stimulate peristaltic activity)...exotic strings of mucous, unbelievable lengths of once-impacted fecal material, and even whole worms [can be] expelled by this method.[26]

If a colonic does not bring immediate improvement, this may indicate that the liver is too impaired to handle the overload of toxins quickly enough. In such cases, liver support protocols are advisable.

The hydrotherapy procedure that Crinnion recommends consists of alternately placing hot and cold packs on the person's back. The therapy is administered not only on the days preceding sauna therapy, but on the days after as well. This increases the body's ability to heal itself by stimulating the dumping of toxins from the blood into the large intestine. Once the toxic material is in the intestine, it can be evacuated. At this point, another colonic irrigation is indicated to help prevent the toxins from being released through the intestinal wall back into the bloodstream.

Dr. Crinnion has also found that three one-hour sessions of low-temperature saunas are better tolerated—and do more for the client—than fewer sessions that are longer and hotter.

Hyperthermia at Integrated Medical Specialists

Sometimes, a serious illness such as cancer requires *hyperthermia*, a body heating method that is much more strenuous than sauna therapy and requires medical supervision (see Chapter 2). At Integrated Medical Specialists in Stockbridge, Georgia, Dr. T. R. Shantha often uses hyperthermia for people with cancer. "We use anything and everything that works," he says, "and which has a scientific basis to it"—so it is not unusual for allopathic drugs to be combined with complementary medicine. Those who need intensive-care treatment stay in a hotel close to the facility and visit the clinic five days a week.

"Body temperature," summarizes Shantha, "can be increased by exposing the person to far infrared rays, putting the person in an enclosed room heated by hot stones, or putting the person in a room filled with steam. Sauna therapy incorporates these three methods. You can also immerse the person in hot water, or parts of the body in heated wax. Finally, you can take the blood out of the body, heat it, and put it back. This last method is known as whole body hyperthermia by extra corporal circulation." He adds that the body can also be heated "by subjecting it to sonic sound (ultrasound), or to electromagnetic energy from radio frequencies or microwaves." Although Dr. Shantha sometimes applies radio frequencies and microwaves locally to destroy tissue or eliminate chronic pain, he generally does not recommend these methods or ultrasound for body heating, since there is no proof of their short– or long–term safety—and in fact, evidence suggests that they are harmful.

One specialty of the clinic is two-cycle Insulin Potentiation Therapy (IPT), originated by the late Dr. Donato Perez Garcia and further developed by Dr. Shantha. The therapy is based on the fact that cancer cells have about 10 times more insulin receptors than do healthy cells. Therefore, when the insulin is administered intravenously, it is absorbed mostly by abnormal cancerous tissue instead of normal body tissue. The insulin acts not only as a carrier but also as a fortifier, augmenting the effects of whatever is being transported with it into the cell—in this case, chemicals that destroy cancerous tissue. "When insulin is used," Shantha explains, "there are very few, if any, toxic reactions to chemotherapy. Since the cancerous cells are much more receptive than the healthy cells to the chemo, we can use small doses." Normally, insulin is produced by the pancreas to escort sugars that are in the bloodstream into the cells to give them energy. During the course of a successful treatment, the atypically high amount of insulin drives so much glucose into the body cells that the blood glucose plummets to abnormally low levels. Therefore, Insulin Potentiation Therapy requires a skilled, highly trained physician who will monitor the subject carefully and continually, raising the blood glucose levels as soon as the treatment is finished. Sometimes, instead of conventional allopathic drugs, Dr. Shantha uses a potentized version of an Austrian herb called Ukraine (familiar to European doctors) to kill the cancer.

Heating the body makes IPT even more effective. For deep-seated cancers, far infrared is utilized, with temperatures ranging from 99°F to 104° F (37.2°C to 40° C). For tumors that can be seen with the eyes and palpated with the fingers, local hyperthermia is administered. The clinic has a special hot pack fueled by a water heater, which can stay hot indefinitely. Other kinds of hot and cold packs, colonics, homeopathy, and additional therapies are also used at Integrated Medical Specialists.

Now that you have read about some detoxification protocols that people find helpful, I will conclude with some practical suggestions on how to stay well, inside and outside the sauna.

GUIDELINES FOR STAYING WELL

During sauna therapy—or at any other time—the following procedures will help you optimally nourish yourself on a physical level so you can remain healthy:

1. *Drink pure, uncontaminated water with a pH of at least 7.0.*

Have your water tested periodically to make sure it is free of the carcinogens chlorine, PCBs, dioxin, and other toxic chemicals; lead and other heavy metals; pesticides; and pathogenic microbes. Use a good quality filter. There are several different types of water purification systems that use charcoal, coconut shell, steam, and other methods of cleaning the water.

You also need to make sure that the water has a pH of at least 7.0, preferably higher. A reading below the neutral 7.0 indicates that the water pH is acidic. A reading above 7.0 indicates that the water pH is alkaline. Drops to test the pH of your water (more reliable than paper test strips), used for aquariums, are available at pet stores. If your water is acidic—or if you have alkaline water that you want to make even more alkaline—consider buying a water electrolysis unit (see the "Products" section in Appendix B). Most people's systems are too acidic. If you change only one thing in your health protocol, drink alkaline water. Over time, you will experience a positive shift in your health.

2. *Eat clean, whole, fresh, unprocessed food.*

This means that vegetables, fruits, legumes, and grains are organically grown without synthetic chemical pesticides—unless you can buy from a farmer you trust (not all farmers who grow clean food can afford to pay to have it certified organic). Animals should be raised without antibiotics or hormones. Grass-fed beef and lamb, and free-range pork, poultry and eggs are ideal, since these conditions are the best and most natural for the animal. Under no circumstances should your food be genetically engineered! Avoid refined carbohydrates (white sugar or white flours); chemicals such as MSG (monosodium glutamate) and other flavorings; preservatives such as sodium nitrate or potassium nitrite; and artificial sweeteners like Aspartame (which can cause neurological disorders). These are all fake foods, not only devoid of nutrition but outright harmful. For more information, see *Nourishing Traditions* and *The Handbook of Rife Frequency Healing* (see Bibliography).

3. *Eliminate toxic chemicals from your environment.*

Most of the cleaning products available today contain poisonous chemicals such as alcohols, detergents (like sodium laurel sulfate), dyes, heavy metals, petrochemicals, solvents, and volatile organic compounds. (The word *organic* is used differently in this context than when describing safe food; here it refers to compounds containing carbon.) Most personal care products also contain harmful ingredients. Clothing should be made of natural fibers, as synthetics such as polyester and nylon do not allow the skin to breathe. The furniture, carpets, and drapes in your home may be emitting fumes from chemicals such as formaldehyde. Vaccines are dangerous because they contain poisonous mercury derivatives and unnaturally altered biological materials against which the body has no evolutionary history for developing a defense. So-called silver fillings used by dentists contain mercury; ask for other types instead. In today's world it is impossible not to have chemicals in your bloodstream, but at least you don't have to add to the toxic load in your home and on your body. See Debra Lynn Dadd's *Home Safe Home: Protecting Yourself and Your Family from Everyday Toxics and Harmful Household Products* (see Bibliography) for more information and solutions to the problem of chemicals in household furnishings.

4. *Avoid overloading your environment with electromagnetic pollution.*

Many researchers (including Becker, Brodeur, Levitt, and Smith and Best; see Bibliography) have proven that the wrong kind of electromagnetic radiation can deplete the body's immune function and even directly cause illnesses including cancer and leukemia. Do not sleep next to an electrical socket. Even if an appliance is turned off, electricity is still running through the wires in the wall. Whenever possible, use appliances that are properly shielded to eliminate harmful electromagnetic fields. As more consumers request such products, manufacturers will start making them.

5. *Breathe fresh air.*

Much of the air we breathe, especially in large cities, is now heavily polluted with hydrocarbons and other synthetic chemicals. Running a good quality air filter and/or ozone generator in your home—and in your car too—can make a huge difference in your health. Some essential oils (eucalyptus, lavender, lemon, peppermint) put into an aromatherapy diffuser or vaporizer can also help freshen and decontaminate indoor air. (See the "Products" section in Appendix B for sources of air purification units and essential oils.)

6. *Get enough sunshine.*

Due to the increasing number of breaches in the upper atmosphere's ozone layer (which ordinarily prevents some of the most harmful ultraviolet rays from reaching us), sunlight in some places is now harsh, and people are getting burned in ways they haven't been burned before. Nevertheless, a moderate amount of sunlight is still healing. Humans thrive under the numerous beneficial electromagnetic rays of the sun, and we need to maintain our connection to this nourishment. Sunlight also helps the skin manufacture Vitamin D_3, a nutrient.

7. *Get enough exercise.*

The amount and type of exercise you need depends on your level of health, body type, and constitution. Some people enjoy, and are more suited to, a heavy aerobic workout, while others do better with gentler movement or stretching. But whatever type of exercise you like, try to do it every day. Even a simple 20- or 30-minute walk four times a week can help keep your bones dense and circulate the lymph. A special small circular trampoline that is easy on the joints can give you an excellent workout in your own home. (For more information, see the "Products" section in Appendix B.)

8. *Get enough sleep.*

Lying down is the position that most minimizes the stressful effects of gravity on the body. Eight hours per night is the amount of sleep that most people need, although some people can function on less and some need more. Darken the room as much as possible; this will help you sleep. The pineal gland produces the bulk of its sleep-inducing melatonin in the absence of light. It is a mistake to think that you're not doing anything during this valuable period. The body repairs itself when you sleep. The brain also processes new material that you have learned, and transfers the information from short-term to long-term memory cells.

9. *Maintain a positive outlook while living as holistically as you can.*

Studies show that the body's immune response operates much more efficiently when people truly release their negative thoughts and emotions, focus on their blessings, and enjoy compassionate, supportive relationships filled with understanding and humor. There is a world of difference between the negative concept "a glass that is half empty," and the positive concept "a glass that is half full." When you read, say or think about these two phrases, observe how they look and sound, and how they feel in your body. Do you feel hollow, or satiated? The emptiness creates a contraction that is fear, and the fullness creates an expansion that is love.

As a healing modality, sauna therapy may be fundamentally simple, but its benefits are almost immeasurable. Without exception, all diseases and chronic conditions of ill health are exacerbated, if not directly caused by, toxic substances inside the body. Once you eliminate what doesn't belong there, you have a much better chance of becoming well. Good health is your birthright. Fortunately, sweating is one therapeutic modality that you can administer to yourself.

Nevertheless, it's important to recognize when you can do it yourself and when you require the assistance of someone else. If you are in doubt, consult a qualified health care provider, be it a conventional doctor, naturopath, chiropractor, or other practitioner. Should you seek medical supervision, this book can still help you, for it will guide you in asking the right questions and knowing what issues need to be addressed.

Whether you decide to administer sauna therapy to yourself or seek the supervision of a health care professional, it's good to know that the detoxification stimulated by body heating can benefit practically everyone. In 1910, Dr. John Harvey Kellogg wrote: "The last few years have witnessed a growing interest in phototherapy and the time will soon arrive when no hospital will be considered completely equipped which does not include in its outfit a full set of electric light appliances for therapeutic use."[27] He was, of course, referring to his own invention. However, I don't think he would object to the updated models. Perhaps it is time for his vision to come true.

Notes

1. Mark Percival, "Nutritional Support for Detoxification," *ANSR—Applied Nutritional Science Reports*, (Advanced Nutrition Publications, Inc.; 1997), 3.

2. "Understanding Free Radicals and Antioxidants," <http://www.healthchecks ystems.com/antioxid.htm> (accessed March 6, 2003).

3. Anthony Cichoke, *The Complete Book of Enzyme Therapy* (Garden City Park, N.Y.: Avery Publishing Group, 1999), 23-24.

4. Ibid., 24

5. Percival, op. cit., 4.

6. Nina Silver, *The Handbook of Rife Frequency Healing: Holistic Technology For Cancer and Other Diseases* (Stone Ridge, N.Y.: The Center for Frequency Education, 2001), 159.

7. Lawrence Wilson, *Nutritional Balancing and Hair Mineral Analysis* (Prescott, Ariz.: L.D. Wilson Consultants, Inc.), 278-279.

8. L. Ron. Hubbard, *Clear Body, Clear Mind: The Effective Purification Program* (Los Angeles: Bridge Publications, Inc.), 98.

9. Ibid., 98-99.

10. Ibid., 99.

11. Ibid.

12. Ibid., 43.

13. Ibid., 51.

14. Ibid., 102.

15. Ibid., 102-103.

16. Ibid., 104.

17. D.W. Schnare et al., "Evaluation of a Detoxification Regimen for Fat Stored Xenobiotics," *Medical Hypotheses* 9: 265-282; reprint, unpaginated.

18. David E. Root, David B. Katzin, and David W. Schnare, "Diagnosis and Treatment of Patients Presenting Subclinical Signs and Symptoms of Exposure To Chemicals which Bioaccumulate in Human Tissue," *Proceedings of the National Conference on Hazardous Wastes and Environmental Emergencies,*

Cincinnati, Ohio (May 14-16, 1985), 152.

19. Jacqueline Krohn and Frances Taylor. *Natural Detoxification, A Practical Encyclopedia: The Complete Guide to Clearing Your Body of Toxins, 2nd Edition, Revised & Expanded* (Pt. Roberts, Wash.: Hartley & Marks Publishers, Inc.), 38.

20. Max Ben, "Is Detoxification a Solution to Occupational Health Hazards?" *National Safety News* (May 1984), 2-3.

21. David E. Root, "Statement before the Presidential Special Oversight Board for Department of Defense Investigations of Gulf War Chemical and Biological Incidents" (November 20, 1998), 1.

22. Krohn, op. cit., 16.

23. David E. Root, personal interview, September 11, 2002.

24. William J. Rea, *Chemical Sensitivity, Volume 4: Tools of Diagnosis and Methods of Treatment* (Boca Raton: Lewis Publishers, 1997), 2590.

25. Walter Crinnion, personal conversation, October 27, 2002.

26. Nina Silver, op. cit., 102.

27. John Harvey Kellogg, *Light Therapeutics: A Practical Manual of Phototherapy for the Student and the Practitioner, Revised Edition* (Battle Creek, Mich.: The Good Health Publishing Co., 1910), 4.

A Brief Summary of Ozone[1]

Remember to cure the patient as well as the disease.

ALVAN BARACH, MD (DIED DECEMBER 15, 1977), THE FIRST PHYSICIAN TO
SYSTEMATICALLY EMPLOY OXYGEN FOR THE TREATMENT OF BACTERIAL
PNEUMONIA; AN ADVOCATE OF BREATHING THERAPY FOR PEOPLE WITH
OBSTRUCTIVE LUNG DISEASE; AND MODIFIER OF THE FIRST OXYGEN TENT,
MAKING IT PRACTICAL FOR REGULAR USE.

For a couple of decades, various opinions have circulated regarding the levels of oxygen in Earth's atmosphere today compared to levels thousands or millions of years ago. Research has been reportedly based on many types of geological testing, from samples of air inside the pyramids to polar ice cores. The most concrete data suggesting increased oxygen levels is from an article, "Gas Bubbles in Fossil Amber as Possible Indicators of the Major Gas Composition of Ancient Air." The authors write:

> [W]e present data that…suggest that the major gas composition of air (N_2/O_2 ratio) has changed appreciably during the past 90 million years.…[C]alculation of original oxygen concentrations…appear to have changed from greater than 30 percent O_2 during one part of the late Cretaceous (between 75

and 95 million years ago) to 21 percent during the Eocene-Oligocene and for present-day samples, with possibly lower values during the Oligocene-Early Miocene.[2]

The above interpretations, and even the data itself, have been contested by some researchers. They assert that when the ratio of oxygen to other gases is at 25%, the humidity must not drop below 50%; otherwise, numerous materials will easily combust. Therefore, they conclude, it is impossible for the ratio of oxygen to have ever been 25%. This discussion is beyond the scope of this book—but whether our planet once had much higher concentrations of oxygen or not, it is clear that within the last century, it has become harder and harder to breathe. One whiff of city air is all we need to know this. In the 21st century, especially in industrialized cities with unbelievably high amounts of pollution, we are literally starving for oxygen. It is no surprise that Tokyo—not only with its high air pollution levels but with more people per square mile than any other city in the world—opened "oxygen bars" recently, where people congregate (as some do here in liquor bars), and inhale oxygen. Oxygen bars have now opened in the United States.

The diminishing quality of our oxygen supply has cost us dearly in terms of our health. Dr. Otto Warburg, who won the Nobel Prize for medicine twice (1931 and 1944), believed that the fundamental cause of all degenerative disease, including cancer, is oxygen starvation at the cellular level. It is irrefutable that oxygen is an important factor in remaining healthy. A sufficient oxygen supply confers more efficient bodily metabolism, which means better mental and physical abilities. Oxygen also provides more natural immunity to disease, since most pathogenic microbes are anaerobic (that is, they cannot survive in an aerobic [oxygen-rich] environment). Even those microbes that are aerobic—or which are adaptable enough to switch from being anaerobic to aerobic—are less likely to survive if the person receives ozone therapy. There are two reasons for this. First, the therapy has a beneficial effect on the body's immune response. Second, properly administered ozone therapy can destroy the cell wall of even aerobic microorganisms.

Oxygen therapy is not new. Various forms of oxygen used for therapy—hydrogen peroxide, ozone, and oxygen in its hyperbaric (pressurized) form—have been used for 100 years or longer. The antiseptic properties of hydrogen peroxide are familiar to every child who ever skinned a knee and watched bubbles emerge from the wound as the hydrogen peroxide was applied. Hyperbaric oxygen was used to treat deep sea divers who came to the surface too quickly, and later its medical applications were realized. In this Appendix, I will be focusing on ozone and how it is used in sauna therapy. First, however, I want to discuss how ozone is formed and dispel the poor public image that it often receives.

Oxygen is found in nature in a diatomic form (two atoms together), and thus has the chemical designation of O_2. Ozone, also found in nature, is triatomic (three atoms together), and thus has the chemical designation of O_3. O_3 is much more reactive than O_2: the extra atom of oxygen easily leaves its two partners and, in a process called oxidation, combines with other substances that have a suitable charge. Inside the body, this oxidation process commonly occurs with lipid (fat) molecules, bacteria, viruses, fungi, and toxins.

The word *ozone* comes from the Greek word *ozein*, which means "to smell." You may remember being outside and smelling ozone created by lightning after a thunderstorm. However, more commonly ozone is created by the sun's ultraviolet radiation, "produced constantly in the upper atmosphere as long as the sun is shining," writes health care practitioner and ozone specialist Saul Pressman in *The Story of Ozone*.

> [S]ince ozone is heavier than air, it begins to fall earthward. As it falls, it combines with any pollutant it contacts, cleaning the air—nature's wonderful self-cleaning system. If ozone contacts water vapor as it falls, it forms hydrogen peroxide, a component of rainwater, [which is] the reason why rainwater causes plants to grow better than irrigation with ground water.[3]

Ozone was discovered and named in 1840 by a German chemist working at the University of Basel in Switzerland. In 1856, the gas was used to disinfect operating rooms, and in 1870 it was reported to purify blood in test tubes. Monaco was the first country to build a water treatment plant using ozone in 1860, followed by Holland, Germany and France. The Germans began injecting ozone into the blood of sick people in 1898. Meanwhile in America, the Florida Medical Association published a work explaining how to use ozone therapeutically. And Dr. John Harvey Kellogg first used ozone in sauna steam cabinets in 1881 at his sanitarium in Battle Creek, Michigan, having written in his 1880 book *Diphtheria: Its Causes, Prevention, and Proper Treatment* that "Probably, no agent…for the purpose of purifying the air of the sick-room…is so useful for this purpose as ozone, one of the most powerful disinfectants known."[4] In 1896, "free energy" scientist Nikola Tesla patented his first ozone generator, and in 1900 sold ozonated olive oil to doctors for medical use. Throughout the first half of the 20th century, numerous physicians and dentists published detailed accounts of successfully using ozone to treat a wide variety of diseases and conditions, including anemia, asthma, gout, hay fever, syphilis, many kinds of cancers, chemical poisoning, diabetes, influenza, pneumonia, gangrene, wounds, and even insomnia and strokes. A 1904 volume of chemist Charles Marchand's *The Medical Uses of Hydrozone* [ozonated water] *and Glycozone* [ozonated olive oil] is still in the Library of Congress, the ozonated products having been approved by the U.S. Surgeon General. On June 22, 1909, Dr. William D. Neel of Chicago was awarded a patent for a device that was designed to treat numerous medical conditions by combining ozone with aromatic (essential) oils for inhalation. And during World War I, as was reported later in German medical journals, the Germans used ozone to treat many conditions including chlorine gas burns, gangrene, influenza, and trench foot.

Despite the efforts of certain prominent people in the medical-pharmaceutical establishment to eliminate ozone therapy as a viable medical treatment, respected doctors continued working with ozone and reporting their successes. As of this writing, ozone is a medically recognized therapy in Brazil, Bulgaria, Cuba, the Czech Republic, France, Germany, Hungary, Israel, Italy, Japan, Mexico, Poland, Romania, Russia, Singapore, Yugoslavia, four Canadian provinces, and fourteen U.S. states.

A few companies have managed to bind the unstable ozone with other substances such as magnesium or calcium to form a powder, which when mixed in water for drinking releases the ozone (and, like its cousin hydrogen peroxide, has a taste and sensation that some people find unpalatable). Other products are called "stabilized oxygen." However, in most cases, ozone is taken in its gaseous form.

There has been considerable negative publicity concerning ozone near the earth's surface. The United States Environmental Protection Agency has stated that ozone works fine where it belongs—in the upper atmosphere to (presumably) shield us from the sun's UV rays (more about that later)—but, it claims, no amount of ground-level ozone is good for you. (The agency "settles" for .08 parts per million as acceptable, since there will always be some ozone at ground level.) Ozone amounts are most likely to be elevated from around noontime through early evening on hot, sunny days, we are told—a true enough statement, considering that the UV rays from the sun produce ozone, and the sun shines most strongly in the afternoon. But this information is used to persuade people to stay indoors!

The likeminded weather services in the United States and Canada issue a daily "ozone health advisory," which warns the public when these levels are "too" high. We constantly hear reports alleging the adverse effects of ozone, which include all kinds of respiratory irritation from shortness of breath and coughing to chest pain and asthma. It's hard to ignore allegations such as: "Automobile exhaust is the primary cause of ground level ozone and the most serious air pollution problem in the northeast" from the New York State Department of Environmental Conservation.[5] Or consider this statement from the Rhode Island Public Transit Authority: "The poor air quality is due to elevated ground level ozone concentrations. Ozone is a major component of smog and is formed by the photochemical reaction of pollutants emitted by motor vehicles, industry and other sources in the presence of elevated temperatures and sunlight."[6] Even those sympathetic to the medical uses of ozone sometimes misinform, saying for instance that there is "good" ozone and "bad" ozone. All of these statements indicate a gross misunderstanding of what ozone is and how it works.

The best article on ozone that I have ever seen that explains why there are such opposing opinions about the gas is called "The Toxicity of Ozone: A Report and Bibliography." It first appeared in the February 1950 edition of *Industrial Medicine and Surgery* and was written by Clark E. Thorp, acting Chairman of the Department of Chemistry and Chemical Engineering at the Armour Research Foundation of the Illinois Institute of Technology. After conducting an extensive review of all the literature on ozone to date, Dr. Thorp pointed out that the reason researchers differed was that *they were not analyzing the same gas.* Ozone in one study was created very differently from the "ozone" in another study. *Investigators who reported intrinsically high toxicity levels for ozone were creating the gas with air instead of oxygen,* and/or were also using comparatively high current densities in the machines that created the gas. Investigators who reported no, or intrinsically low, toxicity levels for ozone were creating the gas with pure oxygen from cylinders instead of mixed-gas air, and/or were also using low current densities in the machines that created the gas. *It was this difference in the production of ozone that determined whether or not the final product was pure ozone, or contained harmful nitrogen oxides that appear when ozone is not made properly. It is these nitrogen compounds that are toxic, not the ozone itself.*

Unfortunately, many of the researchers whose papers Thorp read did not know the difference. "The majority of the reports claiming ozone to be a highly toxic gas are a direct result of the use of [certain] equipment in making toxicity studies." And despite the fact that several different scientists "called attention to the harmful effects of nitrogen oxides in ozone as early as 1913…no direct study of the influence of nitrogen oxides on the toxicity of ozone was published until 1941."[7] One researcher even misreported and later recanted, Thorp explained.

> After noting the work of Thorp previously mentioned [the author is referring to himself here in the third person], Hill, *realizing that oxides of nitrogen had been present in his previous test,* decided to rerun the test on an identical basis to determine if pure ozone had higher toxic limits. *These later tests showed that pure ozone was definitely non-toxic in concentrations as high as 50 parts per million.* As a final result of his work, Hill states: "*Pure ozone is not poisonous in any sense of the word as it breaks down in contact with the mucous membrane and oxygen only remains. For this reason, there are no cumulative effects and pure ozone may be breathed for long periods of time without harm,* provided, of course, that immediate irritation of strong concentrations is avoided."[8] [emphasis added]

Thorp's review of the literature clearly shows that research subjects were quite comfortable with pure ozone of concentrations of up to 20 ppm, whereas when ozone was mixed with nitrogen compounds levels of 5 ppm could not be tolerated. Also, ozone's irritation of tissues is quite different from an *inherent* toxicity. As for the effects of inhaling ozone, the issue is more complex than one might think. I will say more about this shortly.

Thus, most mainstream literature on ozone is incorrect. What is called "ozone" is actually *contaminants* that occur in the *production* of ozone and which *accompany* ozone that is not properly made. Depending on how ozone is produced (if cathode rays, radioactive emissions or high-voltage charge are present), and the composition of the feed gas (whether it is air or pure oxygen), highly toxic nitrogen oxides and other compounds can exist along with the ozone. Pure ozone is O_3. If ozone contains contaminants, it is no longer O_3, but something else! "Broadly saying 'Ozone is toxic' is an uninformed opinion, due to oversimplification," ozone expert Ed McCabe comments. "It's what you hear from the media, which usually only has time for 'one-liners.'…If [the ozone is] contaminated, the contaminants are the toxins, not the ozone used at proper levels!"[9]

Other contaminants that can exist alongside ozone, and which are falsely accused of somehow being caused or exacerbated by ozone, include carbon monoxide, sulfur dioxide, and nitric oxide. These compounds are actually caused by burning hydrocarbons in oxygen in the internal combustion engine. Ozone has been incorrectly blamed for smog, Pressman writes; it is not physically possible to produce ozone in an internal combustion engine. The ozone that occurs in smog "is produced by the photoelectric effect of the sun's energetic photons acting on polluting gases." These do not pose any danger, since the single oxygen molecules that split off from these gases reattach themselves "in seconds" to the other gases, "which is part of nature's system for cleaning the atmosphere." In fact, Pressman concludes, "The problem is not one of too much ozone in smog, but not enough. If sufficient amounts existed, the pollutants would all be oxidized and rendered harmless."[10]

Thus the pollutants around ozone have nothing to do with the intrinsic qualities of ozone itself. It's like leaving a bowl of beef stew out in the hot sun for many hours where it becomes contaminated with *Bacillus botulinus*, eating it, contracting food poisoning, and then deciding that stew is bad for you instead of acknowledging that you got sick because you let the food spoil. Neither the mainstream media, nor scientists at our government agencies, have seemed very willing to investigate the fact that pure ozone does not contain any contaminants or poisonous compounds.

Thus the phenomenon of "ozone contamination"—more accurately called "toxic contaminants"—simply indicates the need for clean sources of power, and for the manufacture of good quality ozone equipment that does not produce harmful chemical contaminants. Some manufacturers of commercial ozone generators use inferior components in an effort to save money, resulting in machines that deliver toxic compounds along with the ozone. Ethical manufacturers install the proper components, ensuring that pure ozone is produced.

Now I want to discuss the concern about ozone inhalation. Detractors of ozone like to point out that inhaling even uncontaminated ozone at too high a concentration through the nose or mouth over long periods may cause lesions or other damage in the delicate mucous membrane lining of the respiratory tract. However, this is a half-truth, isolated out of context and used as a tactic to scare people away from a highly beneficial healing modality. First, as stated in *Medical Applications of Ozone*, ozone is indeed "toxic if inhaled," but "it is only a local toxicity"—and the studies concluding that ozone had negative effects on animals "were done by only observing respiratory tract lesions after *long-term* inhalation of ozone."[11] [emphasis added] Second, as Pressman points out, even this information from a sympathetic source is misleading, because rats and mice—the most commonly used laboratory animals—are affected adversely only because their lungs are unable to clear fluid as rapidly as animals with more advanced lung protection mechanisms. Physician George Freibott further clarifies the issue:

> All I can say about ozone therapy is good things, as I have never seen it do harm to any patient yet. Even the Armour Report done in the 1950s states the following (this is the report that most governments and many scientists base their *horror* stories about ozone and its *supposed* harmfulness on): "Mice put in an *extremely* high flow of *concentrated ozone* developed pulmonary edema for 2 days, but by the third day the mice grew *strangely resistant* to the ozone and *no more pulmonary edema was evident.*"

The reason no more pulmonary edema was evident was because the *toxicity* or toxic elements *coating* the lungs of these mice was fully oxidized, neutralized and eliminated by day three! The substances being fully oxidized left nothing more for the ozone to oxidize, thus the pulmonary edema and the "sensitivity" disappeared. We have seen it work likewise in patients that have had different respiratory dysfunctions.

Personally, I oftentimes work in atmospheres of ozone (in our laboratories) that exceeds the allowable EPA and FDA standards of allowable ppm (parts per million) by 52,000 times! I suffer *no* diminution in lung capacity (in fact it has increased over the years).

We have given IA [intra-artery], IV [intra-venous], IM [intra-muscular], and by inhalation, doses of ozone and oxygen therapies to patients for over 25+ years personally, without any untoward side effects, ever.[12] [all emphases in the original]

The third twist to the particle of truth promoted by ozone detractors is that (as always) the source of the ozone is critical. If the gas is made improperly and contaminated with toxic chemicals, lesions on the lungs may indeed form. But again, that is not the fault of the ozone.

Ironically, it should be noted that *the inhalation of raw ozone was never meant to be used as a medical therapy* anyway. Physicians and informed laypersons who use ozone for inhalation make sure that it is first passed through olive oil or a suitable essential oil. The title of the patent for the aforementioned aromatic inhaler device invented by Dr. Neel was called "Process of Producing a Medicament [medication]" because the ozone, combined with high-terpene oils (Neel used juniper, pine and eucalyptus) atomized the oils into an unstable terpene gas that penetrated the lungs without causing an oxidative reaction. Thus 10 times more ozone than usual was present in the lung tissue, without any irritation whatsoever. The device was so effective, Neel wrote in his patent application, that

My experiments covering this long period [of time] have convinced me of its efficacy in curing consumption [tuberculosis], asthma and other diseases of the respiratory organs, as well as diseases of the blood. I find that this medicament, when properly administered, increases the red blood corpuscles and hemoglobin and has a general beneficial action upon the system. . . .

> Briefly stated, my invention may be said to consist in bringing
> an active oxidizing agent [ozone] into proximity to or in contact
> with…[an] oil of the terpene group, the resultant product being
> administered to the patient in an inhalable form.[13]

Variations of Neel's original device are used today by physicians, clinics, and laypeople worldwide. However, the most popular ozone-producing technology appears to be larger generators.

Generally, there are three types of units that safely produce ozone. The first is a low powered generator containing a specially designed short wave ultraviolet lamp. This unit creates ozone from ordinary air by duplicating the action of a narrow band of UV radiation from the sun (which produces ozone by reacting with oxygen). With this type of device, the production of ozone is limited by the UV wavelength that must be used to produce ozone (as in nature). Such devices are excellent for air purification or light water purification—although since there is no way to increase the strength of a UV bulb, the ozone concentrations remain far below what is necessary for most laboratory or clinical purposes.

The other ozone technologies are usually called *cold plasma* and *cold corona discharge* (although the word "cold" is a bit misleading, since due to the use of electricity some heat does exist). Both technologies can be used for medical applications if they are supplied with oxygen from an oxygen tank or oxygen concentrator (the latter extracts oxygen from ordinary air). Sending pure oxygen rather than mixed-gas air through these ozone generators guarantees that only oxygen and/or ozone are produced, instead of ozone and toxic nitrogen compounds, or ozone and other harmless (but unwanted) gases. The *cold plasma* design (invented by Nikola Tesla) consists of glass rods filled with noble gases excited by high voltage. The *cold corona* discharge technology consists of a double walled glass tube, around which an electrical field is generated. In both cases, the oxygen fed to the equipment becomes so energized that it splits apart and recombines to form ozone.

How does ozone operate as a scavenger and de-contaminant? A good description can be found in *Medical Applications of Ozone*, where one scientist defines ozone as an "oxygen atom in the body on a rapid transit."[14] And a "rapid transit" it is indeed, whether in the body, in water, or in air.

Ozone's high oxidative energy allows it to neutralize toxins that the body can then eliminate, often through sweat. Ozone's powerful disinfectant properties account for its huge success in the treatment of all kinds of conditions, including serious infections. The electrical charge that ozone carries is so strong that it can literally blast a hole through the outer cell wall of a microbe and kill even aerobic pathogens. However, as with all substances, ozone must be dispensed in the correct amounts to be safe. To kill aerobic pathogens, the concentration of the gas must be high enough without exceeding the capacity of human cells to contain it. Therefore, manufacturers of ozone equipment either have the output set for a single safe level, or include controls that regulate the ozone flow.

There are many types of ozone-producing units, which can range in price from $300 to $6000. Many readers are familiar with air purifiers that emit ozone to help clean up contaminants in their homes. Other ozone generators emit ozone that flows through tubing into a special nylon body sack, which covers the person (except for the head and hands) to allow the ozone to be absorbed transdermally, or through the skin. Some units have attachments that can pass ozone through oil to make it safe to inhale. Olive oil is commonly used, although the essential oils of eucalyptus, peppermint, spearmint, and tea tree can be added too. Inhaling modified ozone in this way has proven to be an effective treatment for asthma, bronchial infections, and even emphysema. Aside from the special care required with inhalation, in the proper amounts ozone can be safely administered through all of the bodily orifices. It can also be injected into the blood vessels and muscles in people who are very ill with cancer, AIDS, and numerous degenerative illnesses. In Germany and other European countries, doctors remove the person's blood, infuse it with ozone, and inject it back into the body. This process is called *Major Autohemotherapy* or MAHT. In Appendix B, I list some doctors who perform ultraviolet blood irradiation or photoluminescence, a procedure in which the blood is irradiated with a narrow band of UV light and then returned to the body. The reason this procedure helps eliminate serious infections such as AIDS-related conditions and cancer is that the UV light creates ozone.

Ozone can also be dispersed into drinking water. If kept in the refrigerator at 40°Fahrenheit (7.2°Celsius) after being bubbled into water for 45 minutes, the ozone will remain intact in the water for three to four days. Frozen in a plastic container, the water can be stored for several months. Another unique way of storing ozone consists of bubbling it continuously through extra virgin olive oil for about three weeks (following Nikola Tesla's original recipe), which first bleaches the oil and then gels it into a paste-like consistency. When kept refrigerated, German researchers have found, the salve retains its effectiveness for over 10 years. "When used during massage," Pressman reports, "the ozonide [the altered ozone in the olive oil salve] enters the tissue and oxidizes lactic acid and toxins, and this has proven to be an effective treatment for many skin problems"[15] including burns, dry skin, fungal infections, insect bites, sunburn, sweat gland infections, and wounds.

One health-related but industrial use of ozone is the decontamination of swimming pools and hot tubs, a much more popular practice in Europe than in the United States. In fact, it is so common in Europe that when the Olympics were held recently in America, visiting overseas swimming teams, knowing how poisonous chlorine is, insisted on having ozone instead of chlorine to disinfect the swimming pools. (This was done; although once the Olympics ended, the ozone equipment was removed and chlorine was reinstated.) For most industrial uses, the ozone can be created with plain air, whereas for medical uses, oxygen is always the feed gas.

This brings me to the growing popularity of including ozone as a feature in steam cabinets. (A sauna *room* should never be used, since as I mentioned earlier, ozone should not be inhaled except through olive or other oils.) According to the health care providers I consulted who use ozone in their practice, the wetness of the steam allows the ozone to seep through the skin, as ozone does not enter the body at all if the skin is dry. (Also, the heat from the steam might help the person perspire.) Once the skin is wet, the ozone is readily absorbed into all the bodily tissues, including the lymph and fat, which hold the majority of the body's toxins. (Transdermally applied ozone is especially helpful for cleansing the lymphatic tissue—which, as I explained in Chapter 2, needs plenty of support since it does not have an independent pump to make the lymph flow.) After the bloodstream reaches its natural saturation point, the body simply does not accept any more.

Although ozone has traditionally been used with steam sauna cabinets, I see no reason why ozone cannot also be combined with a FIR sauna cabinet, as long as you are able to perspire. If you have trouble perspiring, shower and leave some moisture on your skin before entering the cabinet. This allows your body to accept the ozone. Or you can exercise to begin the sweating process. As of this writing, I am aware of only one FIR sauna cabinet that is made with suitably ozone-resistant materials and can therefore accommodate an ozone generator. However, I believe that this will soon change, since both FIR sauna cabinet manufacturers and a better informed public are becoming eager for the benefits of both ozone and far infrared. *Remember, you can use outboard ozone equipment only if the cabinet is constructed of an ozone resistant material such as fiberglass.* Place the ozone generator near the cabinet and run the tube from the generator to the inside of the sauna through the hole at the top where the neck sticks out. To avoid breathing the ozone, wrap a towel around the opening.

Be aware that ozone can cause intense cleansing reactions (also known as a healing crisis), which can feel quite uncomfortable and even scary, especially for people who are not used to detoxification programs and don't understand how to interpret the symptoms they feel when the body is expelling toxic waste. Cleansing reactions typically resemble the flu, although any symptoms can manifest from waste materials that the body is trying to expel. The body often tries to eliminate waste materials through the skin, which can cause very itchy skin rashes. The rashes can be helped by taking orally liberal amounts of protease enzymes and applying soothing creams. It is true, as Pressman writes, that "the more frequent the treatments, the more rapid the healing, and the more severe the healing reactions will be. It may become so uncomfortable that the person will need to reduce the frequency of treatments from once daily to once weekly."[16] Some people follow Pressman's suggestion of once a day for a half hour. However, other health care practitioners as well as some laypeople prefer a more moderate approach, such as 20 minutes three times a week. Rather than push the body so hard in the first place, you might simply reduce the treatments before reaching that level of discomfort. If toxins have to emerge through the skin, it means they are circulating in the bloodstream; and if toxins are that plentiful in the bloodstream, they might be putting an extra strain on the body to eliminate them. Since many people who are ill already have a weak liver and/or kidneys, it seems wise to proceed slowly. This is good advice for any detoxification program.

Pressman advises people with heart conditions to stay in the ozone sauna cabinet for only 15 minutes at a lower temperature for the first few sessions, and gradually increase their sauna sessions to 30 minutes over time as the body adjusts to the thermal stress. (Note, however, that there is considerable debate among practitioners about frequency of use.) He does not advise ozone saunas at all for those with a history of strokes, due to the heat that causes dilation of the blood vessels and could potentially loosen another clot. (On the other hand, the administration of ozone via another delivery system is recommended.) For those who wish to focus on specific organs or areas of the body while in the cabinet, the ozone can be projected through silicone tubing (which resists corrosion from ozone) to a funnel over the area. "This is especially effective with hepatitis, diverticulitis, pancreatitis and cancer," writes Pressman. "It also involves the person in actively taking responsibility for initiating the healing process." He adds that ozone, when combined with hyperthermia, works particularly well to arrest and reverse cancer because

> Cancer tumor cells are tightly packed as they try to force their way in between other cells, and they are thus less able to shed heat. This accounts for the effect that heat stress has in killing cancer. Both heat stress and ozone kill cancer, so this treatment offers the best opportunity to eliminate cells which are fermenting sugar anaerobically, [and to] halt metastasis and restore healthy aerobic function. Ozone is able to seek out and destroy all the cancer cells with more certainty than the surgeon's crude scalpel. In addition, ozone will oxidize the toxins which caused the original problem, and thus prevent recurrence of the problem. This is in contrast to chemotherapy which is massively immune-suppressive, and radiation which causes cancer.[17]

In his *Let's Talk Health* newsletter, Dr. Kurt Donsbach summarizes that oxygen therapies:

- Increase tissue oxygenation, which brings about improvement in metabolic rate

- Stimulate production of white blood cells, which are necessary to fight infection
- Decrease blood carbon monoxide load, which frees hemoglobin to carry oxygen
- Increase hemoglobin disassociation [the ability of hemoglobin in the red blood cells to let go of the oxygen they are carrying], thus increasing delivery of oxygen from blood to cells
- Increase red blood cell flexibility, thus allowing them to squeeze through the smallest blood vessels more easily
- [Break down] petrochemicals
- [Inhibit] the growth of new tissues such as tumors
- Increase the production of interferon and tumor necrosis factor, used to fight infection and cancer
- Increase the efficiency of the antioxidant enzyme system, which scavenges excess free radicals[18]

Although some of ozone's effects replicate or overlap with the effects of heat alone, clearly the combination of ozone with conventional body heating methods provides additional benefits. Many people who use ozone along with body heating have serious illnesses—and for them, ozone is a necessity rather than a luxury, well worth the extra cost. However, if you cannot afford ozone, don't worry about it. Simulating most of the effects of a fever solely through heat is very powerful, particularly if it's done repeatedly. While ozone and body heating are synergistically quite potent, heat by itself can accomplish wonders.

There are many ways to take a sauna.

NOTES

1. Adapted and excerpted from Nina Silver, *The Handbook of Rife Frequency Healing: Holistic Technology For Cancer and Other Diseases* (Stone Ridge, N.Y.: The Center for Frequency Education, 2001), 106-113.

2. Robert A. Berner and Gary P. Landis, "Gas Bubbles in Fossil Amber as Possible Indicators of the Major Gas Composition of Ancient Air," *Science* 239 (March 18, 1988), 1406.

3. Saul Pressman, *The Story of Ozone* (British Columbia: Plasmafire International, 2001), 1.

4. John Harvey Kellogg, *Diphtheria: Its Causes, Prevention, and Proper Treatment* (Battle Creek: The Good Health Publishing Co., 1880), 56.

5. Ozone Health Advisory for the New York City Metropolitan Area, New York State Department of Environmental Conservation <www.dec.state.ny.us/website/dar/bts/ozone/advise.html>.

6. Rhode Island Public Transit Authority database (untitled) <www.ripta.com/contentmgr/showdetails.php?id=219>.

7. Clark E. Thorp, "The Toxicity of Ozone: A Report and Bibliography," reprint from *Industrial Medicine and Surgery* 19:2 (February, 1950), 3, 5.

8. Ibid.

9. Ed McCabe, *Oxygen Therapies: A New Way of Approaching Disease* (Morrisville, N.Y.: Energy Publications, 1988), 92-93.

10. Saul Pressman, *The Owner's Manual for the Human Body* (British Columbia: Plasmafire International), 1-2.

11. R.M. Mattassi, F. D'Angelo, A. Franchina, and P. Bassi, "Ozone as Therapy in Herpes Simplex and Herpes Zoster Diseases," in *Medical Applications of Ozone,* ed. Julius LaRaus (Norwalk, Conn.: The International Ozone Association, ca. 1983), 135.

12. George Freibott, "29 May 1997 Re: Ozone generators" quoted on <www.thefinchleyclinic.co.uk/nojavascript/therapies/ozone/safe.htm> (accessed August 31, 2002).

13. William D. Neel, "Process of Producing a Medicament," patented June 22, 1909, Patent # 925,590.

14. LaRaus, op. cit., 3.

15. Pressman, *Owner's Manual,* op. cit.. 44.

16. Pressman, *Story of Ozone,* op. cit.. 25.

17. Ibid.

18. Kurt Donsbach, *Let's Talk Health Newsletter* 5 no. 1 (March/April 2002), 3.

Resources

The more you sweat in peace, the less you bleed in war.

ADMIRAL HYMAN G. RICKOVER,
AT HIS US NAVY 1983 RETIREMENT SPEECH

The inclusion of a particular doctor, facility, organization, service, spa, or sauna manufacturer does not imply unconditional endorsement by the author. The listings are provided solely for the convenience of the reader, who is responsible for investigating and evaluating these entries.

Please note: The 011 code in front of all the international phone numbers is *only if you're calling from the United States.*

CLINICS, DOCTORS, AND MEDICAL TREATMENT CENTERS

Most of these facilities are equipped to handle people with serious problems such as allergies, arthritis, cancers, cardiovascular disease, environmental illness, hard-to-treat infections, and neurological disorders. They administer sauna sessions, hyperthermia, or other heat treatments as part of a supervised, systematic detoxification program. Resort spas and a few medically-oriented spas are on pages 287 to 304.

Aquavitae Hydrotherapy and Physiotherapy Centre
6501 Campeau Drive, Suite 100
Kanata, Ontario K2K 3E9
Canada
    contact: Nadine Bellman, Physiotherapist
    phone: 613-592-2222
    fax: 613-592-0284
    website: www.aquavitae.ca

People with arthritis, rheumatism, chronic pain, fibromyalgia, neurological conditions, injuries, tendonitis, pre- and post- surgical conditions such as joint replacements, and repetitive stress injuries are treated with physiotherapy, exercise therapy, massage, and many forms of hydrotherapy.

Austin Rejuvenation Center
911 W. Anderson Lane #205
Austin, Texas 78757
    contact: Vladimir Rizov, MD
    phone: 512-451-8149

Detoxification treatments include chelation with EDTA. DMSO, enzymes, homeopathy, laetrile, oxygen, and vitamins are also used. Hyperthermia treatments are in electric heater saunas to 120°F (48.9°C), with ozone added.

Ayurvedic Institute
11311 Menual Boulevard NE
Albuquerque, New Mexico 87112
    contact: Pancha Karma Department
    phone: 505-291-9698
    fax: 505-294-7572
    website: www.ayurveda.com

Therapies include diet, lifestyle recommendations, synchronized oil massage, Shirodhara (a mind-balancing treatment), and Pancha Karma, which balances body, mind and spirit through the elimination of toxins so the body can return to its normal healthy state. The institute offers herbal steam treatments.

Battle Creek Lifestyle Health Center
101 N. 20th Street
Battle Creek, Michigan 49015
    contact: **Jeff Gates, MD, and Bruce R. Hyde, MD**
    phone: **888-255-3180 or 269-963-0368**
    fax: **269-963-3305**
    website: **www.bclifestylecenter.com**

In this descendent of Dr. John Harvey Kellogg's spa, treatments include alpha stimulation, herbs, massage, nutrition, physical therapy, sunlight treatments, and hydrotherapy. Sauna therapy is given in one of Kellogg's original electric light baths.

Black Hills Health & Education Center
PO Box 19
Hermosa, South Dakota 57744
    contact: **Dick Nunez, FT, SFT, CPT**
    phone: **800-658-5433 or 605-255-4101**
    fax: **605-255-4687**
    website: **www.bhhec.org**

People with autoimmune disorders, arthritis, diabetes, heart disease, and obesity receive a 6-day non-medical program or a 13-day or 20-day medical program. Modalities include exercise equipment, hot and cold contrast treatments, hydrotherapy, and massage. The sauna uses steam.

Celebration of Health Center
122 Thurman Street
Bluffton, Ohio 45817
    contact: **Dr. L. Terry Chappell, MD**
    phone: **419-358-4627**
    fax: **419-358-1855**
    website: **www.healthcelebration.com**

People with allergies, arthritis and joint pain, autism (in children), cardiovascular problems, and yeast infections are treated with various healing modalities including IV chelation, nutrition, and prolotherapy. The sauna uses steam with ozone.

Center for Occupational and Environmental Medicine
7510 Northforest Drive
North Charleston, South Carolina 29420
   contact: Allan D. Lieberman, MD
   phone: 843-572-1600
   website: www.coem.com

Specialties include allergies and food sensitivities, children with learning disabilities or other special needs, occupational and environmental medicine (including chemical injury/sensitivity), preconception care, and yeast problems. Treatments include chelation, nutrition, and detoxification. The sauna uses dry heat.

Clinque La Prairie SA Medical & Revitalization Center
CH-1815 Clarens
Montreux, Switzerland
   phone: 011+41+21+989 3311
   fax: 011+41+21+989 3333
   website: www.laprairie.ch

Medical services include cardiology, dental care, dermatology, endocrinology, general surgery, gynecology, neurology, opthalmology, plastic surgery, and psychiatry. The staff beauticians, dermatologists, and massage therapists administer hydrotherapy, lymphatic drainage, massage, and ozone. The facility has a dry sauna and Turkish bath.

The Cole Center for Healing/Cincinnati Hyperbarics
11974 Lebanon Road, Suite 228
Cincinnati, Ohio 45241
   contact: Theodore J. Cole, DO, NMD
   phone: 800-667-5395 (toll-free) or 513-563-4321
   fax: 513-563-3131
   website: www.drhealth.net

Modalities include acupuncture, chelation, herbs, homeopathy, nutritional therapy, all oxygen therapies, psychological modalities, and photoluminescence (UV blood irradiation) to combat infections like HIV and hepatitis. (Blood is drawn, subjected to UV light, and then returned to the body.) The sauna cabinet uses steam with ozone.

Comprehensive Health Association
9910 Long Point Road
Houston, Texas 77055
    contact: **Robert Battle, MD**
    phone: **713-932-0552**
    fax: **713-932-0551**
    website: **www.chamd.com**

People with allergies, arthritis, autism, cancer, chemical sensitivities, chronic fatigue, environmental illness, and other conditions are treated with chelation (oral and IV), homeopathy, nutrition, and neural, oxidative and pain therapies. The two saunas use steam with ozone, and FIR.

Ealing Natural Therapies
108 Westcott Crescent
Hanwell, London W7 1PB
England
    contact: **Enrida Kelly, Dip, ANP (Naturopathy)**
    phone: **011+44+0208 933 4520**
    website: **www.natpath.co.uk**

Services include ear acupuncture, herbs, homeopathy, iridology, metabolic typing, mineral analysis, nutrition, and ozone cupping and insufflations. The sauna uses steam with ozone.

The Edelson Center for Environmental & Preventive Medicine
3833 Roswell Road, Suite 110
Atlanta, Georgia 30342
    contact: **Stephen Edelson, MD**
    phone: **404-841-0088**
    fax: **404-841-6416**
    website: **www.edelsoncenter.com**

People with chronic diseases such as ALS, autism, cancer, chronic fatigue, lupus, multiple chemical sensitivity, multiple sclerosis, and Parkinson's are given chelation (oral and IV), nutrition, ozone therapy (including injections), and photoluminescence (UV blood irradiation). The two saunas use FIR and convection heat.

Élan Vitál Medical Centers and Spas
21 West Street
Worcester, Massachusetts 01609
  contact: **Abbas Qutab, MD**
  phone: **508-753-0006**
      and
7 Whittier Place, Suite 108
Boston, Massachusetts 02114
  phone: **617-227-6573**
  website: **www.spadocs.com**

Specialities are women's health, aging problems, and hormone regulation. An adrenal stress index, food allergy profile, Ayurvedic pulse diagnosis, and cardiovascular, parasite, and urine tests are given. Treatments include Ayurvedic medicine, chiropractic, herbs, homeopathy, and nutrition. Heat treatments consist of smooth, hot lava stones soaked in essential oils and massaged onto the body.

Environmental Health Center
8345 Walnut Hill Lane, Suite 220
Dallas, Texas 75231
  contact: **William J. Rea, MD**
  phone: **214-368-4132**
  fax: **214-691-8432**
  website: **www.ehcd.com/chemsens.html**

This is the first environmentally safe residential clinic constructed in the U.S., by the award-winning Dr. Rea, with organic foods, safe water, and rooms containing only natural, scent-free materials. The detoxification program uses dry and steam saunas.

Environmental Health Center of Western New York
65 Wehrle Drive
Buffalo, NY 14225-1021
  contact: **Kalpana D. Patel, MD**
  phone: **716-833-2213**

Specialties include adolescent, pediatric and geriatric medicine; allergies; clinical immunology; environmental medicine; metabolic disorders; and preventive medicine. Treatments include chelation and nutrition. The sauna is Finnish.

Fun Fit Studio
Noellenstrasse 15a, CH-9443
Widnau, Switzerland
>   contact: **Dorit Boehme, Government approved massage therapist**
>   phone: **011+41+71+722 5250**
>   fax: **011+41+71+722 5205**
>   website: **www.fun-fit.ch**

People with allergies, back pain, cellulitis, headaches, and other conditions are treated with acupuncture, massage, spine corrections, and the F-Scan and Theraplex energy devices to kill microbes and impart restorative frequencies to the body. There is a Finnish sauna and steam aroma shower.

Health Care for the 21st Century
875 Walnut Street, Suite 370
Cary, North Carolina 27511
>   contact: **Joan Amtoft-Nielsen, MD, PhD**
>   phone: **919-467-5770**
>   fax: **919-469-2971**
>   website: **www.drnielsen.net**

People with hard-to-treat conditions, including arthritis, cancer, cardiac disease, Cushing's disease, digestive problems, mold, and yeast infection are treated with many modalities including environmental medicine, homeopathy, orthomolecular medicine, and nutrition. The sauna uses steam with ozone.

HealthMed
5501 Power Inn Road, Suite 130
Sacramento, California 95820
>   contact: **David Root, MD**
>   phone: **916-387-8252**
>   fax: **916-387-6977**
>   website: **www.healthmeddetox.org**

People afflicted by environmental illness, chemical exposure, alcoholism, and drug abuse (of either prescription or street drugs, but not crack cocaine or heroin) are given the Hubbard detox protocol. The all-tile sauna rooms use dry heat.

HealthMed of New York
139 Fulton Street, Suite 515
New York, New York 10038
    contact: Apryl McNeil, MD
    phone: 212-587-3994, 212-587-3998, or 212-587-3761
    fax: 212-587-3760
    website: www.healthmeddetox.org

This facility was created to administer the Hubbard detox protocol
to people who worked at Ground Zero, including police, firefighters,
Emergency Medical Technicians, and custodial staff at Stuyvesant High
School (which became an impromptu infirmary), and now experience
neurological and pulmonary disorders from the dangerous chemicals
they absorbed. See HealthMed listing above.

Health Tools
3736 Mount Diablo Boulevard, Suite 202
Lafayette, California 94549
    contact: Wootie McAdams, ND
    phone: 415-925-1831

People with allergies, digestive disorders, fatigue, heavy metal and
chemical toxicity, immune dysfunction, muscular and skeletal pain,
TMJ syndrome, and other chronic illnesses are treated with cell therapy, herbs, homeopathy, massage, neural therapy, orthomolecular nutrition, oxygen therapies, and local and whole body hyperthermia. The
saunas use steam and FIR.

Healthy By Nature
126 Laurel Road
East Northport, New York 11731
    contact: Christopher J. Fischer, ND
    phone: 631-757-3366
    fax: 631-757-3385
    website: www.webndny.com

Services include naturopathy, homeopathy, nutritional and herbal consultations, and constitutional hydrotherapy. The sauna cabinet uses
steam.

Holos Center
2211 Corinth Avenue, #301
Los Angeles, California 90064
>   contact: **Nadine Cutright, MBA, CtH**
>   phone: 310-345-8649
>   website: **www.holoscenter.com**

Holos provides information, education, services, and products that encourage clients to be proactive in their own lives and make enjoyable, informed choices about their health care. Modalities include biofeedback, hypnotherapy, and cleansing protocols. The sauna is FIR.

Integrated Medical Specialists
115 Eagle Spring Drive, Suite A
Stockbridge, Georgia 30281
>   contact: **Dr. T. R. Shantha, MD, PhD, FACA**
>   phone: 770-474-4029
>   fax: 770-474-2038
>   website: **www.iptmd.com**

People with AIDS, ALS, arthritis, cancer, chronic fatigue, cardiovascular disorders, Crohn's, diabetes, heavy metal and environmental poisoning, hepatitis, lupus, and multiple sclerosis receive holistic and allopathic care that includes acupuncture, chelation, herbs, nutritional supplements, colonics, drugs, hormone replacement, Hyperbaric Oxygen Therapy (HBOT), and Insulin Potentiation Therapy (IPT). A FIR sauna is used for hyperthermia.

Johnson Medical Associates
317 Dal-Rich Village
Richardson, Texas 75080
>   contact: **Alfred R. Johnson, DO**
>   phone: 972-479-0400
>   fax: 972-479-0400
>   website: **www.johnsonmedicalassociates.com**

Specialties include allergy testing and desensitization, environmental and internal medicine, and toxicology. Treatments include chelation, homeopathy, nutrition, oxygen therapies, and intravenous and oral supplementation. The saunas are dry.

Klinikzentrum Bad Sulza GmbH
Multidisziplinäre REHA- und AHB Klinik
Rudolf-Gröschner-Str. 11
D-99518 Bad Sulza
Germany
    phone: 011+49+(0)36461-90
    fax: 011+49+(0)36461-91890

Specialities include allergies, dermatology, cardiology, orthopedics, pediatrics, sports, and environmental medicine. Modalities include phototherapy, and electrotherapy, and mineral and mud baths. The saunas use both dry heat and steam.

Longevity Institute Indiana
9292 North Meridian Street, Suite 300
Indianapolis, Indiana 46260
    contact: Arthur Sumrall, MD
    phone: 317-574-1677
    fax: 317-574-1688
    website: www.longevity-inst.com

People with chronic fatigue, fibromyalgia, and heavy metal toxicity receive electrodermal screening, chelation (oral and IV), herbs, homeopathy, live cell analysis, nutrition, oxygen therapies, and photoluminescence (UV blood irradiation). The dry heat sauna capsule dispenses aromatherapy and vibrating massage. The low-EMF, FIR sauna cabinet is used for intensive detox.

Magaziner Center for Wellness
1907 Greentree Road
Cherry Hill, New Jersey 08003
    contact: Alan Magaziner, MD
    phone: 856-424-8222
    fax: 856-424-2599
    website: www.drmagaziner.com

People with allergies, arthritis, autism, ADD, cancer, cardiovascular disease, chronic fatigue, diabetes, fibromyalgia, and heavy metal toxicity are treated with chelation (oral, IV, rectal), herbs, homeopathy, and nutrition. The sauna uses FIR.

New Hope Health Clinic
7320 South Yale Avenue
Tulsa, Oklahoma 74136
    contact: Kent R. Bartell, ND, DC
    phone: 877-544-HOPE (4673), toll-free
    website: www.newhopehealthclinic.com

People with arthritis, cancer, fatigue, heavy metal toxicity, heart disease, fibromyalgia, digestive disorders, immune system suppression, osteoporosis, hormonal problems, and endocrine dysfunction are treated with homeopathy, intravenous chelation and nutrition, naturopathy, and oxygen therapies. The sauna cabinet uses steam with ozone.

The Oxygen Spa
14346 Cape May Road
Silver Spring, Maryland 20904
    contact: Marian Porter, ND
    phone: 301-879-0212
    website: www.oxygensauna.com

People with many conditions, including heavy metal and chemical toxicity, come here for detoxification. The session begins with 30 minutes in a steam cabinet with ozone, followed by 15 minutes of oxygen inhalation, or ozone inhaled through olive oil or olive with essential oils.

Queen Elizabeth Hospital
Whakaue Street (mail only: PO Box 13421)
Rotorua, New Zealand
    phone: 011+64+7+348 0189
    fax: 011+64+7+348 4266
    website: www.qehospital.co.nz

Specialities include rheumatism, arthritis, and other locomotor disorders. Treatments are modern, combined with older, more traditional "spa cures" including massage and mud packs. The spa area of the hospital, which is open to the public as a regular day spa, has a steam bath, and mineral water pool at temperatures of 98.6° to 104°F (37° to 40°C).

Robbins Environmental Medicine Center
400 South Dixie Highway
Boca Raton, Florida 33432
    contact: Albert Robbins, MD
    phone: 561-395-3282
    fax: 561-395-3304
    website: www.allergycenter.com

Specialities include allergies, asthma, chemical sensitivity, chronic fatigue, and occupational and environmental medicine. Modalities include optimal dose immuno-therapy, massage, and nutrition with IV vitamin therapy. The sauna is dry.

Sanoviv Medical Institute
2602-C Transportation Avenue (satellite office)
National City, CA 91950
    contact: Cynthia Tercha, ext. 6005
    phone: 800-SANOVIV or 801-954-7600
    fax: 561-395-3304
    website: www.sanoviv.com

This holistic Mexican hospital provides anti-aging and spa services, and treats people with serious conditions including cancer, chronic fatigue, fibromyalgia, lupus, Lyme disease, Parkinson's, and multiple sclerosis. Therapeutic modalities include biological dentistry (removing silver-mercury fillings), chelation, colonics, nutrition, and psychotherapy. Hydrotherapy is in sea water pools. The sauna is dry.

SpiritMed
16534 37th Avenue NE
Seattle, Washington 98155
    contact: Walter Crinnion, ND
    phone: 206-361-5600
    fax: 206-367-1888

Dr. Crinnion teaches health care providers how to recognize and treat toxic overload, and how to use the sauna therapeutically. He also teaches environmental medicine as a full professor at the Southwest College of Naturopathic Medicine in Tempe, Arizona.

StressBusters Body Therapy Center
26548 Moulton Parkway, Suite D
Laguna Hills, California 92653
    contact: Mikki M. Anderson, LMT
    phone: 949-831-1988
    fax: 949-831-2689

Nearby hospitals refer high-risk, pregnant women to this center. Special massage techniques correct potential breech births—giving the baby more room to return to a normal head-first position—and rehabilitate the postpartum woman's stomach muscles and back. Induction massage, given to mothers who are due or overdue for delivery, stimulates labor. Ms. Anderson also offers infant massage classes for parents, and emotional release and cognitive therapy to people with cancer. A chiropractor on staff treats injuries. The sauna is Finnish.

Zdraviliš e Laško
Zdraviliska 4
Lasko 3270, Slovenia
    phone: 011+386+3+734 5555
    fax: 011+386+3+734 5298
    website: www.zdravilisce-lasko.si

People who want to relax, or with serious and degenerative conditions such as burns, rheumatism, or locomotor/neurological difficulties, come for Aryuvedic and underwater massage, electrotherapy, hot pumice stone therapy with essential oils, menthol and pearl baths with medicinal herbs, exercise, and post-operative physiotherapy. Staff includes doctors, nurses, and surgeons. The facility has a thermal spring 89.6° to 95°F (32° to 35°C), solarium, whirlpool, Roman bath, and Turkish steam bath. The sauna is Finnish.

Health-Related Organizations

American Academy of Environmental Medicine (AAEM)
c/o The American Financial Center
7701 E. Kellogg, Suite 625
Wichita, Kansas 67207
  phone: 316-684-5500
  fax: 316-684-5709
  website: www.aaem.com

This group will send you a list of physicians who practice environmental medicine in your area.

HEAL (Human Ecology Action League)
PO Box 49126
Atlanta, Georgia 30359-0629
  phone: 404-248-1898
  fax: 404-248-0162

HEAL provides information on environmental illness, environmental testing for toxic chemicals, and safe substitutes for toxic products. Publications include a reading list and a guide to environmentally-related health care practitioners. There are also support groups for members across the country.

International Clinical Hyperthermia Society
12099 W. Washington Boulevard, #304
Los Angeles, California 90066
  contact: James I. Bicher, MD
  phone: 310-398-0013
  website: www.hyperthermia-ichs.org

The Society was organized to provide a forum for members to discuss their ideas on the use of hyperthermia and present their clinical experience at meetings. The website contains abstracts of articles by the presenters, plus a list of treatment facilities (many of them holistic) worldwide that provide hyperthermia.

The Weston A. Price Foundation for Wise Traditions
PMB #106-380
4200 Wisconsin Avenue NW
Washington, DC 20016
    contact: Sally Fallon, MA
    phone: 202-333-HEAL
    web site: www.WestonAPrice.org

This organization shares the research of 20th century dentist Weston Price, who found that the healthiest, cavity-free people ate traditional, local foods (animal and vegetable) that were either raw or pre-digested (fermented, sprouted, soaked or slow cooked); while the sickest ate refined carbohydrates, sugars, and fake foods that caused tooth decay and malformed dental arches in the malnourished offspring of nutrient-deprived mothers. Publications include a quarterly magazine with articles on food, healing, and nutrition politics.

Products

ALKALIZER-DETOXIFIER, AND HEALTHY TANNING SYSTEM

Healing Arts & Wellness Centre Inc.
#3–3911 51st Avenue
Lloydminster, Alberta T9V 2Z2, Canada
    contact: Noel and Pat Livingston, independent distributors
    phone: 888-870-3933 (toll-free)
    websites: www.thehealthreview.com

Microbiologist Robert O. Young, PhD, who formulated these products from Inner Light, Inc., says that SuperGreens—an enzyme-rich powder of grasses, herbs, and vegetables (1 teaspoon equals about 5 pounds of greens)—when mixed with Prime pH alkaline drops, raises the pH of the system. This facilitates detoxification of the liver, flushes the kidneys and the intracellular fluid, and helps eliminate fat and cellulite. His company's StarTan air brush system confers a lovely bronzed tan. But it is very different from a conventional tanning bed, Dr. Young notes: it is safe enough to be used weekly for a year-round tan (at a fraction of the cost) because it nourishes, rejuvenates, and improves the skin with DHA, essential fatty acids, and oxygen (nutrients for the skin and brain).

CHAPPARAL CAPSULES, LOTION, AND SPRAY

Energy Medicine Association
15639 Four Seasons Drive
Houston, Texas 77084
    contact: **Paddy McAlister**
    phone: **281-463-1026**
    website: **www.shegoi.net/naturalhealth**

One of the most popular herbs in the Native American medical repertoire is chapparal, or *Larrea tridentata. Larrea* produces numerous compounds to protect itself against bacteria, fungi, viruses, insects, rodents, and weeds. The very phytochemicals that enable a single *Larrea* plant to survive up to 11,000 years in the hot, dry, southwestern United States desert—without being riddled with microorganisms, or eaten by insects or animals—are desirable to humans. Five patents were granted to a doctor for extracting and purifying the plant's beneficial constituents while eliminating those that could be toxic to the liver. *Larrea* is available in capsules, or in lotion and spray for the skin.

CLEANERS, BOTANICAL

Safer Cleaner
7015 Elfin Oaks Road
Elfin Forest, California 92029
    contact: **Kirby Hughes**
    phone: **888-241-6089 toll-free**
                760-744-3454 local and international
    fax: **760-744-8593**
    website: **www.theSaferSolution.com**

These liquid soaps—completely safe even for chemically sensitive people—clean dishes, furniture, laundry, body and hair, pets, vegetables, and saunas. The ingredients (pure water, amino acids, minerals, enzymes, and edible plant extracts) contain an electrical charge, which allows the fluid to easily engulf grease and oil. The cleaners are anti-fungal and anti-bacterial. There are no hazards from inhalation, ingestion, or skin and eye exposure. Properly used, the products are not chemically reactive, corrosive, flammable, fuming, or poisonous.

COFFEE, HERBAL ALTERNATIVE TO

Teeccino Caffé, Inc.
PO Box 42259
Santa Barbara, California 93140
>   contact: **Customer Service**
>   phone: **800-498-3434 (toll-free) or 805-966-0999**
>   fax: **805-966-0522**
>   website: **www.teeccino.com**

Coffee is addictive and dangerous. Even the 7% caffeine in "decaf" causes blood sugar swings and heart arrhythmia, and releases stress hormones. Ground roasted herbs, fruits, grains, and nuts in caffeine-free Teeccino brew (and look) just like coffee, but taste better. Bitter herbs promote digestion; chicory root contains inulin (a soluble fiber that nourishes digestive flora); roasted barley has no detectable gluten levels; and there are 65 mg. of alkalizing potassium per cup. Teeccino is also nationally distributed to natural foods stores, the food service industry, holistic health practitioners, and spas.

ESSENTIAL OILS AND PERSONAL CARE PRODUCTS

A Natural Hi
PO Box 1033
South Bend, Indiana 46624
>   contact: **Val Lang, herbalist/consultant**
>   phone: **574-286-5834**
>   fax: **775-248-0851**
>   website: **www.anaturalhi.com**

This company provides excellent quality, organic and wild-crafted pure essential oils, as well as hundreds of plant-based spa and beauty products. Ms. Lang also creates custom skin care items, essential oil blends, and unusual combination homeopathic and medicinal herbal tinctures. She is very careful about not using synthetic toxic ingredients like sodium laurel sulfate, mineral oil, etc.

EXERCISE EQUIPMENT: MINI-TRAMPOLINE (THE CELLERCISER™)

Center for Cellular Health, LLC
2255 North University Parkway
Provo, Utah 86404
>   contact: **David Hall, inventor**
>   phone: **800-856-4863 (toll-free) or 435-835-5867**
>   fax: **435-835-5869**
>   website: **www.cellercise.com**

The body's dense lymphatic fluid must be moved to eliminate dead cells, infectious microbes, heavy metals, and other waste. Bouncing on the Cellerciser™ utilizes the three-fold forces of gravity, acceleration, and deceleration to provide an aerobic, weight loss-promoting, body contouring workout that is more complete and beneficial than regular exercise (weight training, running, or swimming). David Hall's portable folding Cellerciser™ is not a typical mini-trampoline or rebounder. Its exceptionally "easy" bounce protects your knees and joints while literally massaging every cell, and revitalizing bones, blood vessels, connective tissue, glands, internal organs, and skin.

LYMPHATIC PATCHES

Health Gems
1330 Booker T. Washington Highway, #35
Moneta, Virginia 24121
>   contact: **Kae Thompson-Liu**
>   phone: **540-297-6485**
>   website: **www.health-gems.com**

Square compresses from the Orient, usually placed on the soles of the feet, draw out heavy metals, chemicals, and other wastes from the body. Bamboo sap vinegar, wood vinegar, ionic particles, agarikus mushroom, chitosan, eucalyptus, *hottuynia cordata*, and *saururus chinesis*—with the FIR emitted by crushed tourmaline—complement any detox program.

Fawcett Research
19689 7th Avenue N.E. #138
Poulsbo, Washington 98370
    contact: Dale Fawcett or Carol Fawcett
    phone: 866-315-1838 (toll-free) or 360-598-6585
    fax: 360-697-6595
    website: www.LivingNow.net; www.AboutRoyalRife.com

This international networking center provides information on holistic treatments for research scientists, clinicians, journalists, and seekers of holistic health care. Transfer factor, the immune modulator in colostrum (produced by a nursing mammal)—and a critical part of many detoxification and wellness programs—is also available.

Better Way Health
2029 Kramer Way
Marietta, GA 30062-5476
    contact: Dave Perkins, owner
    phone: 877-461-4463 toll free; 678-560-1808 local
    fax: 678-560-1961
    website: www.betterwayhealth.com

Dave Perkins used ionized alkaline water as part of his protocol to recover from medically diagnosed Stage IV cancer. His water filter uses a .03 micron, silver impregnated filter to decontaminate microbes, and comes with a 30-day money back guarantee.

Saunas—Build Your Own, Instructions

Aaland, Mikkel. *Sweat* (Santa Barbara, California: Capra Press, 1978). The book is currently out-of-print. But instructions are available at www.cyberbohemia.com, or can be ordered from Cyberbohemia, 539 Greenwich Street, San Francisco, CA 94133.

Jalasjaa, Bert Olavi. *Art of Sauna Building* (Key Industries, 1981).

McVicker, Marilyn. *Sauna Detoxification Therapy: A Guide for the Chemically Sensitive* (McFarland & Company, Inc., 1997).

Virtanen, John O. *The Finnish Sauna: Peace of Mind, Body and Soul* (O-W Enterprise, Withee, Wisconsin 54498; 1998).

Wilson, Lawrence. Dr. Wilson offers plans for building a crude infrared light bulb sauna with detailed assembly instructions, as well as a kit of parts for an infrared bulb heating unit. Write to PO Box 54, Prescott, Arizona 86302, or visit the website www.drlwilson.com.

SAUNAS—CUSTOM BUILDERS

Custom companies build saunas individually cut to fit any space, from blueprints, floor plans, or given dimensions. The customer can purchase prefabricated saunas, liners for rooms, or modular, freestanding sauna kits. Saunas can be installed for home or public use; indoors or outdoors; and as part of a room, or as a separate room. Most custom builders also supply heaters, steam baths, and accessories. Some manufacture their own heaters, controls, and doors. The woods vary. Each builder is unique, so ask what they do. Most are willing to travel.

Am–Finn Sauna Company
PO Box 29406
Greensboro, North Carolina 27429
    contact: **Ed Gideon, owner**
    phone: **800-237-2862 (toll-free) or 336-854-1991**
    fax: **336-854-3677**
    website: **www.saunasolutions.com**

Finlandia *(in Canada)* **/ Saunafin** *(in the U.S.)*
115 Bowes Road, Unit 2
Concord, Ontario L4K 1H7, Canada
    phone: **800-387-7029 (toll-free) or 905-738-4017**
    fax: **905-738-2486**
    website: **www.saunafin.com**

Finnleo Sauna, Steam and Infrared
575 East Cokato Street
Cokato, Minnesota 55321
    contact: **Mark Raisanen, owner**
    phone: **800-346-6536**
    fax: **320-286-6100**
    website: **www.finnleo.com**

Helo Sauna, Steam and Infrared *(sells to other dealers and installers only)*
575 East Cokato Street
Cokato, Minnesota 55321
   contact: John Oster, national sales manager
   phone: 800-882-4352
   fax: 800-528-9665
   website: www.helosaunas.com

Northernlight Sauna
167 Clinton Street
Kingston, New York 12401
   contact: Stephen Johnson, owner
   phone: 800-344-0513 (toll-free) or 845-340-9934
   website: www.northernlightsaunas.com

Solhem Sauna LLC
Box 880
Moretown, Vermont 05660
   contact: Nils Per Shenholm, owner
   phone: 802-244-6460
   website: www.saunavermont.com

SAUNA AND SAUNA ACCESSORY MANUFACTURERS

In this section, portability means wheels, a relatively small size, relatively lightweight, or a unit that can easily be broken down after each use.

Aran Aqua Pollution Control Systems, Inc.
PO Box 288
Chippewa Lake, Ohio 44215
   contact: Ted Trikilis, president
   phone: 866-272-6247 (toll-free) or 330-769-4844
   fax: 330-769-1755
   website: www.aranizer.com

The Aranizer™ is an unusual air purification unit that regroups the atmospheric oxygen molecule (O_2) into allotropic, high-energy molecules containing four or more atoms of oxygen (O_4, O_5, O_6, O_7, etc.) called Aran™, which does not contain dangerous nitrogen compounds, kills bacteria and microbes, removes dust, pollen, and mold; and produces beneficial negative ions.

Arrowhead HealthWorks
PO Box 950
Twin Peaks California 92391
    contact: **Carolyn Bormann, ND**
    phone: **909-338-3533**
    fax: **909-338-7343**
    website: **www.arrowheadhealthworks.com**

Brand name of sauna: (a) BioTherm, (b) Silver Bullet.

Type of sauna and body position: (a) Cabinet; horizontal, (b) Tent; horizontal.

Materials from which sauna is constructed: (a) Mahogany lined with fiberglass and carbon, (b) Silver metallic mesh lined with fiberglass and carbon.

Any glues or adhesives used in construction: No.

Price: (a) $2495 to $3095, (b) $795 to $995.

Portability: (a) Yes (connecting modular units), (b) Yes.

Type of heater: (a) FIR, (b) FIR.

Noteworthy features: No plastics, PVC, neoprene, or styrofoam. Domes in the ozone/oxygen compatible BioTherm, available in multiple sizes, can be used separately for selected areas. The FIR-emitting carbon panels were patented by NASA. Personal and tech support from a medical hyperthermist is available for a fee.

BNH Corporation
16000 Phoenix Drive
City of Industry, California 91745
    contact: **Sales**
    phone: **800-622-4316 (toll-free) or 626-336-8800**
    fax: **626-369-7800**

Brand name of sauna: (a) Infra Therapist, (b) Aurora Infrared Sauna, (c) Aroma N Steam.

Type of sauna and body position: (a) Cabinet; horizontal, (b) Room; seated, (c) Room; seated.

Materials from which saunas are constructed: (a) Plastic, (b) Wood (cedar, aspen, poplar, basswood), (c) Plastic.

Any glues or adhesives used in construction: No.

Price: (a) $2000 to $2500, (b) Wholesale only, (c) $2000 to $3000.

Portability: (a) Yes, (b) No, (c) Yes.

Type of heater: (a) FIR, (b) FIR, (c) Steam.

Noteworthy features: No additional information provided.

Heavenly Heat
1106 Second Street
Encinitas, California 92024
  contact: **Bob Morgan, owner**
  phone: **800 MY SAUNA (800-697-2862)**
  fax: **760-634-1268**
  website: www.heavenlyheatsaunas.com
Brand name of sauna: Heavenly Heat Saunas.

Type of sauna and body position: Room; seated or (for the larger models) lying down.

Materials from which sauna is constructed: White poplar, exclusively, and glass for the windows.

Any glues or adhesives used in construction: No.

Price: $2675 to $4900.

Portability: No for all units except the narrowest, one-person model, which is on wheels.

Types of heaters: Two heating systems in each sauna: Far Infrared, and electric stone-filled upon which water can be thrown.

Noteworthy features: Saunas come in seven sizes, as modular room kits. All saunas contain filters to eliminate noxious fumes, and vents to allow fresh air in the room. The FIR models have individual heating controls for each bather.

High Tech Health, Inc.
2695 Linden Drive, Suite 200
Boulder, Colorado
  contact: **Bill Johnson, president**
  phone: **800-794-5355 or 303-413-8500**
  fax: **303-449-9640**
  website: www.hightechhealth.com.
Brand name of sauna: Thermal Life Far Infrared Sauna.

Type of sauna and body position: Room; seated.

Materials from which sauna is constructed: Poplar.

Any glues or adhesives used in construction: Small amount, water-based.

Price: $2800 to $3800.

Portability: No.

Type of heater: FIR.

Noteworthy features: Assembles in 15 minutes without tools; heater has single degree setting increments. Company president will give support and answer questions while customer detoxifies. Offices in England (phone: 011+45+787 3429) and Australia (phone: 011+61+75+448 8367).

Longevity Resources Inc.
2412 Beacon Ave, Suite A
Sidney, British Columbia
Canada V8L 1X4
>   contact: **Roger Chown, owner**
>   phone: **877-543-3398 or 250-654-0092**
>   fax: **888-543-3439 (toll-free)   or 250-654-0093**
>   website: **www.ozonegenerator.com**

Brand name of sauna: Hyperthermic Chamber.

Type of sauna and body position: Cabinet; seated.

Materials from which sauna is constructed: Fiberglass.

Any glues or adhesives used in construction: No.

Price: $2199 to $2399 (US).

Portability: Yes (on wheels).

Type of heater: Steam generator.

Noteworthy features: A patented "curing" process virtually eliminates outgassing from fiberglass. Steam generators and piping are made of food grade copper to eliminate unwanted degradation (electrolysis) that can occur when copper is combined with stainless steel. Company also manufactures ozone generators.

Nippa Sauna Heaters by Bruce Enterprises, Inc.
5125 US 45 North
Bruce Crossing, Michigan 49912
>   contact: **Christine Bowers, owner**
>   phone: **906-827-3906**
>   fax: **906-827-3889**
>   website: **www.nippa.com**

Wood stoves: heavy duty steel; between 190 and 250 pounds; hold up to 150 pounds of rock; priced from $589.

Gas stoves: heavy duty steel; 160 pounds and up; hold 150 pounds of rock; priced from $1199.

Electric heaters: stainless steel with triple insulation walls; weigh between 35 pounds and 75 pounds; hold between 50 and 150 pounds of rock; priced from $478.

All of the heaters accommodate rocks on which water can be thrown to create steam.

Plasmafire Intl.
7186-205th Street
Langley, British Columbia
Canada V2Y 1T1
  contact: **Dr. Saul Pressman, DCh**
  phone: **604-532-9596**
  fax: **604-532-9596**
  website: **www.plasmafire.com**
  Brand name of sauna: Omega
  Type of sauna and body position: Cabinet; seated.
  Materials from which sauna is constructed: Fiberglass.
  Any glues or adhesives used in construction: No.
  Price: $2500 (US).
  Portability: Yes (on wheels).
  Type of heater: Steam from stainless steel boiler.
  Noteworthy features: Steam sauna is ozone-ready with Teflon fittings.
    Company also manufactures medical ozone generators (sold separate-
    ly) based on Tesla's "cold plasma" design, with a lifetime warranty.

PLH Products, Inc.
16000 Phoenix Drive
City of Industry, California 91745
  contact: **Sales**
  phone: **800-946-6001 (toll-free) or 626-961-0700**
  fax: **626-968-0444**
  website: **www.healthmatesauna.com**
  Brand name of sauna: Healthmate.
  Type of sauna and body position: Room; seated.
  Materials from which sauna is constructed: Cedar, aspen, poplar, bass-
    wood.
  Any glues or adhesives used in construction: No.
  Price: $3000 to $6000.
  Portability: No.
  Type of heater: FIR.
  Noteworthy features: No additional information provided.

U.S. Health Equipment Co., Inc.
138 Maple Hill Drive
Kingston, New York 12401
> contact: **Bernarr Schaeffer, president or**
>   **James Schaeffer, engineering and marketing manager**
> phone: **877-7-SAUNEX (or 877-772-8639, toll-free) or**
>   **845-658-7576**
> fax: **845-658-7224**
> website: **www.saunex.com**

Brand name of sauna: Saunex.

Type of sauna and body position: Cabinet; seated.

Materials from which sauna is constructed: ABS plastic.

Any glues or adhesives used in construction: No.

Price: $2895.

Portability: Yes (on wheels).

Type of heater: FIR.

Noteworthy features: The less than three-quarter-inch thick patent pending FIR heaters lie flush against cabinet and line all sides. Heater covers contain grooves that prevent the user from being burned. The design eliminates nearly all harmful EMF (electromagnetic fields). A smaller-size seat that clips onto the regular seat to accommodate children is also available.

SPA ASSOCIATIONS

The popularity of spas has grown in the last decade, thanks to the educational and outreach efforts of spa organizations. Over 50 countries are represented by these organizations, with thousands of members that include-besides day spas, medical spas and resort spas—body care product companies, cruise ships, fitness centers, hotels, medical clinics, mineral spring facilities, spa consulting firms, spa equipment manufacturers, spa magazine publishers, and trade show organizations. Service providers such as physicians, massage therapists, nutritionists, and wellness instructors also may belong to spa associations, as well as any interested consumer.

These associations are devoted to influencing policy for the spa industry, as well as promoting a positive spa experience to the public. They accomplish these goals through educational literature, seminars, and websites. They may offer information on spa history and etiquette; spa travel specials and cuisine; and members' products and services, which can include acupuncture, aromatherapy, herbal wraps, homeopathy, massage, and sauna therapy as well as conventional spa services like hair and nail care. The websites of most spa organizations include a search engine that finds a specific type and location of a member facility, and helps match consumers to a suitable spa.

The Day Spa Association / The Medical Spa Association
310 17th Street
Union City, New Jersey 07087
   contact: **Hannelore R. Leavy, executive director**
   phone: **201-865-2065**
   fax: **201-865-3961**
   website: **www.spaassociation.com**

The International SPA Association (ISPA)
2365 Harrodsburg Road, Suite A325
Lexington, Kentucky 40504
   contact: **Debra Locker, director of public relations**
   phone: **888-651-4772 (toll-free) or 859-226-4374**
   fax: **859-226-4445**
   website: **www.experienceispa.com**

Spa Finder
91 Fifth Avenue
New York, New York 10003
   phone: **212-924-6800 (magazine subscriptions)**
                800-255-7727 (toll-free) or
                757-382-4380 (spa information and reservations)
   website: **www.spafinder.com**

Spa Index
1511 M Sycamore, Suite 104
Hercules, California 94547
   contact: **Kristina J. Fitzhugh, editor**
   phone: **877-832-6169 (toll-free)**
   fax: **707-598-7653**
   website: **www.spaindex.com**

SPAS

A spa provides facilities and services pertaining to beauty, fitness, and health. This listing contains a very small sample of English-speaking facilities that have dry saunas, steam, and/or some type of therapeutic pool. Services can include aromatherapy and oil infusions; body and herbal wraps (using Aryuvedic plants, algae, seaweed or other botanicals); electrolysis; exercise, fitness and yoga classes; facials; hair and scalp care; hydrotherapy (moving water in a pool, often containing therapeutic liquids); many types of massage; mineral water pools; mud or clay baths; nail care; specialized skin care, and more. Resort spas are connected to overnight-stay hotels. Day spas may have similar, and as many, features as resort spas, but they do not accommodate overnight guests. Medical spas can be affiliated with homeopaths, naturopaths, nurses, physicians, and/or medical centers; and in addition to traditional spa fare they offer more medically-oriented services such as acupuncture, Aryuvedic medicine treatments, chiropractic, dermatology, homeopathy, nutritional consultations, oxygen therapy, and plastic surgery. Medical spas may accommodate either overnight or day guests.

In the entry that notes which type of sauna is used, "dry" indicates non-steam heat—usually conventional electric or far infrared, though not always—to distinguish it from heavy steam (although some of the dry saunas are made to accommodate hot rocks onto which water can be poured). "Steam" can indicate the dissemination of steam from a capsule, so-called "steam shower," large room, tent, or cabinet. Hydrotherapy, hot tubs, whirlpools, waterfalls, and hot and cold plunge pools are referenced as well; but swimming pools are not. Be aware that some state laws in the US require that whirlpools and similar tubs be decontaminated with chlorine, which is poisonous and can cause respiratory and skin problems in many people.

It is impossible to list every establishment that has a sauna, so consult your local phone directory under "YMCA" (or "YWCA," "YMHA," or "YWHA") and "Health Clubs." I did not list the chain health clubs such as The Equinox or Health and Racquet Club, or spas found in the following well-known chain hotels: the Biltmore, Doral, Hilton, Hyatt Regency, La Quinta, Loews, Marriott, Plaza, Radisson, Ritz-Carlton, and St. Regis—partly because these facilities can be found easily in the phone book, and partly because many of the larger chain hotels no longer open their facilities to people who are not guests of the hotel. See the beginning of this Appendix for strictly medical treatment facilities that administer to people with serious conditions such as cancer and environmental illness.

Be an informed consumer. Whether you want a day spa, resort, or medical spa, be clear about what is offered before you visit. Due to the widespread use of poisonous chemicals for hair and nail care, I tried not to list establishments with a major focus on "beauty" (unless precautions are taken to use safe ingredients)—but please, since everyone has a different tolerance of chemicals and scents, for your own safety and peace of mind, double check. Prices at these facilities can vary widely. Search the internet to see if the spa has a website; a quick look may help you decide whether or not that facility is for you.

Guide to fees

NFG = No Fee for Guests. This pertains to *resort spas* only. If the spa is part of a resort, people staying at the resort may use the spa sauna, steam, and other facilities without having to pay an additional fee.

FG = Fee for Guests. This pertains to *resort spas* only. If the spa is part of a resort, people staying at the resort must pay an additional fee if they want to use the spa sauna, steam, and other facilities.

DP = Day Pass. This pertains to *day spas* (non-resort), and to *resort spas* that allow *non-resort guests for the day*. For a (usually) moderate fee, the customer may use the sauna (and other facilities such as exercise equipment or swimming pool) as much as desired, without having to pay for a special spa service.

PS = Purchase a Service. The facility allows the use of the sauna or steam room if the customer buys other spa services such as a facial or massage.

SF = Separate fee. There is a separate fee for use of the sauna, steam, whirlpool, etc., independent of other services. (This separate fee usually arises in spas that don't issue a Day Pass.) There might be a time restriction with this option, so check with the facility; otherwise, an hour-long sauna can be rather expensive. However, I tried to include only those spas that are generous with their time and reasonably priced.

NFR = No Fee for Residents. This pertains to *residential spas* only. They do not allow outside guests to use their facilities.

United States

ALABAMA

Fairhope

Hideaway in Fairhope Medi-Spa. 251-929-2114. Medical. Steam, aromatherapy, oxygen. By appointment only. PS or SF.

Mobile

Lynn Cary's Holistic Day Spa. 251-450-0002. Steam, aromatherapy, oxygen. PS or SF.

ARIZONA

Scottsdale

Slender Elegance Body & Soul Spa. 480-368-0022. Medical. Hydrotherapy, steam with ozone. DP, time restriction for ozone.

The Spa at Gainey Village. 480-609-6980. Dry. DP.

The Stress Less Step. 480-945-1579. Dry, steam. DP.

Tucson

Canyon Ranch Health Resort. 800-742 9000. Medical (four-night minimum stay). Dry, steam, eucalyptus steam, whirlpool. NFR.

ARKANSAS

Hot Springs

Andrea Rose Salon. 501-623-6449. Steam. SF or PS.

Arlington Resort Hotel & Spa. 800-643-1502. Dry, steam. PS (guests and non-guests).

CALIFORNIA

Burbank

Burbank Spa & Garden. 818-845-1251. Dry. SF or PS.

Calistoga

Dr. Wilkinson's Hot Springs Resort. 707-942-4102. Hot springs. NFG (guests of resort only).

Calistoga Village Inn & Spa. 707-942-0991. Dry, hot springs. NFG; PS (non-guests).

Mount View Hotel & Spa. 707-942-6877; 800-816-6877. Hydrotherapy with herbs, hot stone massage. SF (guests and non-guests).

	Indian Springs Resort & Spa. 707-942-9035. Steam, mineral pool. PS.
	Lavender Hill Spa. 707-942-4495, 800-528-4772 . Mineral salt bath, hot stone massage. SF.
Carlsbad	**La Costa Resort and Spa.** 760-438-9111. Dry, steam, whirlpool. DP.
Carmel Valley	**Spa at Bernardus Lodge.** 831-658-3514. Dry, steam, whirlpool. FG, PS (non-guests).
Corona	**Glen Ivy Hot Springs Spa.** 888-258-2683. Dry, steam. DP.
Desert Hot Spgs	**Desert Hot Springs Spa Hotel.** 800-808-7727. Dry, hot mineral pools. NFG; DP.
Encino	**Skin Spa, Inc.** 818-995-3888. Dry, steam. DP.
Escondido	**Bellissima Day Spa.** 760-480-9072. Steam. SF or PS.
Fallbrook	**Los Willows Inn & Spa.** 888-731-9400. Dry, steam, whirlpool. NFG; DP or PS.
June Lake	**Double Eagle Resort & Spa.** 760-648-7134. Steam, whirlpool. DP.
La Jolla	**The Spa at Torrey Pines.** 858-777-6690. Dry, steam, eucalyptus steam. NFG; DP.
Lodi	**Bodyspa.** Medical. 800-269-5167. Dry, steam. SF or PS.
Los Angeles	**Beverly Hot Springs.** 323-734-7000. Dry, steam. DP.
Napa	**Spa at Silverado.** 707-257-5555. Dry, steam, whirlpool. DP.
Ojai	**The Oaks at Ojai.** 805-646-5573. Medical (two-night minimum stay; nutritional consulting only from nurse on staff). Dry, steam.
	Ojai Valley Inn & Spa. 805-640-2020. Dry, steam, whirlpool. NFG; DP.
Olympic Valley	**Spa at Squaw Creek.** 530-583-6300. Dry, whirlpool. NFG; DP.
Palm Springs	**The Palms.** 760-325-1111. Dry. PS.

Pasadena	**New Beginning Day Spa.** 626-449-1231. Medical. Steam. SF.
Pebble Beach	**Spa at Pebble Beach.** 888-565-7615. Dry, steam. DP or PS.
Rancho Mirage	**Spa at Mission Hills.** 760-328-5955. Steam. DP or PS (for both overnight and day guests).
San Diego	**Paradise Point Resort & Spa.** 800-344-2626. Dry, eucalyptus steam, hot tub. PS.
	Rancho Bernardo Inn, Buena Vista Spa. 858-675-8471. Dry, steam, whirlpool. DP.
	World Spa Resorts, Inc. 619-624-0506. Dry, steam. DP or PS.
San Francisco	**Kabuki Springs & Spa.** 415-922-6000. Dry, steam, hot and cold plunge pools. DP, or a small additional charge with service. (Call first; men and women are sometimes admitted on different days.)
	Nob Hill Spa. 415-345-2807. Dry, steam, whirlpool. DP (M-Th only), PS (weekend).
	Re:Fresh, A Day Spa. 415-563-2316. Dry. PS.
Santa Monica	**Aqua Day Spa.** 310-899-6222. Dry, steam, whirlpool. SF or PS.
	Burke Williams Day Spa & Massage Center. 310-587-3366. Dry, steam, whirlpool. DP (Mon-Th), PS (Fri, Sat and Sun).
Sonoma	**Garden Spa at MacArthur Place.** 707-933-3194. Steam, whirlpool. PS.
	Raindance Spa. 707-931-2031. Dry, eucalyptus steam, mineral bath. DP or PS.
Woodland Hills	**Allen Edwards Serenity Spa.** 818-593-7094. Dry. SF or PS.

COLORADO

Aspen	**Aspen Club.** 970-925-8900. Dry, steam. Members, no charge; non-members, PS.

Buena Vista	**Cottonwood Hot Springs Inn & Spa.** 800-241-4119 or 719-395-6434. Dry, hot mineral springs, cold plunge pool. NFG; DP.
Lakewood	**A+ European Body & Health.** 303-233-0712. Steam, hydrotherapy. SF.
Ward	**Gold Lake Mountain Resort & Spa.** 303-459-3544. Dry, whirlpool, hot pools. DP.

CONNECTICUT

Branford	**By the Sea Inn & Spa.** 203-483-3333. Dry. SF (guests and non-guests call ahead for appointment).
Norwich	**The Spa at Norwich Inn.** 860-886-2401. Dry, steam, whirlpool. NFG; DP or PS.

FLORIDA

Fort Lauderdale	**Wyndham Bonaventure Resort & Spa.** 954-349-5515. Dry, steam, whirlpool, warm and cool plunge pools. NFG; DP.
Key Biscayne	**Sonesta Beach Resort & Spa.** 305-365-2949. Dry, steam. NFG; DP.
Key West	**Pier House Resort and Caribbean Spa.** 305-296-4600. Medical. Dry, steam, whirlpool. DP (guests and non-guests).
Miami	**Bellezza Spa Salon and Boutique.** 305-665-3656. Dry. PS.
N. Miami Beach	**Aventura Holistic Day Spa.** 305-957-8814. Medical. Steam (aromatherapy), hydrotherapy. SF or PS.
Orlando	**Grand Floridian Spa & Health Club.** 407-824-2332. Dry, steam, whirlpool. DP.
	Papillon Spa. 407-992-2938. Dry, steam, whirlpool. DP or PS.
Palm Beach	**Babor Institut.** 561-832-9385. Steam, hydrotherapy. Steam no fee; hydrotherapy SF.
	Spa at the Breakers. 561-653-6656. Dry, steam, whirlpool. NFG; PS.

Ponte Vedra Bch	Spa at the Ponte Vedra Inn & Club. 904-273-7700. Dry, steam, whirlpool. DP.
Safety Harbor	Safety Harbor Resort & Spa. 727-726-1161. Dry, steam and whirlpool. DP.
Wesley Chapel	Spa at Saddlebrook Resort. 800-729-8383. Dry, steam, whirlpool. FG; PS (non-guests).

DELAWARE

Rehoboth Beach	Life Force Massage & Wellness Center. 302-227-6818 or 866-676-2437. Hot stone massage. SF.

GEORGIA

Braselton	Spa at Chateau Elan. 678-425-6064. Dry, steam, whirlpool. NFG; DP or PS.
Marietta	Renew Day Spa. 770-998-8592. Dry, hydrotherapy. DP or PS.

HAWAII

Honolulu	Abhasa Waikiki Spa. 808-922-8200. Steam, whirlpool. DP or PS.
Kapolei	Ihilani Resort & Spa. 808-679-0079. Dry, steam, whirlpool. PS.
Lanai City	Manele Bay Hotel. 808-565-2086. Dry, steam. DP or PS.
Wailea (Maui)	Spa Kea Lani. 808-875-4100. Steam. NFG; PS.

IDAHO

Lava Hot Spgs	Aura Soma Lava. 208-776-5221. Hot spring pool. NFG.
	State of Idaho Foundation Pools. 208-776-5221. Hot springs, cold plunge, private hot tub. DP, season pass, family pass, multiple-admission card.
Moscow	Pure Energy Elements Day Spa. 208-882-3401. Dry (combined with vibrational massage), hydrotherapy. SF.

Sun Valley	**Solavie Spa & Salon.** 208-726-7211. Dry, steam, hot tub, cold plunge pool, waterfall. SF for each modality.

ILLINOIS

Chicago	**Betty O. Day Spa.** 773-752-3600. Hydrotherapy with different liquids. SF.

IOWA

Vedic City	**The Raj Resort.** 800-248-9050. Medical. Primarily residential, although individual daily services are also available. Steam, hot oil massage. SF.

LOUISIANA

Bossier City	**The Horseshoe Casino Spa.** 800-895-0711. Dry, steam. SF (½ price for hotel guests) or PS.
Hammond	**Paris Parker.** 888-990-2468. Dry, steam. SF or PS.
Houma	**Allie's Figure & Day Spa.** 985-917-0009. Steam. SF or reduced rate as PS.

MAINE

Augusta	**Senator Inn & Spa.** 207-622-5804. Dry, hot tub, salt water pool. NFG; DP or PS.

MARYLAND

Baltimore	**Total Body Concept Day Spa.** 410-663-1010. Steam. PS.

MASSACHUSETTS

Lenox	**Canyon Ranch in the Berkshires.** 800-326-7080. Medical. Dry, steam, eucalyptus steam, whirlpool. Three-night minimum stay, NFR.

MICHIGAN

Ann Arbor	**Bellanina Day Spa.** 734-747-8517. Dry, steam. DP.
Farmington Hills	**Tamara.** 248-855-0474. Dry, steam, hydrotherapy. DP.
Gaylor	**Heart to Heart Massage Spa.** 989-705-1717. Dry. SF.

Great Falls	**Linda Michaels Day Spa.** 406-727-3287. Dry. SF or PS.
Petoskey	**Spa at the Inn at Bay Harbor.** 231-439-4046. Hydrotherapy with mineral water. SF.

MINNESOTA

Litchfield	**Birdwing Spa.** 320-693-6064. Dry, steam, whirlpool. Residential only. NFR.
Marsh	**A Center for Balance and Fitness.** 952-935-2202. Dry, steam. NFG; DP or PS.
Oakdale	**Body Rhythms Therapeutic Day Spa.** 651-739-6388. Dry. SF or PS.

MISSISSIPPI

Biloxi	**The Spa at Beau Rivage.** 228-386-7472. Dry, steam. FG, PS.

MISSOURI

Clayton	**The Face & The Body.** 314-725-8975. Dry. PS.
Excelsior Spgs	**Elms Resort and Spa.** 800-THE-ELMS. Dry, steam, hot and cold plunge pools, hot tub. NFG; DP or PS.
Jefferson City	**Riversong Spa & Salon.** 573-636-5438. Dry, steam, hot tub, whirlpool. SF or PS.
Lake Ozark	**Spa Shiki.** 800-THE-LAKE. Dry, steam, whirlpool, hydrotherapy. DP (guests and non-guests), PS (non-guests).

MONTANA

Big Sky	**Moonlight Spa.** 406-995-7700. Steam. NFG; DP or PS.
Bozeman	**Spa at Bozeman Hot Springs.** 406-522-9563. Dry, steam, hot and cold plunge pools. DP.

NEVADA

Las Vegas	**Dolphin Court Salon & Day Spa.** 702-949-9999. Steam, whirlpool. DP or PS.

<table>
<tr><td></td><td>Mirage Spa. 702-791-7472. Dry, steam, whirlpool. NFG; DP or PS.</td></tr>
<tr><td>Reno</td><td>Reverse Aging Club. 775-327-4878. Medical. Dry. SF, or monthly or longer memberships (members use saunas as often as desired).</td></tr>
</table>

NEW HAMPSHIRE

Jaffrey	**The Grand View Inn & Resort.** 603-532-9880. Dry, steam. NFG; DP or PS.

NEW JERSEY

Hackensack	**Beyond.** 201-996-4500. Dry, steam. PS.
Princeton	**Spa Therapia.** 609-921-9510. Steam. SF or PS.

NEW MEXICO

Albuquerque	**Betty's Bath and Day Spa.** 505-341-3456. Dry, hot tub. SF or PS.
Santa Fe	**La Posada de Santa Fe Resort & Spa.** 505-954-9630. Eucalyptus steam, whirlpool. NFG; DP or PS.
	The Sterling Institute. 505-984-3223. Dry. SF.
Taos	**Casa de las Chimeneas.** 877-758-4777. Dry, hot tub. For guests only; NFG.

NEW YORK

Accord	**Hudson Valley Spa & Resort.** 845-626-8888. Dry, steam, whirlpool. NFG; DP or PS.
Cornwall	**A-NU-U Spa.** 845-534-3656. Dry. SF or PS.
East Meadow	**Nassau County Aquatic Center.** 516-572-0501. Dry, whirlpool, unusually large (25-by-68 meter / about 82-by-223 foot) swimming pool. Membership or DP.
Lake Placid	**Mirror Lake Inn Resort & Spa.** 518-523-2544. Dry, steam, whirlpool. NFG; PS.
Montauk	**Gurney's International Health & Beauty Spa.** 631-668-2345. Dry, steam. NFG; DP or PS.

Moriches	**Luna Mesa Day Spa.** 631-874-4114. Steam. SF or PS.
Mt. Tremper	**The Emerson Spa.** 845-688-7900, ext. 380. Dry, steam, whirlpool. NFG; DP or PS.
New York	**Beauty & Wellness Day Spa.** 212-983-9577. Steam. SF or PS.
	Pratima Ayurvedic Skin Care. 212-581-8136. Steam. SF or PS.
	Soho Sanctuary. 212-334-5550. Dry, steam. Dry, SF; Steam, PS or SF.
Skaneateles	**Mirbeau Inn and Spa.** 315-685-5006. Dry, steam. NFG; DP or PS.
Woodstock	**River Rock Health Spa.** 845-679-7800. Dry, steam. PS.

NORTH CAROLINA

Asheville	**Grove Park Inn Resort.** 800-438-5800. Dry, steam, mineral pool, waterfall pool, hot and cold plunge pools. DP (guests and non-guests) or PS (guests and non-guests).
Duck	**Spa at the Sanderling.** 800-701-4111, ext. 744. Steam, hot tub. NFG; DP or PS.
High Point	**Ambiance European Salon.** 336-883-7778. Steam. SF or PS.
Marshall	**Madison Medical Massage.** 877-839-0125. Medical. Dry. SF or reduced fee with service.
Pinehurst	**The Spa at Pinehurst.** 910-235-8320. Dry, steam, whirlpool. PS (must have 3-day advance reservation).

OHIO

Chagrin Falls	**Martha's La Look Medi-Spa.** 440-543-2797. Medical. Dry, steam. SF.
Shaker Heights	**Charlotte's Day Spa-Salon.** 216-283-2400. Dry, steam, whirlpool. SF.
Toledo	**Bella Via Therapeutic Wellness Spa.** 419-534-6552. Hydrotherapy. SF.

OKLAHOMA

Oklahoma City   Face Beautiful Medi Spa. 405-840-3223. Hydrotherapy. SF.

OREGON

Detroit   Breitenbush Hot Springs Retreat & Conference Center. 503-854-3314. Steam, hot mineral pools. NFG; DP.

Hillsboro   The Pointe at Hawthorn Farm Athletic Club. 503-640-6404. Dry, steam, whirlpool. DP or PS.

Portland   Avalon Hotel and Spa. 888-556-4402 (toll-free) or 503-802-5800. Dry, steam. NFG; DP or PS.

PENNSYLVANIA

Farmington   Nemacolin Woodlands Resort & Spa. 724-329-6930. Dry, steam, whirlpool, hot tubs. DP (guests and non-guests) or PS (guests and non-guests).

Wyomissing   Bell Tower Salon & Spa. 610-372-6379. Steam. SF or PS.

RHODE ISLAND

East Greenwich   Kenneth Cote Renewal Center. 401-884-2810. Steam. SF or PS.

SOUTH CAROLINA

Charleston   Charleston Hotel Place Spa. 843-937-8522. Dry, whirlpool. NFG; PS.

SOUTH DAKOTA

Hot Springs   Springs Bath House. 605-745-4424 or 888-817-1972. Hot mineral pool, steam, hydrotherapy, hot stone massage. SF or PS.

TENNESSEE

Hendersonville   Yana's Salon & Spa. 615-822-9551. Steam, whirlpool. PS.

Knoxville	**Bella Spazio.** 865-670-0998. Steam. SF or PS.
Memphis	**French Riviera Spa.** 901-368-1871. Dry, steam. DP.

TEXAS

Austin	**Barton Creek Resort & Conference Center.** 512-329-4559. Dry, steam, whirlpool. NFG; PS.
	YouTopia Day Spa. 512-5506-9864. Steam. SF or PS.
Dallas	**The Spa at the Crescent.** 214-871-3200. Dry, steam, whirlpool, cool plunge. FG, PS (guests and non-guests).
Galveston	**Moody Gardens Hotel Spa.** 409-744-4673. Dry. NFG; PS.
Lubbock	**Avalon Day Spa.** 806-785-7546. Steam. SF or PS.
San Antonio	**Alamo Plaza Spa at the Menger Hotel.** 210-223-5772. Dry, steam, whirlpool. PS (guests and non-guests).

UTAH

Snowbird	**Cliff Spa at Snowbird.** 801-933-2267. Dry, eucalyptus steam, hot tub. FG, DP or PS.

VERMONT

Killington	**Woods at Killington.** 802-422-4302. Dry, steam hot tub. NFG; DP or PS.
Stowe	**Stoweflake Mountain Resort & Spa.** 802-253-7355. Dry, steam, whirlpool. NFG; DP or PS.
	Topnotch at Stowe Resort & Spa. 802-253-8585. Dry, steam, whirlpool, waterfall pool. NFG (but with some restrictions—contact the resort); DP or PS.

VIRGINIA

Fairfax	**Comfort & Joy Wellness Spa.** 571-331-7333. Steam. DP.
Hot Springs	**Homestead Spa.** 540-839-7547. Dry, steam. DP, PS with day and time restrictions for both guests and non-guests.

Williamsburg	**Kingsmill Resort.** 757-253-8230. Dry, steam, whirlpool. NFG; PS.
Wintergreen	**Wintergreen Spa & Fitness Center.** 800-266-2444. Dry, steam, whirlpool, hot tubs. NFG; DP or PS.

WASHINGTON

Anacortes	**Watersedge Health Club & Spa.** 360-299-2180. Dry, eucalyptus steam. DP.
Bellingham	**Chrysalis Inn & Spa.** 360-756-1005. Steam. NFG; PS.
Monroe	**Kathleen's Salon & Day Spa.** 360-794-3395. Steam with aromatherapy. SF.
Port Townsend	**Annapurna Center for Self-Healing.** 800-868-2662. Dry, steam. NFG; DP.
Snoqualmie	**Salish Lodge & Spa.** 425-888-2556. Dry, steam, hot tub, waterfall. NFG; PS.

WEST VIRGINIA

Berkeley Springs	**Coolfont Health Spa & Resort.** 304-258-4500. Dry. NFG; DP or PS.

WISCONSIN

DePere	**The Day Spa.** 920-339-5250. Dry, steam. Dry SF; steam SF or PS.
Kohler	**Kohler Water Spa/American Club.** 920-457-7777. Dry, steam, whirlpool, hot and cold plunge pools, waterfall pool. DP (guests and non-guests), PS.

WYOMING

Jackson Hole	**Amangani Resort.** 307-739-0333. Steam. PS.
Teton Village	**Snake River Lodge and Spa.** 800-445-4655. Dry, steam, hydrotherapy, hot tubs. NFG; DP (includes one treatment).

Austria

**Loipersdorf,
 Styria**   Thermalquelle Loipersdorf GmbH & Co KG. 011+43+
33+828 2040. Medical. Dry, steam, herbal steam, mineral pool, waterfall. NFG; DP.

Belize

Placencia   Soulshine Resort. 011+501+523 3347. Herbal and mineral baths, whirlpool, hot and warm pools. Residential only. NFR.

Bermuda

Somerset Parish   The Ocean Spa at Cambridge Beaches. 800-468-7300 (toll-free, US and Canada) or 441-234-3636. Dry, steam, hot mud. Residential only. NFR.

**Southampton
 Parish**   The Spa at Sonesta Beach Resort. 441-238-1226. Dry, steam and whirlpool. DP (guests and non-guests).

Brazil

Gramado   Kurotel Longevity Center and Spa. 011+55+54+286 2133, ext. 189. Medical. Dry, steam, hydrotherapy. Residential only; program of one week or more. Saunas included in treatments.

Canada

ALBERTA

Canmore   Bodyworks Salon & Day Spa. 403-678-5746. Steam. Residential only. Saunas included in treatments.

Satori Day Spa. 403-678-9388. Steam. SF or PS.

BRITISH COLUMBIA

Clinton	**Echo Valley Ranch & Spa.** 800-253-8831. Steam. Residential only. Saunas included in treatments.
Victoria	**Nature's Spectrum Far Infrared Sauna Center.** 888-262-4477. Dry. SF.

ONTARIO

Grafton	**St. Anne's Country Inn & Spa.** 888-346-6772. Dry, steam, eucalyptus steam. Residential only. PS.
Kingston	**Spa at the Mill.** 613-544-1166. Hydrotherapy. SF.
London	**Fayez Beauty Spa.** 519-652-2780. Dry, whirlpool. SF.
Port Hope	**The Hillcrest Victorian Inn & Spa.** 888-346-6772. Dry. Residential only.

Canary Islands

Lanzarote	**Terapia Natural España (Natural Therapy Center).** 609 010 231 928 513505. Medical. Sauna in the arthritis and back pain clinic. NFG; PS or SF.

Germany

Baden-Baden	**Brenner's Park-Hotel & Spa.** 011+49+7221+900 0. Dry, steam, aromatherapy pool. NFG; PS.
	Schlosshotel Bühlerhöhe. 011+49+7226+55 0. Dry, steam, whirlpool. DP.

Puerto Rico

Puerto Vuevo	**Nouvelle D'Spa.** 787-783-9492. Steam. SF or PS.

Scotland

Fife	**The Old Course Hotel, Golf Resort & Spa.** 011+44+334+474 371. Dry (oven), moist heat. NFG; PS.

South Africa

Hermanus   **AltiraSpa.** 011+27+28+284 0000. Dry sauna with ozone, steam, hydrotherapy, brine pool, whirlpool. NFG; DP (outside guests must call ahead).

Switzerland

Interlaken   **Grand Hotel Victoria-Jungfrau.** 011+41+33+828 2710. Sauna, steam, whirlpool. NFG; DP (non-guests on selected days)

Mont Pelerin   **Le Mirador Resort Hotel and Spa.** 011+41+21+925 1111. Dry, steam, whirlpool, NFG; PS (non-guests).

Wales

Newport   **Forum Health Club and Spa at Celtic Manor Resort.** 011+44+1633 410326. Steam (heated coals plus water). PS.

Note to clinics, manufacturers, product providers and spas:

If you are listed and there are errors in your entry, or if you are not listed and think you should be in the next edition of this book, please contact the author.

BIBLIOGRAPHY

*Genius is one per cent inspiration
and ninety-nine per cent perspiration.*

THOMAS ALVA EDISON
U.S. INVENTOR 1847–1931, REMARK MADE ABOUT 1903

Aaland, Mikkel. *Sweat*. Santa Barbara: Capra Press, 1978. [Though the book is out of print, excerpts from it are online at www.cyberbohemia .com/Pages/sweat.htm.]

Abbott, George Knapp, Fred B. Moor, and Kathryn L. Jensen–Nelson. *Physical Therapy in Nursing Care*. Washington, D.C.: Review and Herald Publishing Association, 1941.

Ahonen, E., and U. Nousiainen. "The Sauna and Body Fluid Balance." *Annals of Clinical Research* 20 (1988): 257–261.

Amidon, Robert B. "Chemical Hazards in Law Enforcement." *Journal of California Law Enforcement* 18, no. 3 (Summer 1984).

Anders, Nedda Casson. *Complete Cookbook for Infra-Red Broiler and Rotisserie.* New York: M. Barrows & Co. Inc., 1953.

Asimov, Isaac. *Understanding Physics, 3 Volumes in 1.* New York: Barnes & Noble, 1993.

Baird, Deborah N., and William J. Rea. "The Temporomandibular Joint Implant Controversy: Its Clinical Implications." *Journal of Nutritional and Environmental Medicine* 9 (1999): 209–222.

Batmanghelidj, Fereydoon. *Your Body's Many Cries for Water.* 2nd ed. Falls Church, Va.: Global Health Solutions, Inc., 1997.

Becker, Robert O. *Cross Currents: The Perils of Electropollution, The Promise of Electromedicine.* New York: Jeremy P. Tarcher, 1990.

Ben, Max. "Is Detoxification a Solution to Occupational Health Hazards?" *National Safety News* (May 1984).

Bennett, Homer Clark. *The Electro-Therapeutic Guide, or A Thousand Questions Asked and Answered.* 9th ed., rev. and enl. Lima, Ohio: Literary Dept. of the National College of Electro-Therapeutics, 1912.

Berner, Robert A., and Gary P. Landis. "Gas Bubbles in Fossil Amber as Possible Indicators of the Major Gas Composition of Ancient Air." *Science* 239 (March 18, 1988): 1406–1409.

Brodeur, Paul. *Currents of Death: Power Lines, Computer Terminals, and the Attempt to Cover Up Their Threat to Your Health.* New York: Simon and Schuster, 1989.

Carter, K. Codell. "Nineteenth-century treatments for rabies as reported in the Lancet." *Medical History* 26 (1982): 67–78.

Chien, C.H., J.J. Tsuei, S.C. Lee, Y.C. Huang, and Y.H. Wei. "Effect of Emitted Bioenergy on Biochemical Functions of Cells." *The American Journal of Chinese Medicine* 19, no. 3–4: 285–292.

Christy, Martha M. *Your Own Perfect Medicine.* Scottsdale: Self Healing Press, 1994.

Cichoke, Anthony. *The Complete Book of Enzyme Therapy.* Garden City Park, N.Y.: Avery Publishing Group, 1999.

Cohn, James R.. and Edward A. Emmett. "The Excretion of Trace Metals in Human Sweat." *Annals of Clinical and Laboratory Science* 84 (1978): 270–275.

Collins, Kenneth. "Thermal Effects." In *Clayton's Electrotherapy 10E*, ed. Sheila Kitchen and Sarah Bazin. London: W.B. Saunders Company Ltd., 1996.

Dadd, Debra Lynn. *Home Safe Home: Protecting Yourself and Your Family from Everyday Toxics and Harmful Household Products.* New York: Jeremy P. Tarcher/Putnam, 1997.

de Langre, Jacques. *Seasalt's Hidden Powers: The Biological Action of All Ocean Minerals on Body and Mind.* Magalia, Calif.: Happiness Press, 1994.

Dong, Zhang Jian. *Conybio F.I.R.: Health Knowledge.* Luala Lumpur, Malaysia: Conybio (n.d.).

Donsbach, Kurt. *Let's Talk Health Newsletter* 5, no. 1 (March/April 2002).

Drury, Nevill and Susan. *The Illustrated Dictionary of Natural Health.* New York: Sterling Publishing Co., Inc., 1989.

Edelson, Stephen. *What Your Doctor Won't Tell You About Auto-Immune Disease.* New York: Time Warner, 2003.

Egyptian Orthopedic Assocation. *The Edwin Smith Papyrus.* Online at www.eoa.org.eg/edwintxt.htm [accessed April 27, 2003].

Eisalo, A., and O.J. Luurila. "The Finnish Sauna and Cardiovascular Diseases." *Annals of Clinical Research* 20 (1998): 267–270.

Enig, Mary. *Know Your Fats: The Complete Primer for Understanding the Nutrition of Fats.* Silver Spring, Md.: Bethesda Press, 2000.

Environmental Protection Agency. *Proceedings of the 1998 International Radiological Post-Emergency Response Issues Conference.* Washington, D.C.: EPA, 1998.

————. Office of Toxic Substances. *National Human Adipose Tissue Survey Broad Scan Analysis: Population Estimates from Fiscal Year 1982 Specimens.* EPA 560/5–90–001. Arlington, Va.: EPA, 1989.

Ernst, E., E. Pecho, P. Wiry, and T. Saradeth. "Regular Sauna Bathing and the Incidence of Common Colds." *Annals of Medicine* (1990): 224–227.

Fallon, Sally, with Pat Connolly and Mary G. Enig. *Nourishing Traditions: The Cookbook that Challenges Politically Correct Nutrition and the Diet Dictocrats*. San Diego: ProMotion Publishing, 1995.

Finnerty, Gertrude Brentano, and Theodore Corbitt. *Hydrotherapy*. New York: Frederick Ungar Publishing Co., 1960.

Finnish Sauna Society. "Development of the Finnish Sauna." Article online at www.sauna.fi/pages/develpt.htm [accessed March 3, 2003].

Fitzgerald, Patricia. *The Detox Solution: The Complete Cleansing Plan to Remove Toxins from Your Environment, Body, Mind, and Spirit*. Santa Monica: Illumination Press, 2001.

Fletcher, D.J. "Warming Up to Far-Infrared." *Alternative Medicine* (January 2001).

Flickstein, Aaron. "Infrared Thermal System for Whole-Body Regenerative Radiant Therapy." PDF document online at www.spaequipmentintl.com/indexfolder/formostar/info.pdf [accessed April 27, 2003].

Ford–Martin, Paula. "Hydrotherapy." In *The Gale Encyclopedia of Alternative Medicine*, Farmington Hills, Mich.: The Gale Group, Inc., 2000.

Forest, Waves. "AIDS, Cancer Cured by Hyper-Oxygenation." *Now What* Newsletter, no. 1. Monterey, Calif.: 1987.

Foster, Harold. "Aluminum and Health." *The Journal of Orthomolecular Medicine* 7, no. 4 (Fourth Quarter 1992).

Foundation for Advancements in Science and Education Research. "Fate and Distribution of Cocaine, Diazepam, Phencyclidine PCP and THC Marijuana: A Technical Review." *FASE Bulletin* (August 1985).

———. "A Review of Scientific Literature Supporting the Detoxification Method 'Purification Program' Developed by L. Ron Hubbard." FASE report (Fall 1991).

Free, Valerie H. "Far-Infrared: Technologies that Harness the Sun." *Complementary Healing* (1998).

Freeman, Jeffrey. "Why We Use Hyperthermia." Handout. Twin Peaks, Calif.: Europa Institute of Integrated Medicine, 1999.

Freibott, George A. "Ozone Generators." Article online at www.thefinch leyclinic.co.uk/nojavascript/therapies/ozone/safe.htm [accessed August 31, 2002].

Freudenrich, Craig C. "How Sweat Works." Article online at www .howstuffworks.com/sweat1.htm [accessed July 29, 2001].

Gard, Zane R., and Erma J. Brown. "Literature Review and Comparison Studies of Sauna/Hyperthermia in Detoxification." *Townsend Letter for Doctors & Patients* (August/September 1999).

Gautherie, M., ed. *Whole Body Hyperthermia.* New York: Springer–Verlag New York, Inc., 1992.

Guyton, Arthur C., and John E. Hall. *Textbook of Medical Physiology.* 10th ed. Philadelphia: W.B. Saunders Company, 2000.

Hannuksela, M., and A. Väänänen. "The Sauna, Skin and Skin Diseases." *Annals of Clinical Research* 20 (1988): 276–278.

Hannuksela, Minna L., and Samer Ellahham. "Benefits and Risks of Sauna Bathing." The *American Journal of Medicine* 110, no. 2 (February 2001).

Hawke, Jenny. "Uncovering the Facts on Toxic Carpet." *Nexus* 9, no. 6 (November/December 2002).

HealthCheck Systems. "Understanding Free Radicals and Antioxidants." Article online at www.healthchecksystems.com/antioxid.htm [accessed March 6, 2003].

HealthComm International, Inc. "Detoxification Biochemistry." Technical Bulletin. 2000.

Helamaa, E., and E. Äikäs. "The Secret of Good 'Löyly'." *Annals of Clinical Research* 20 (1988): 224–229.

Hermans–Killam, Linda. "Infrared Astronomy: Near, Mid and Far Infrared." Article online at www.ipac.caltech.edu/Outreach/Edu/Regions/ irregions.html [accessed October 7, 2001].

Herriott, Eva. "Steam and Sauna Therapy: Applications with Massage." *Massage Magazine* 67 (May–June 1997).

Hillila, Bernhard. *The Sauna Is. . . .* Iowa City: Penfield Press, 1988.

Horsley, Victor. "On Hydrophobia and Its 'Treatment': Especially by the Hot-Air Bath, Commonly Termed the Bouisson Remedy." *British Medical Journal* (June 9, 1888): 1207–1211.

Hubbard, L. Ron. *Clear Body, Clear Mind: The Effective Purification Program.* Los Angeles: Bridge Publications, Inc., 1990.

———. *Purification: An Illustrated Answer to Drugs.* Los Angeles: Bridge Publications, Inc., 1990.

Hussein, M. Kamel. "The Oldest Surgical Treatise in the World." Introduction to *The Edwin Smith Papyrus* (Egyptian Orthopedic Association). Online at www.eoa.org.eg/oldest.htm [accessed April 27, 2003].

Imamura, Masakazu, Sadatoshi Biro, Takashi Kihara, Shiro Yoshifuku, Kunitsugu Takasaki, Yutaka Otsuji, Shinichi Minagoe, Yoshifumi Toyama, and Chuwa Tei. "Repeated Thermal Therapy Improves Impaired Vascular Endothelial Function in Patients with Coronary Risk Factors." *Journal of the American College of Cardiology* 38, no. 4 (October 2001).

Incropera, Frank P., and David P. DeWitt. *Fundamentals of Heat and Mass Transfer.* 4th ed. New York: John Wiley and Sons, 1996.

Inoué, Shojiro, and Morihiro Kabaya. "Biological Activities Caused by Far–Infrared Radiation." *The International Journal of Biometeorology* 33 (1989):145-150.

Isomäki, H. "The Sauna and Rheumatic Diseases." *Annals of Clinical Research* 20 (1988): 271–275.

Jalasjaa, Bert Olavi. The *Art of Sauna Building: The Complete Sauna Book.* Waterloo, Ontario: Key Industries, 1981.

Jokinen, E., E.L. Gregory, and I. Välimäki. "The Sauna and Children." *Annals of Clinical Research* 20 (1988): 283–286.

Junaid, A.J. "Treatment of Cutaneous Leishmaniasis with Infrared Heat." *International Journal of Dermatology* 25, no. 7 (Sept. 1986): 470–72.

Jurasunas, Serge. "A Far Infrared Ray Emitting Stone SGES to Treat Cancer and Degenerative Diseases." *Townsend Letter for Doctors & Patients* (June 2000).

Kellogg, John Harvey. *Diphtheria: Its Causes, Prevention, and Proper Treatment.* Battle Creek: The Good Health Publishing Co., 1880.

———. *Light Therapeutics: A Practical Manual of Phototherapy for the Student and the Practitioner.* Rev. ed. Battle Creek: The Good Health Publishing Co., 1910.

Kihara, T., S. Biro, M. Imamura, S. Yoshifuku, K. Takasaki, Y. Ikeda, Y. Otuji, S. Minagoe, Y. Toyama, and C. Tei. "Repeated Sauna Treatment Improves Vascular Endothelial and Cardiac Function in Patients with Chronic Heart Failure." *Journal of the American College of Cardiology* 395 (Mar. 6, 2002): 754–9.

Kilburn, Kaye, Raphael H. Warsaw, and Megan G. Shields. "Neurobehavioral Dysfunction in Firemen Exposed to Polychlorinated Biphenyls PCBs: Possible Improvement after Detoxification." *Archives of Environmental Health* 44, no. 6 (November/December 1989).

Kime, Zane. *Sunlight Could Save Your Life.* Penryn, Calif.: World Health Publications, 1980.

Kitchen, Sheila, and Sarah Bazin. *Clayton's Electrotherapy 10E.* London: W.B. Saunders Company Ltd., 1996.

Kleiner, Susan M. "Can '8-a-Day' Keep Cancer Away? The Latest News on Water, Health and Performance." Article online at www.nutrifit .org/nutr_info/8aday.html [accessed September 26, 2001].

———. "Water: An Essential but Overlooked Nutrient." *Journal of the American Dietetic Association* 99, no. 2 (February 1999).

Kočka, Miloš. "Vinzenz Priessnitz, Founder of Modern Hydrotherapy." Online at www.afx.cz/Priessnitz/EN/Default.htm [accessed November 21, 2002].

Kovács, Richard. *Electrotherapy and Light Therapy with Essentials of Hydrotherapy and Mechanotherapy.* Philadelphia: Lea & Febiger, 1949.

Krohn, Jacqueline, and Frances A. Taylor. *Natural Detoxification, A Practical Encyclopedia: The Complete Guide to Clearing Your Body of Toxins.* 2nd ed., rev. and expanded. Point Roberts, Wash.: Hartley & Marks Publishers, Inc., 2000.

————, Frances A. Taylor, and Jinger Prosser. *The Whole Way to Natural Detoxification: The Complete Guide to Clearing Your Body of Toxins*. Point Roberts, Washington: Hartley & Marks Publishers, Inc., 1996.

Krop, J. "Chemical Sensitivity after Intoxication at Work with Solvents: Response to Sauna Therapy." *Journal of Alternative Complementary Medicine* 41 (Spring 1998):77–86.

Krusen, Frank H. "The Blood Picture before and after Fever Therapy by Physical Means." *The American Journal of the Medical Sciences* 193 (April 1937), 470–474.

Kukkonen–Harjula, K., and K. Kauppinen. "How the Sauna Affects the Endocrine System." *Annals of Clinical Research* 20 (1998): 262–266.

Langer, Stephen E., and James F. Scheer. *Solved: The Riddle of Illness*. New Canaan, Conn.: Keats Publishing, Inc., 1984.

Laitinen, L.A., A. Lindqvist, and M. Heino. "Lungs and Ventilation in Sauna." *Annals of Clinical Research* 20 (1998): 244–248.

Laraus, Julius, ed. *Medical Applications of Ozone: Based on Papers Presented at the Medical Seminar, May 24–25, 1983, in Washington, D.C., at the Sixth World Ozone Conference*. Norwalk, Conn.: The International Ozone Association, 1983.

Lark, Susan M., and James A. Richards. *The Chemistry of Success: Secrets of Peak Performance*, San Francisco: Bay Books, 2000.

Lee, Richard H. *Scientific Investigations into Chinese Qigong*. San Clemente: China Healthways Institute, 1999.

Leppäluoto, J. "Human Thermoregulation in Sauna." *Annals of Clinical Research* 20 (1998): 240–243.

Levitt, B. Blake. *Electromagnetic Fields: A Consumer's Guide to the Issues and How to Protect Ourselves*. San Diego: Harcourt Brace & Company, 1995.

Liberman, Jacob. *Light: Medicine of the Future*. Santa Fe: Bear and Company Publishing, 1991.

Licht, Sidney, with Herman L. Kamenetz. *Therapeutic Heat and Cold*, 2nd ed. Vol. 2 of the Physical Medicine Library. New Haven: Elizabeth Licht, Publisher, 1972.

Lovejoy, H.B., Zeb G. Bell, Jr., and T.R. Vizena. "Mercury Exposure Evaluations and Their Correlation With Urine Mercury Excretions." *Journal of Occupational Medicine* 15, no. 7 (July 1973).

Macfadden, Bernarr. *The Encyclopedia of Health and Physical Culture*, vol. 6. New York: MacFadden Book Company, Inc., 1937.

McCabe, Ed. *Oxygen Therapies: A New Way Of Approaching Disease*. Morrisville, N.Y.: Energy Publications, 1988.

McVicker, Marilyn. *Sauna Detoxification Therapy: A Guide for the Chemically Sensitive*. Jefferson, N.C.: McFarland & Company, Inc., Publishers, 1997.

Montagu, Ashley. *Touching: The Human Significance of the Skin*. New York: Harper & Row, 1986.

Mott, Lawrie, and Karen Snyder. *Pesticide Alert: A Guide to Pesticides in Fruits and Vegetables*. San Francisco: Sierra Club Books, 1987.

Neel, William D. "Process of Producing a Medicament." Patent # 925,590, patented June 22, 1909.

Niwa, Y., O. Lizawa, K. Ishimoto, X. Jiang, and T. Kanoh. "Electromagnetic Wave Emitting Products and 'Kikoh' Potentiate Human Leukocyte Functions." *International Journal of Biometeorology* 375 (Sept. 1993): 133–8.

Oschman, James L. *Energy Medicine: The Scientific Basis*. Edinburgh: Churchill Livingstone, 2000.

Ott, John N. *Light, Radiation, and You: How to Stay Healthy*. Old Greenwich, Conn.: The Devin–Adair Company, 1982.

Papp, A. "Sauna-Related Burns: A Review of 154 Cases Treated in Kuopio University Hospital Burn Center 1994–2000." *Burns* 281 (Feb. 2002): 57–59.

Parpalei, I.A, L.G. Prokofeva, and V.G. Obertas. "The Use of the Sauna for Disease Prevention in the Workers of Enterprises with Chemical and Physical Occupational Hazards." *Vrachebnoe Delo* 5 (May 1991): 93–5.

Percival, Mark. "Nutritional Support for Detoxification." Applied Nutritional Science Report. Gig Harbor, Wash.: Advanced Nutrition Publications, Inc., 1997.

———. "Phytonutrients and Detoxification." Applied Nutritional Science Report. Gig Harbor, Wash.: Advanced Nutrition Publications, Inc., 1997.

Peräsalo, J. "Traditional Use of the Sauna for Hygiene and Health in Finland." *Annals of Clinical Research* 20 (1988): 220–223.

Porter, Marian. *Dr. Porter's Health Notes* (November 17). Silver Spring, Md.: The Oxygen Spa, 2001.

Pressman, Saul. *The Owner's Manual for the Human Body.* Langley, British Columbia: Plasmafire International, 1997.

———. *The Story of Ozone.* Langley, British Columbia: Plasmafire International, 2001.

Puranen, M., K. Syrjanen, and S. Syrajanen. "Transmission of Genital Human Papillomavirus Infections is Unlikely through the Floor and Seats of Humid Dwellings in Countries of High-Level Hygiene." Scandinavian Journal of Infectious Disease 283 (1996): 243–246.

Rapp, Doris. *Is This Your Child? Discovering and Treating Unrecognized Allergies in Children and Adults.* New York: William Morrow, 1991.

Rea, William J. *Chemical Sensitivity, Vol. 4: Tools of Diagnosis and Methods of Treatment.* Boca Raton: Lewis Publishers, 1997.

Rea, W.J., Y. Pan, and A.R. Johnson. "Clearing of Toxic Volatile Hydrocarbons from Humans." *Boletin—Asociacion Medica de Puerto Rico* 837 (July 1991): 321–4.

Rehunen, S. "The Sauna and Sports." *Annals of Clinical Research* 20 (1988): 292–294.

Reilly, Harold J., and Ruth Hagy Brod. *The Edgar Cayce Handbook for Health Through Drugless Therapy.* New York: Berkeley Publishing Group, 1986.

Rissmann, A., J. Al–Karawi, and G. Jorch. "Infants' Physiological Response to Short Heat Stress During Sauna Bath." *Klinische Padiatrie* 214, no. 3 (May–June 2002): 132–5.

Robins, H. Ian, Anders Hugander, and Justin D. Cohen. "Whole Body Hyperthermia in the Treatment of Neoplastic Disease." *Radiologic Clinics of North America* 27 (May 1989): 603–610.

Rogers, Sherry A. *Detoxify or Die.* Sarasota, Fl.: Sand Key Company, Inc., 2002.

———. *Total Wellness* Newsletter (May 2000).

Root, David E. Statement before the Presidential Special Oversight Board for Department of Defense Investigations of Gulf War Chemical and Biological Incidents, November 20, 1998.

———, David B. Katzin, and David W. Schnare. "Diagnosis and Treatment of Patients Presenting Subclinical Signs and Symptoms of Exposure to Chemicals Which Bioaccumulate in Human Tissue." Proceedings of the National Conference on Hazardous Wastes and Environmental Emergencies, Cincinnati, Ohio, May 14–16, 1985.

Saul, Andrew. "What is in Second Hand Cigarette Smoke?" *The Doctor Yourself Newsletter* 1, no. 19 (July 15, 2001). Article online at www.doctoryourself.com/news/v1n19.txt [accessed November 20, 2002].

Schittek, Birgit, Rainer Hipfel, Birgit Sauer, Jürgen Bauer, Hubert Kalbacher, Stefan Stevanovic, Markus Schirle, Kristina Schroeder, Nikolaus Blin, Friedegund Meier, Gernot Rassner, and Claus Garbe. "Dermcidin: A Novel Human Antibiotic Peptide Secreted By Sweat Glands." *Nature Immunology* 2, no. 12:1133–1137.

Schnare, David W., Max Ben, and Megan G. Shields. "Body Burden Reductions of PCB, PBBs and Chlorinated Pesticides in Human Subjects." *Ambio* 13, no. 5–6 (1984): 378–380.

———, Gene Denk, Megan G. Shields, and S. Brunton. "Evaluation of a Detoxification Regimen for Fat Stored Xenobiotics." *Medical Hypotheses* 9 (1982): 265–282.

———, Max Ben, Peya Carmi Robinson, Megan G. Shields, and Gene Denk. "Reduction of Human Organohalide Body Burdens." Final Research Report, Foundation for Advancements in Science and Education, July 1983.

Schwartz, Richard W. *John Harvey Kellogg, M.D.: Father of the Health Food Industry*. Berrien Springs, Mich.: Andrews University Press, 1970.

Sheridan, P., and N. Shilton. "Application of Far Infra-Red Radiation to Cooking of Meat Products." *Journal of Food Engineering* 41, no. 3–4 (August 9, 1999): 203–208.

Shields, Megan, Shelley Beckmann, Forest Tennant, and R. Michael Wisner. "Reduction of Drug Residues: Applications in Drug Rehabilitation." Paper presented at the 123rd Annual Meeting of the American Public Health Association.

Silver, Nina. *The Handbook of Rife Frequency Healing: Holistic Technology for Cancer and Other Diseases.* Stone Ridge, N.Y.: The Center for Frequency Education, 2001.

Sinatra, Stephen. "Sweat Your Way to Detoxification with a Far Infrared Sauna." *The Sinatra Health Report,* August 2003.

Smith, Cyril W., and Simon Best. *Electromagnetic Man: Health & Hazard in the Electrical Environment.* London: J.M. Dent and Sons Ltd., 1990.

Solar Products Inc. *Infrared Heat: A Simplified Approach.* Pompton Lakes, N.J.: Solar Products Inc. (n.d.)

Sorri, P. "The Sauna and Sauna Bathing Habits—A Psychoanalytic Point of View." *Annals of Clinical Research* 20 (1988): 236–239.

Steinman, David. *Diet For A Poisoned Planet.* New York: Harmony Books, 1990.

Svoboda, Terese. "Every Breath She Takes." *Utne Reader* (March–April 1997).

Tei, C., Y. Horikiri, J.C. Park, J.W. Jeong, K.S. Chang, Y. Toyama, and N. Tanaka. "Acute Hemodynamic Improvement by Thermal Vasodilation in Congestive Heart Failure." *Circulation* 9110 (May 15, 1995): 2582–90.

Thorp, Clark E. "The Toxicity of Ozone: A Report and Bibliography." Reprint from *Industrial Medicine and Surgery* 19, no. 2 (February 1950): 45–57.

Tortora, Gerard J., and Nicholas P. Anagnostakos. *Principles of Anatomy and Physiology.* 6th ed. New York: Harper & Row, 1990.

Trattler, Ross. *Better Health Through Natural Healing: How to Get Well Without Drugs or Surgery.* New York: McGraw–Hill Book Company, 1985.

Tretjak, Ziga, Shelley Beckmann, Ana Tretjak, and Charles Gunnerson. "Occupational, Environmental, and Public Health in Semic: A Case Study of Polychlorinated Biphenyl PCB Pollution." Reprint from Post-Audits of

Environmental Programs and Projects, Proceedings/Environmental Impact Analysis Research Council/ASCE, New Orleans, Louisiana, October 11, 1989.

Tsyb, A.F., E.M. Parshkov, J. Barnes, V.V. Yarzutkin, N.V. Vorontsov, and V.I. Dedov. "Rehabilitation of a Chernobyl Affected Population Using a Detoxification Method." Proceedings of the 1998 International Radiological Post-Emergency Response Issues Conference, Washington, D.C, September 9–11, 1998.

Vähä–Eskeli, K., and R. Erkkola. "The Sauna and Pregnancy." *Annals of Clinical Research* 20 (1988): 279–282.

Valtakari, P. "The Sauna and Bathing in Different Countries." *Annals of Clinical Research* 20 (1988): 230–235.

Vance, Judi. *Beauty to Die For: The Cosmetic Consequence*. San Diego: Pro-Motion Publishing, 1998.

Virtanen, John O. *The Finnish Sauna: Peace of Mind, Body and Soul*. Withee, Wisc.: O–W Enterprise, 1998.

Vuori, Ilkka. "Healthy and Unhealthy Sauna Bathing." *Annals of Clinical Research* 20 (1988): 217–219.

———. "Sauna Bather's Circulation." *Annals of Clinical Research* 20 (1988): 249–256.

———, and Heikki Vapaatalo. "The Finnish Sauna: Is It Safe for Patients?" *Annals of Clinical Research* 20 (1988): 215–216.

Wakim, K.G., C.S. Wise, and F.B. Moore. "Basic Fundamentals and Clinical Applications of Heat and Cold." *Medical Arts and Sciences* 13 (1959): 126–138.

Whang, Sang. *Reverse Aging*. Miami: JSP Publishing, 1999.

Wilford, John Noble. "Before Rome's Baths, There Was the Maya Sweat House." *The New York Times* (March 20, 2001): F5.

Wilson, Lawrence. "Far Infrared Sauna Therapy." *Townsend Letter for Doctors & Patients* (November 2002). Also available as "Detox in the Sauna," online at www.mercola.com/2002/aug/14/sauna.htm [accessed October 20, 2002].

———. *Nutritional Balancing and Hair Mineral Analysis.* Prescott, Ariz.: L.D. Wilson Consultants, Inc., 1998.

Winter, Ruth. *A Consumer's Dictionary of Food Additives.* 4th ed. New York: Three Rivers Press, 1994.

Winterfeld, H.J., H. Siewert, D. Strangfeld, J. Bohm, R. Aurisch, U. Engelmann, and R. Frenzel. "Sauna Therapy in Coronary Heart Disease with Hypertension after Bypass Operation, in Heart Aneurysm Operation and in Essential Hypertension." *Zeitschrift fur Die Gesamte Innere Medizin und Ihre Grenzgebiete* 485 (May 1993): 247–250.

Wisner, R. Michael, and the HealthMed Clinics. "Drug and Alcohol Rehabilitation." *Complementary Medicine* (July/August 1986).

———, G. Megan Shields, and Shelley L. Beckmann. "Treatment of Children with the Detoxification Method Developed by Hubbard." Proceedings of the American Public Health Association National Conference, San Diego, 1995.

Wolff, Mary S., Henry A. Anderson, and Irving J. Selikoff. "Human Tissue Burdens of Halogenated Aromatic Chemicals in Michigan." *Journal of the American Medical Association* 247, no. 15 (April 16, 1982): 2112–2116.

Yiamouyiannis, John. *Fluoride: The Aging Factor; How to Recognize and Avoid the Devastating Effects of Fluoride.* Delaware, Ohio: Health Action Press, 1993.

Ylikahri, R., E. Heikkonen, and A. Suokas. "The Sauna and Alcohol." *Annals of Clinical Research* 20 (1988): 287–291.

Young, Robert O. and Shelley Redford Young. *Sick and Tired.* Pleasant Grove, Utah: Woodland Publishing, 2001.

Zamm, Alfred V., and Robert Gannon. *Why Your House May Endanger Your Health.* New York: Simon and Schuster, 1980.

T

About the Author

Nenah Sylver has enjoyed a rich and varied career as a Reichian psychotherapist, a holistic health educator, and an internationally published writer. In 1996 she received her doctorate in Transformational Psychology, an interdisciplinary program of bodymind psychotherapy, holistic health, and gender studies, from the Union Institute.

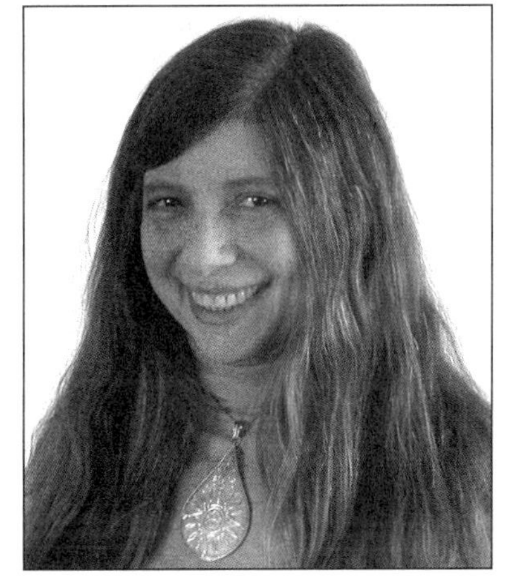

Dr. Sylver's last book, *The Handbook of Rife Frequency Healing: Holistic Technology for Cancer and Other Diseases* (Stone Ridge, New York: The Center for Frequency Education, 2001), explores a safe, non-invasive modality developed in the 1930s that uses frequencies, combined with the latest research in many areas of complementary health. Forthcoming books include a work integrating feminism, depth psychology, and the bodymind principles of Wilhelm Reich; and a handbook that studies poisonous chemicals in the home, and presents safe, effective substitutes.

Formerly published under the name "Nina Silver," her writings in holistic health, psychology, feminism, sexuality, and social change have appeared in *Natural Food & Farming, Natural Living Today, The New Internationalist,*

Nexus, Off Our Backs, Beiträge zum Werk von Wilhelm Reich (Contributions to the Work of Wilhelm Reich), and the anthologies *Journeys of the Heart: Perspectives on Intimacy in America* (Bruner-Mazel, 1999), *An Introduction to Women's Studies* (Simon & Schuster, 1997), *Women, Culture, and Society: Readings in Women's Studies* (Simon & Schuster, 1994), *Transforming a Rape Culture* (Milkweed Editions, 1993), and *Closer To Home: Bisexuality and Feminism* (Seal Press, 1992). Her volume of poetry, *Birthing,* was published in 1996 by Woman in the Moon Publications. Dr. Sylver has also been cited in *Utne Reader* (now called *Utne* magazine) and *The New Yorker,* and listeners have enjoyed her holistic health discussions on the radio.

In addition to her scholarly pursuits, Dr. Sylver is also a lifelong musician and award-winning songwriter. She looks forward to recording an album of original songs.

THE HANDBOOK OF RIFE FREQUENCY HEALING
Holistic Technology for Cancer and Other Diseases

ORDER FORM

Book Price: USD $60 each

Shipping/Handling:
(shipping prices subject to change without notice)

Country	First book	Ea. add'l bk.
United States (including US territories): Priority Mail (2 to 3 day delivery) Media Mail (8 to 21 day delivery)	 $15 $9	 $10 $7
Canada: Air (7 to 10 day delivery)	$16	$9
Mexico: Air (7 to 10 day delivery)	$23	$14
South America, Central America, & adjacent Islands: Air (7 to 10 day delivery)	$32	$10
Eastern & Western Europe (including Scandinavia, & the Republic of Ireland): Air (7 to 10 day delivery)	 $33	 $15
United Kingdom (England, Scotland, Wales, & Northern Ireland): Air (7 to 10 day delivery)	 $33	 $18
Australia, New Zealand, Africa, & the Middle East: Air (7 to 10 day delivery)	 $35	 $11
Asia: Air (7 to 10 day delivery)	$35	$19

Number of books ordered _____ x $60 per book = $ __________

TOTAL SHIPPING (from chart above) + __________

Subtotal __________

New York State residents only: multiply subtotal by .0825 + __________

GRAND TOTAL __________

Payment Options:

1. Visa/MasterCard (supply credit card information below)
2. Check or money order in US funds only, payable to The Center for Frequency
3. PayPal, through our online storefront at www.NenahSylver.com

For check, money order, or credit card orders, fill out this form and mail it to:
The Center for Frequency ■ PO Box 952 ■ Stone Ridge, New York 12484-0952 ■ USA
Phone: 845-687-0963

To read Dr. Sylver's essays, send email, and buy books and other products online,
go to her website: www.NenahSylver.com

PLEASE PRINT !

Name: ____

Address (street, apartment number, city, state, country, and zip or postal code):

____

____

Telephone (specify home, work, cell): ________________________________

Email/Second Phone:____

If paying by Visa or MasterCard:

Card Number_______________________________ Expiration Date ______________

Name on Card _________________________________

Billing Address for Card (if different from Shipping Address)

____

____

Bulk orders anywhere over 10 copies, please inquire.

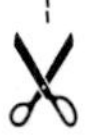

THE HOLISTIC HANDBOOK OF SAUNA THERAPY

ORDER FORM

Book Price: USD $34.95 each

Shipping/Handling:
(shipping prices subject to change without notice)

Country	First book	Ea. add'l bk.
United States (including US territories): Priority Mail (2 to 3 day delivery) Media Mail (8 to 21 day delivery)	$14 $8	$9 $6
Canada: Air (7 to 10 day delivery)	$18	$11
Mexico: Air (7 to 10 day delivery)	$20	$14
South America, Central America, & adjacent Islands: Air (7 to 10 day delivery)	$28	$13
Eastern & Western Europe (including Scandinavia, & the Republic of Ireland): Air (7 to 10 day delivery)	$28	$11
United Kingdom (England, Scotland, Wales, & Northern Ireland): Air (7 to 10 day delivery)	$23	$17
Australia, New Zealand, Africa, & the Middle East: Air (7 to 10 day delivery)	$28	$14
Asia: Air (7 to 10 day delivery)	$28	$19

Number of books ordered _____ x $34.95 per book = $ _________

TOTAL SHIPPING (from chart above) + _________

Subtotal _________

New York State residents only: multiply subtotal by .0825 + _________

GRAND TOTAL _________

Payment Options:

1. Visa/MasterCard (supply credit card information below)
2. Check or money order in US funds only, payable to The Center for Frequency
3. PayPal, through our online storefront at www.NenahSylver.com

For check, money order, or credit card orders, fill out this form and mail it to:
The Center for Frequency ■ PO Box 952 ■ Stone Ridge, New York 12484-0952 ■ USA
Phone: 845-687-0963

To read Dr. Sylver's essays, send email, and buy books and other products online,
go to her website: www.NenahSylver.com

PLEASE PRINT !

Name: ____

Address (street, apartment number, city, state, country, and zip or postal code):

____

____

Telephone (specify home, work, cell): ____________________________

Email/Second Phone:____

If paying by Visa or MasterCard:

Card Number______________________________ Expiration Date _________

Name on Card _____________________________

Billing Address for Card (if different from Shipping Address)

____

____

Bulk orders anywhere over 24 copies, please inquire.